TELEHEALTH ESSENTIALS

for
Advanced Practice Nursing

TELEHEALTH ESSENTIALS
for
Advanced Practice Nursing

Patty A. Schweickert, DNP, FNP-C
Adjunct Faculty, College of Health Sciences, School of Nursing
Old Dominion University
Norfolk, Virginia
Strategic Consultant for Advanced Practice Providers, Karen S. Rheuban Center for Telehealth
Nurse Practitioner and Clinical Faculty, Department of Radiology, School of Medicine
University of Virginia Health System
Clinical Faculty
University of Virginia School of Nursing
Charlottesville, Virginia
Contributing Faculty, College of Health Sciences
Walden University School of Nursing
Minneapolis, Minnesota

Carolyn M. Rutledge, PhD, FNP-BC
Professor and Associate Chair of Nursing, School of Nursing
Co-Director, Center of Telehealth Innovation, Education, and Research
Old Dominion University
Professor, Department of Family Medicine
Eastern Virginia Medical School
Norfolk, Virginia

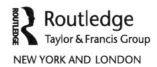
Routledge
Taylor & Francis Group

NEW YORK AND LONDON

Instructors: *Telehealth Essentials for Advanced Practice Nursing Instructor Guidebook* is available. Don't miss this important companion to *Telehealth Essentials for Advanced Practice Nursing*. To obtain the Instructor's Manual, please visit http://www.routledge.com/9781630916053

First published 2020 by SLACK Incorporated

Published 2024 by Routledge
605 Third Avenue, New York, NY 10158

and by Routledge
4 Park Square, Milton Park, Abingdon, Oxon OX14 4RN

Routledge is an imprint of the Taylor & Francis Group, an informa business

Cover Artist: Katherine Christie

Library of Congress Cataloging-in-Publication Data

Library of Congress Control Number: 2020937371

ISBN: 9781630916053 (pbk)
ISBN: 9781003526728 (ebk)

DOI: 10.4324/9781003526728

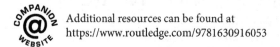

Additional resources can be found at
https://www.routledge.com/9781630916053

DEDICATION

This book is dedicated to all nurses, health care providers, and first responders who are on the front lines addressing the COVID-19 pandemic; who are selflessly caring for others while risking their own lives; and who are embracing telehealth to overcome barriers to health care.

CONTENTS

Patty Alane Schweickert, DNP, FNP-C

Rebecca A. Bates, DNP, FNP-C; Kristi Henderson, DNP, FNP-BC,
FAAN, FAEN; and Carolyn M. Rutledge, PhD, FNP-BC

Carolyn M. Rutledge, PhD, FNP-BC; Katherine E. Chike-Harris, DNP,
APRN, CPNP-PC, NE; Susan V. Brammer, PhD, RN, CNE; and
Patty Alane Schweickert, DNP, FNP-C

Richard L. Rose II, CTC, CWTS; Patty Alane Schweickert, DNP, FNP-C;
David Cattell-Gordon, MDiv, MSW; Samuel Collins, MSc; Rebecca L. Steele,
MSN, RN, CNL; Christianne Nesbit, DNP, AGNP, PMHNP;
Michele L. Bordelon, MSEd; and Brian Gunnell, BS, CTC

Karen S. Rheuban, MD and Kathy H. Wibberly, PhD

Katherine E. Chike-Harris, DNP, APRN, CPNP-PC, NE

Patty Alane Schweickert, DNP, FNP-C; Lynn Wiles, PhD, RN;
Katherine E. Chike-Harris, DNP, APRN, CPNP-PC, NE; R. Lee Tyson, DNP,
PMHNP-BC, ANP-BC; Tonya L. Hensley, DNP, FNP; Kathryn B. Reid,
PhD, FNP-C; Rosalyn Perkins, MNSc, CNP, WHNP-BC; Rebecca A. Bates,
DNP, FNP-C; S. Craig Thomas, MSN, NP, ACNP-BC, ACNS-BC, CHFN;
Teresa Gardner Tyson, DNP, FNP-BC; Brian Myers, MBA, MTS; and
Allison Kirkner, MSN, RN, ACNP-BC

ACKNOWLEDGMENTS

A rich variety of experiences, opportunities, and relationships have created the inspiration for this book and enabled it to come to fruition. Growing up in Appalachia has allowed me to experience firsthand the health care challenges for rural and underserved populations. Telehealth offers significant opportunities to address these existing care disparities and increase access to care for those to whom it might otherwise be unavailable. Nursing is about improving health, and improving nursing's ability to assimilate telehealth into everyday practice is my goal. I would therefore like to thank and provide acknowledgment to those who have allowed me to contribute to nursing knowledge in telehealth. First, I am grateful for the opportunity to have known and cared for patients throughout my nursing career, from intensive care units to rural ambulatory care settings, who have taught me the meaning of nursing, presence, and empathy. Next, I would like to acknowledge those who have mentored, guided, and supported me in my nursing journey, to include my colleagues, friends, and family. I would like to express my deep admiration for David Cattell-Gordon and Karen S. Rheuban, for their unwavering support. Thank you, David, for your expert guidance and mentorship for my doctoral project on telehealth stroke education, as well as for providing ongoing support toward my creative expressions of telehealth nursing ideas. Thank you, Karen, for demonstrating what knowledge, qualities, and behaviors are needed in a telehealth champion and for demonstrating what telehealth leadership looks like. I am also eternally grateful for your support for me as a student member of the American Telemedicine Association Board of Directors (2010-2012). This experience helped to shape my future in telehealth nursing.

I would also like to express my gratitude and respect by thanking:

- All of the nurses and advanced practice registered nurses who came before me who innovatively used telehealth technology, for providing the foundation for telehealth nursing practice
- Jesse Gallo, for his insight and understanding of the importance of nursing in telehealth and for providing me immeasurable opportunities to promote telehealth nursing
- My distinguished colleagues at the University of Virginia (UVA) Department of Telemedicine and the UVA Karen S. Rheuban Center for Telehealth for engaging with me on telehealth nursing
- The American Telemedicine Association Board of Directors (2010-2012), for allowing me to learn from you and with you
- Mary Elizabeth "Lee" Jensen, my trusted friend, mentor, and colleague, for sharing your immense knowledge and expertise with me over the past 20 years, as well as for extending to me your insight, nurturing professionalism, and expert leadership, which has enabled me to expand my horizons of advanced practice nursing
- Lady Swinfen, for sharing her vast knowledge of telehealth with me and for sharing the Swinfen telehealth experiences in e-consults
- Teresa Gardner Tyson and Paula Hill-Collins at The Health Wagon, for engaging with me on educational programs and clinical practice in telehealth, and for sharing examples of telehealth nursing
- The 23 contributors who partnered with Carolyn Rutledge and me to write this book
- Julia Dolinger, for her expertise and guidance on many levels throughout the development and writing of this book, including unwavering support and patience to our group of busy health care professionals
- Kayleigh Bateera, for contributing her excellent photography to this book
- My husband, Louie Christopher Schweickert III, for his support and ongoing encouragement; my son, Adam Schweickert, for his immeasurable assistance in preparing manuscript references; and my son, Dylan Schweickert, for his advice with technical details of the manuscript preparation

Finally, I would be remiss if I did not mention my unending thankfulness, appreciation, and gratitude for my mentor, colleague, and friend, Carolyn Rutledge, with whom I partnered for this book. Carolyn, I could not have immersed myself in telehealth nursing so fully without your guidance, expertise, and insight.

Patty Alane Schweickert, DNP, FNP-C

I wish to acknowledge and thank those who have been with me on my quest to better understand and promote activities to improve health care. First, I must thank the individuals who helped me find my voice in the health care arena. Through the support of my mother, Dorothy Morcom, I learned about the needs of rural populations and to say "yes" to opportunities that could improve their situations even if they tended to be daunting. Through my exposure to the needs of rural and underserved populations as a child and through the experiences of my family, I have seen the value of using health care technology to provide access to those at a distance. Teaching has allowed me to empower my students in the use of telehealth technologies to address the health care barriers many individuals encounter. Not only have I been able to impact students, they have impacted me with their visions and passions. I must specifically thank one student and friend, Patty Schweickert, who constantly challenged me to champion telehealth, including through the partnership in writing of this book. Her insight, drive, and passion have been an inspiration.

I must thank those who have been part of the vision for developing the Center for Telehealth Innovation, Education, and Research (C-TIER) at Old Dominion University: Tina Gustin, Michele Bordelon, and Karen Karlowicz. Without their untiring dedication and work, C-TIER would only be a dream. I also want to thank members of the National Organization of Nurse Practitioner Faculties (NONPF) for embracing the need to educate advanced practice registered nurses in telehealth and asking me to lead the development of their position paper on telehealth. I must acknowledge Julia Dolinger, the acquisitions editor from SLACK Incorporated, for her patience and for having the vision for this book.

My greatest appreciation is for my husband, Jim Rutledge, my best friend and greatest supporter. He has always believed in me, listened to me, and encouraged me to pursue my dreams.

Carolyn Morcom Rutledge, PhD, FNP-BC

ABOUT THE EDITORS

Patty Alane Schweickert, DNP, FNP-C, is an experienced nurse educator with a well-rounded foundation in telehealth practice and telehealth nursing education. Dr. Schweickert has over 32 years' experience in a variety of nursing arenas, including critical care, emergency/trauma care, ambulatory care, family practice, neuroradiology, nursing education, and telehealth. For the past 20 years, Dr. Schweickert has been a nurse practitioner at the University of Virginia (UVA), caring for neurovascular patients as a member of the neurovascular team. Dr. Schweickert received her Bachelor of Science in Nursing from Wheeling Jesuit College, Master of Science in Critical Care Nursing from UVA, Post-Master's Primary Care Family Nurse Practitioner Certification from UVA, and Doctor of Nursing Practice from Old Dominion University (ODU). Her DNP project implemented the first patient focused stroke tele-education program. Dr. Schweickert was a student member of the American Telemedicine Association board of directors from 2010 to 2012 and was presented with the American Telemedicine Association Student Paper Award in 2011 for her work in tele-education.

Since graduating with her DNP in 2011, Dr. Schweickert has focused on educating nurses in telehealth practice as well as developing and participating in a variety of telehealth programs to address rural health care needs, including a 2015 Health Resources and Services Administration (HRSA) grant award for a preceptor education program titled "Advanced Practice Nurse-Preceptor Link and Clinical Education (APN-PLACE)," and a 2016 HRSA grant award for a school telehealth program titled "Better Health Care for Kids, Parents, and Communities (eBACKPAC)." Dr. Schweickert was program director of APN-PLACE from 2015 to 2018.

Dr. Schweickert is the Strategic Consultant for Advanced Practice Providers to the UVA Karen S. Rheuban Center for Telehealth and is on the UVA Center for Telehealth's board of directors. Dr. Schweickert is clinical faculty at the UVA School of Nursing, where she teaches telehealth. She is contributing faculty at Walden University College of Health Sciences, teaching in the DNP program, and adjunct faculty at ODU College of Health Sciences, collaborating with colleagues to promote and teach telehealth nursing. As a member of the National Organization of Nurse Practitioner Faculties work group, which developed the position paper on educating nurse practitioners in telehealth, Dr. Schweickert disseminates support for telehealth nursing education. She is a founding member of the international telehealth Millennia2015 WeHealth Task Force. She is a contributing editor to the UVA Telehealth Village. She lectures and mentors within UVA and has lectured locally, nationally, and internationally on telehealth nursing and neuroradiology nursing. She is a published researcher in nursing telehealth education, telehealth stroke education, neuroradiology, and a variety of nursing topics. Dr. Schweickert lives in rural Virginia with her husband, Louie Christopher Schweickert, and has 2 sons, Adam and Dylan.

Carolyn Morcom Rutledge, PhD, FNP-BC, is professor and Associate Chair of the School of Nursing at Old Dominion University (ODU). In addition to her academic role, Dr. Rutledge holds the position of professor of family medicine at Eastern Virginia Medical School, where she has maintained an active clinical practice as a family nurse practitioner for 32 years. She was instrumental in the development of the Center for Telehealth Innovations, Education and Research at ODU. This is one of the first Telehealth Centers in the nation that is led by nursing and has a truly interprofessional focus. Dr. Rutledge is a national speaker on telehealth and has published numerous articles and served as an investigator on over 25 grants that have focused on developing new models to provide care to rural and underserved populations. Since 2010, Dr. Rutledge has focused on improving the way health care is delivered in remote areas, using telehealth to enhance patient care and communication. She has advocated for the use of telehealth as a means for interprofessional collaboration and as a must when teaching students to work collaboratively at a distance. She was the lead author in developing the National Organization of Nurse Practitioner Faculties position paper on educating nurse practitioners in telehealth. Dr. Rutledge serves as a national consultant and speaker on telehealth training and implementation. She is consulting with schools of nursing across the country on the development of a national telehealth education toolkit. She serves on the board of the Virginia Telehealth Network, which works closely with the state legislature, broadband providers, and telehealth vendors to break down barriers to the use of telehealth. In 2014, Dr. Rutledge received the State Council of Higher Education for Virginia's Outstanding Faculty Award, the highest honor provided to faculty in the state of Virginia.

Dr. Rutledge lives in Virginia Beach with her husband, Jim Rutledge, her greatest supporter. She has 2 sons, Michael and Carson Rutledge.

Contributing Authors

Rebecca A. Bates, DNP, FNP-C
(Chapters 2 and 7)
Adams Compassionate Healthcare Network
Chantilly, Virginia

Michele L. Bordelon, MSEd (Chapter 4)
School of Nursing
Old Dominion University
Norfolk, Virginia

Susan V. Brammer, PhD, RN, CNE (Chapter 3)
College of Nursing
University of Cincinnati
Cincinnati, Ohio

David Cattell-Gordon, MDiv, MSW (Chapter 4)
Karen S. Rheuban Center for Telehealth
University of Virginia Health System
Charlottesville, Virginia

Katherine E. Chike-Harris, DNP, APRN,
CPNP-PC, NE (Chapters 3, 6, and 7)
College of Nursing
Medical University of South Carolina
Charleston, South Carolina

Samuel Collins, MSc (Chapter 4)
Karen S. Rheuban Center for Telehealth
University of Virginia Health System
Charlottesville, Virginia

Brian Gunnell, BS, CTC (Chapter 4)
Karen S. Rheuban Center for Telehealth
University of Virginia Health System
Charlottesville, Virginia

Tina Gustin, DNP, CNS (Chapters 8 and 9)
School of Nursing
Old Dominion University
Norfolk, Virginia

Kristi Henderson, DNP, FNP-BC, FAAN, FAEN
(Chapter 2)
Ascension Healthcare
Austin, Texas

Tonya L. Hensley, DNP, FNP (Chapter 7)
Health-e-Schools Telehealth Program
School of Nursing
Western Carolina University
Cullowhee, North Carolina

Allison Kirkner, MSN, RN, ACNP-BC
(Chapter 7)
University of Virginia
Charlottesville, Virginia

Brian Myers, MBA, MTS (Chapter 7)
The Health Wagon
Clintwood, Virginia

Christianne Nesbit, DNP, AGNP, PMHNP
(Chapter 4)
School of Nursing
Old Dominion University
Norfolk, Virginia

Rosalyn Perkins, MNSc, CNP, WHNP-BC
(Chapter 7)
Institute for Digital Health & Innovation
University of Arkansas for Medical Sciences
Little Rock, Arkansas

Kathryn B. Reid, PhD, FNP-C (Chapter 7)
School of Nursing
University of Virginia
Charlottesville, Virginia

Karen S. Rheuban, MD (Chapter 5)
Karen S. Rheuban Center for Telehealth
University of Virginia Health System
Charlottesville, Virginia

Richard L. Rose II, CTC, CWTS (Chapter 4)
Karen S. Rheuban Center for Telehealth
University of Virginia Health System
Charlottesville, Virginia

Rebecca L. Steele, MSN, RN, CNL (Chapter 4)
Locus Health
Charlottesville, Virginia

S. Craig Thomas, MSN, NP, ACNP-BC,
ACNS-BC, CHFN (Chapter 7)
University of Virginia Health System
Charlottesville, Virginia

R. Lee Tyson, DNP, PMHNP-BC, ANP-BC
(Chapter 7)
College of Nursing
University of Cincinnati
Cincinnati, Ohio

Teresa Gardner Tyson, DNP, FNP-BC
(Chapter 7)
The Health Wagon
Clintwood, Virginia

Kathy H. Wibberly, PhD (Chapter 5)
Karen S. Rheuban Center for Telehealth
University of Virginia Health System
Charlottesville, Virginia

Lynn Wiles, PhD, RN (Chapter 7)
School of Nursing
Old Dominion University
Norfolk, Virginia

PREFACE

We are experiencing an unprecedented time. The novel virus SARS-CoV-2, or COVID-19, has seemingly overnight changed life on a global scale. Most non-essential businesses have been ordered to close leaving an extraordinary number of people out of work. Community, regional, state, and national sporting events including the 2020 Summer Olympics have been cancelled. Many people are working at home remotely for the first time, instead of traveling to work. Students are out of school, many using online educational platforms for the first time. People throughout the world are mandated to stay home and are only to leave for medical care, emergencies, or outside exercise. This pandemic has placed enormous stress on people, communities, regions, states, nations, and our very existence. Health care systems are overrun with infected patients seeking treatment. Providers are overwhelmed with the care of patients, neighbors, families, friends, and, at times, themselves.

Telehealth was an immediate strategy deployed virtually nationwide overnight to address the care needs of patients, providers, and our health care system during this crisis. Telehealth has a history of effectiveness in epidemics and pandemics, being used to provide care during the Ebola, SARS, and MERS outbreaks over the past several decades.[1] There has been an exponential increase in the use of telehealth since March 2020, with some areas reporting as much as a 600% increase.[2] Telehealth is an obvious answer to this health care crisis, and many previous barriers restricting wide scale use have been waived so that rapid deployment could be implemented. During this pandemic, telehealth has been used effectively to enable: 1) remote monitoring of quarantined persons under investigation for the virus, 2) remote monitoring of quarantined COVID-19 positive but asymptomatic people, 3) remote monitoring of symptomatic patients on home quarantine, 4) provision of care for hospitalized COVID-19 positive symptomatic patients, 5) provision of care for critically ill hospitalized patients in intensive care units, 6) providers to mitigate exposure while providing care to those who are ill with the virus, 7) providers to connect infected patients with specialty providers for consults and care, 8) non-infected patients to safely access care for their existing health care needs, and 9) practitioners who are quarantined to work remotely, thus improving workforce capabilities in this time of need.

However, the express positioning of telehealth to address health care needs in this pandemic brings challenges as well. Safety and privacy when using non-Health Insurance Portability and Accountability Act compliant platforms has already shown to be a problem with the hacking of at least one videoconferencing platform. Importantly, providers are now expected to use telehealth platforms without a foundation of knowledge in telehealth. This is legitimately the age of telehealth, and our desire is for nurses to use this book to gain the knowledge and skills needed for effective transition to advanced practice telehealth nursing. This will allow meaningful nursing response and have a vital impact on the care of people during this crisis and going forward. Telehealth is now part of mainstream health care. It will likely never return to its former state. Advanced practice registered nurses with telehealth knowledge and skills will be well positioned to demonstrate the efficiency of care delivery during this crisis, and beyond.

References

1. Ohannessian, R. (2015). Telemedicine: Potential applications in epidemic situations. *European Research in Telemedicine*. 4, 95–98.
2. Roth, M. (2020). *4 Ways You Haven't Thought About Using Telehealth During The COVID-19 Pandemic*. https://www.healthleadersmedia.com/innovation/4-ways-you-havent-thought-about-using-telehealth-during-covid-19-pandemic. Accessed April 24, 2020.

INTRODUCTION

Intended Audiences

Welcome to *Telehealth Essentials for Advanced Practice Nursing*. This book is a concise source for telehealth education and information designed to fill the gap in practice related to knowledge of this emerging technology and its application and assimilation into nursing practice. This textbook is targeted toward advanced practice registered nurse (APRN) students, including nurse practitioner, clinical nurse specialist, nurse midwife, nurse anesthetist, and Doctor of Nursing Practice students. This book is also for School of Nursing faculty that are seeking to better understand telehealth and/or are involved in educating APRN students in telehealth. Additionally, it is applicable as a resource for practicing APRNs because they may not have been exposed to or gained experience using this important new tool in health care. The information in this book is applicable to other health care professions that are involved in interprofessional collaboration using telehealth technologies. Because telehealth is an interprofessional discipline, students and practitioners in a variety of professions, such as public health, allied health, health information technology, and medicine, can benefit from this book. In essence, this book provides an avenue for practitioners to access a concise telehealth resource.

Why Write a Nursing Telehealth Book?

Telehealth Essentials for Advanced Practice Nursing was written primarily to educate and empower nurses in telehealth by providing them with the knowledge and skills needed to navigate the telehealth arena as a consumer, leader, and advocate. The book will provide readers with insight into the role of telehealth within the health care system, how technology can be operationalized to match specific needs, and how it can be used to provide new and innovative methods of care. The purpose for writing this book was to provide a resource for APRN students, faculty, and practitioners that will allow them to understand and optimize telehealth.

Influences of national health care provider shortages, chronicity of disease, the general aging of our population, and limited access to care require new strategies to effectively address these health care challenges. A unifying solution to our health care dilemmas, and to actualize the Institute of Medicine's nursing goals, is to use telehealth technology. Pursuant to recommendations in the report "The Future of Nursing: Leading Change, Advancing Health," nursing should expand opportunities for nurses to lead collaborative care projects, provide innovative solutions to care using technology, and prepare nurses to provide leadership to advance improvements in health and health care.[1] Telehealth is being incorporated into health care and health care delivery at an ever-increasing rate. Telehealth has reached a tipping point due to decreased costs of technology; adoption of standards-based operations; greater movement to desktop and handheld devices; wearables, the internet of things, and artificial intelligence; and simplification of processes. It is now essential that APRNs be educated in its use. For APRNs to be positioned to serve as leaders in the health care of the future, they must possess the advanced knowledge and skills required to advocate for and use such technologies in practice. We hope that the information in this book serves as a foundation for going forward as a telehealth nursing leader.

Overview of Content

The content in this book includes essential knowledge for APRN proficiency for using telehealth in clinical practice. Content is presented in a multimodal approach to telehealth education (Chapter 3) that was developed by the authors through review of evidence in the literature and testing in APRN educational programs at ODU School of Nursing. Additionally, this approach has been used as the basis for educating APRNs in telehealth at both the UVA School of Nursing and ODU School of Nursing, in the HRSA grant program, in APN-PLACE,[2] and for the NONPF background statement on APRN telehealth nursing education.[3]

The learning audience's general educational knowledge level in telehealth has been gleaned from experience educating students, a variety of publications, personal assessments, and discussions with students, APRNs, APRN nursing faculty, interdisciplinary colleagues, telehealth experts, patients, and practicing APRNs. Overall, this assessment revealed a gap in knowledge of telehealth in practicing nurses, student nurses, and nursing faculty. We therefore begin this book with a brief history of nursing in telehealth and telehealth basics and then delve deeper to include information nurses need to know to be proficient in incorporating telehealth into nursing practice. Chapter 1 presents a history of telehealth nursing, the background of telehealth, and the nursing role in telehealth in some of the first clinical telehealth projects. Chapter 2 introduces the concept of telehealth and the natural partnership between health care and telehealth, the capacity for telehealth, and an overview of telehealth programs. Next, Chapter 3 presents the multimodal approach of telehealth nursing education used throughout the book as a framework for assimilating the various aspects of telehealth knowledge and practice.

In Chapter 4, the fundamentals of telehealth technology are provided, as well as a discussion of the internet of things/medical internet of things to increase awareness of the interconnectedness of health care and assimilation of technology into tomorrow's APRN practice. Chapter 5 focuses on nursing practice considerations within the business of telehealth practice. Awareness of federal and state public policies impacting telehealth services requires the APRN to be acquainted with the laws, policies, and regulations governing APRN telehealth practice. Chapter 6 discusses the role of the APRN in implementing telehealth practice, providing the tangible link to implementing successful telehealth programs and services. The layers of complexities inherent in telehealth must be viewed through the prism of not only improving access and care, but also how technology impacts practice issues such as workforce shortages and the patient care experience.

Chapter 7 on APRN practice modalities explores how APRN telehealth practice exists and is experienced and expressed. This chapter showcases how nurses are developing and participating in new models of telehealth and the importance of participating in workforce planning and policy directives affecting use of telehealth. As APRN practice moves into the telehealth arena, new competencies commensurate to telehealth practice will be needed. Nursing must assess telehealth competencies and practice and the scope of nursing practice to ascertain the alignment and support of telehealth within nursing practice. Additionally, existing nursing skills need to be examined to determine how they can be translated or modified to provide meaningful care in the virtual environment. Chapter 8 focuses on the skills that nurses must possess in order to practice in the virtual environment and deliver care using the technology. These include hands-on skills using the technology, how to care for the patient in the virtual environment, and telehealth etiquette. The ethics of care in the virtual environment are also considered as telehealth brings unique challenges to the telehealth encounter. Chapter 9 concludes the book by focusing on telehealth and interprofessional collaboration: how to practice with an interprofessional team, methods of using telehealth to overcome barriers to interprofessional collaboration, and the role of the APRN in telehealth-enhanced interprofessional collaboration and models of care.

Getting Started: How to Use This Book

This book's content and structure presents information regarding telehealth nursing in a logical, stepwise manner that builds upon each chapter so that the nurse can layer telehealth onto his or her existing knowledge of nursing practice. This book is divided into 9 chapters. Each chapter strategically integrates *For Reflection* prompts and a *Group Exercise*. At the end of each chapter, *Thoughtful Questions* are presented for gaining deeper understanding of the content, followed by a *Case Study* for better application of the materials to actual nursing situations and practice. These *For Reflection, Group Exercise, Thoughtful Questions,* and *Case Study* activities are useful for students as well as for faculty to gain appreciation and understanding of telehealth's role in nursing practice. Further, all the contributed chapters have been judiciously edited and integrated into a framework that provides uniformity in structure and style. Additionally, a faculty manual that provides answers to the *For Reflection, Group Exercise, Thoughtful Questions,* and *Case Study* activities serves as a complement to the text.

To effectively use this book and gain a deeper understanding of telehealth as applied tonursing practice, the reader should progress chronologically, making use of the activites for advanced learning; each provides its own unique benefits and outcomes.

For Reflection

- Provide opportunities to process and think about what was learned
- Enable consideration of additional factors that may influence an outcome or decision
- Help to clarify ideas, values, and beliefs to promote insight
- Foster critical thinking to identify strategies to barriers
- Reinforce and bring relationships into focus

Group Exercise

- Enable collaborative dialogue
- Provide opportunity for shared experiences
- Improve critical thinking using others' opinions, thoughts, beliefs, values
- Improve engagement and add interest
- Foster ability to articulate assimilated information

Thoughtful Questions

- Encourage deeper consideration of factors and issues surrounding telehealth care and practice
- Allow critical thinking of the meaning of technology in nursing practice
- Stimulate consideration of other views and alternative outcomes

Case Study

- Enhance experience of how technology can impact care
- Provide opportunities to apply learned knowledge to use in cases that mirror real life
- Enable critical thinking and integration of learned knowledge in practice

The instructor is encouraged to have students provide written answers to the *For Reflection* activities and collaborate and discuss for the *Group Exercise* activities. For the *Thoughtful Questions* and *Case Study* activities, open discussion, written answers, or short essays could all present learning options.

References

1. Institute of Medicine. *Future of nursing: leading change, advancing health.* Washington, DC: The National Academies Press; 2011.
2. Advanced Practice Nurse-Preceptor Link and Clinical Education Health Resources and Services Administration Grant No. D09HP28668.
3. Rutledge C, Pitts C, Poston R, Schweickert P. NONPF supports telehealth in nurse practitioner education 2018. National Organization of Nurse Practitioner Faculties. https://cdn.ymaws.com/www.nonpf.org/resource/resmgr/2018_Slate/Telehealth_Paper_2018.pdf. Accessed February 8, 2020.

1

Telehealth Nursing

Patty Alane Schweickert, DNP, FNP-C

CHAPTER OBJECTIVES

Upon review of this chapter, the reader will be able to:

1. Identify the nursing telehealth role and issues related to the role of the advanced practice registered nurse in telehealth.
2. Summarize the history of telemedicine program development and consider how the programs aimed to improve outcomes.
3. Explore early telehealth nursing and reflect upon the changing role of the nurse in telehealth practice.
4. Discuss nursing and advanced practice registered nurses as an essential component of telehealth.

Nurses have a natural proximity to patients that necessitates their involvement with integration of new technologies in patient care. The professional role of the nurse is changing to include telehealth nursing. For the purposes of this book, the Health Resources and Services Administration's definition of telehealth and telemedicine serves as the foundation and states:

Telehealth is defined as the use of electronic information and telecommunication technologies to support long-distance clinical health care, patient and professional health-related education, public health, and health administration. Technologies include videoconferencing, the internet, store-and-forward imaging, streaming media, and terrestrial and wireless communications. Telehealth is different from telemedicine because it refers to a *broader scope of remote healthcare services* than telemedicine. While telemedicine refers specifically to remote clinical services, telehealth can refer to remote non-clinical services, such as

Schweickert PA, Rutledge CM, eds.
Telehealth Essentials for Advanced Practice Nursing (pp 1-22).
© 2020 Taylor & Francis Group.

provider training, administrative meetings, and continuing medical education, in addition to clinical services.[1(p1)]

Changes in practice bring new questions about translating the art and science of nursing to this virtual environment. Nursing has been always been an essential component of how society cares for the sick and injured, promoting the health of populations. Evolution of the role of the nurse is, in large part, a response to societal needs. These needs include those related to health care and the status of nurses at a given time. Although the significant problems of inequalities in obtaining health care in rural and underserved areas, provider shortages and misdistribution, and the high cost of health care have changed in context over time, they have not been resolved since being identified as health care issues in the early 1960s and 1970s. We are now positioned to better address these long-standing problems.

Today, our unique societal circumstances and sophisticated, forward-thinking technologic capabilities have reached critical mass and are coalescing to produce radical changes in health care. Factors such as the connected consumer who expects readily accessible health information and education, accountability, and quality outcomes; the economic milieu and concern for health care expenditures; and the extraordinary technologic developments and future potential capacity of the internet of things (IoT) and the medical internet of things (mIoT) into everyday health care are significantly influencing the redesign of health care.[2] Demands for personalization of care will evoke systemic changes in how, when, and where care is delivered. To keep pace and remain relevant, nurses must actively and proactively engage to keep abreast of telehealth knowledge and technologies. Nurses must understand the role of the telehealth nurse and continually explore how to align and integrate telehealth technologies into nursing practice.

The role of the telehealth nurse continues to be shaped and further development of the telenursing role should be examined to discern factors affecting this emerging role. Toward this end, a Telenursing Role Study was performed in 2000 to survey qualities and perceptions about the telenursing role among US nurses using telehealth.[3] Results of this descriptive study revealed that 27% of respondents using telehealth were advanced practice registered nurses (APRNs). Role stress was found to be a concern because a change from physically present practice to virtual practice can create uncertainty about the nursing role leading to burnout, increased role stress, and turnover. This study also found that telenurses have less than average stress related to role confusion and conflict and equivalent satisfaction as compared with other similar nurses. One issue in the report that stood out as increasing the telenurse's satisfaction was autonomy; however, a higher educational level was also associated with higher stress, likely due to the increased responsibility of advanced practice nursing.

Other research looking at the telenursing role includes an international telenursing research study conducted in 2004 among nurses using telehealth in practice or those who worked in a facility that used telehealth.[4] Sixty-six percent of respondents were from the United States, representing all but 1 state. Nurses in this study identified 18 nursing telehealth practice arenas. They reported actualizing their telehealth role via administrative, research, and direct patient care responsibilities. Interestingly, the study showed that the nursing telehealth role and responsibilities were only a part of their overall role, showing assimilation of telehealth into the traditional role of the nurse. Because it is likely that telenursing will be a part of many nursing roles, this is an important area for nursing to explore. Additional research is needed to evaluate the nursing telehealth role in advanced practice nursing and to identify issues that affect practice and support transition to telehealth nursing.

A History of Nursing in Telehealth

The history of nursing in telehealth has, at its foundation, the history of caring in the development of the nursing profession, the history of communicating at a distance, the development of electrical telecommunications, the application of technology to health care, and the role of nursing. The confluence between these entities has allowed us to arrive at the present day, where using technology to communicate is commonplace and where 21st-century technology is transforming health care, including nursing, nurses, and nursing care. The synergy created from current health care needs, the role and scope of practice of the advanced practice registered nurse, and available technology have created a trajectory for advanced practice nursing, creating the telehealth nurse, the nurse virtualist, and the eAPRN.

A History of Caring

Nursing begins with caring. Caring has dual significance to nursing because it refers to both the actions taken by a nurse toward another for the purpose of helping and the kindhearted way of helping, as in the compassionate nurse.[5] This discussion of caring pertains to the latter. The ability to have empathy for others is the first step in a caring relationship, being an inherent component of our humanness. Caring for others is a quality that is associated with empathy and has enabled formation of today's society. Even the earliest humans showed evidence of caring for others. Dmanisi, a site in the country of Georgia, offers clues that early humans were caring for one another as far back as 1.77 million years ago. Evidence there shows a Homo erectus skull that was essentially toothless, but the tooth sockets had been reabsorbed.[6] It was surmised from this evidence that this could only happen if the person was alive during this period, and mostly likely he or she would have needed care to survive. The concept of caring provides the structure and foundation of nursing theory and nursing practice.[7,8] Caring for others is the core, essential element that has given rise to the nursing profession's fundamental principles of practice.[5]

Caring is a universal human quality. The first acts of caring were likely provided by one's family; women, along with servants and slaves, were often designated the role of caregiver in ancient times.[9] It has been suggested that the wet nursing of infants led to a natural caring relationship between women and infants, forming the role of the nurse.[10] Additionally, although evidence of historic nursing is often lacking or obscured, the significance of women and caring can be traced back to the ancient Greeks.[9] Theofanidis and Sapountzi-Krepia[9] present a fascinating and detailed history of nursing and caring that provides a foundation for supporting nursing in the caring role. Sanitariums in ancient Greece had an early organized form of nursing that was provided to patients,[11] in addition to having a type of nurse caretaker for children.[12] Ancient nursing was linked to social position, being the work of women in the household.[9] Ancient Roman civilization gave rise to public health initiatives and to women deaconesses, the likely predecessors of nurses, as they cared for patients, prisoners, and the poor in hospitals and private homes.[13] The Christian Bible also provides mention of nurses as they cared for the sick and poor.[14] Of the many women who laid the foundation for the development of the nurse through caring, one of the earliest nurses was Phoebe, who was the first deaconess of the Christian church.[9] Phoebe is referred to as a visiting nurse, and she is considered by many today to be the first nurse.[15] Another Roman woman named Fabiola founded the first public hospital in the 4th century AD[16] and also founded a sanatorium to care for the ill.[9] Theofanidis and Sapountzi-Krepia[9] cite additional historical examples of women in the role of the caring nurse, such as in Jerusalem where a Roman noblewoman named Paula formed a hospital and is thought to be the first educated nurse who trained other nurses. Interestingly, another Roman noblewoman named Marcella used her home as a monastery where charitable work for patients was offered as she taught the art of nursing.[9,17] Clearly, nursing had multifaceted components of caring at its core from these early beginnings.

During the early Middle Ages, women continued caring for the sick and infirmed. The fall of Rome in 476 AD was the beginning of the Dark Ages, where Roman science, medicine, nursing knowledge, libraries, scientific learning environments and discoveries, and languages to communicate were essentially lost.[9] Over time, the church and religious orders responded and filled this gap by opening numerous hospitals, infirmaries, and monasteries for the sick and the poor.[9] By the

13th century AD, there were 200,000 nuns and peasants providing structured care as organized by the churches.[18] Unfortunately, survival was the daily chore during the Middle Ages, and the loss of basic knowledge about sanitation and germs created the perfect milieu for disaster to strike in the 1300s, when the bubonic plague was introduced to Europe.[9] Beginning in China, the bubonic plague spread through Constantinople trade routes leading to Europe, causing the death of up to two-thirds of the European population.[19] As nursing deteriorated throughout much of Europe during this time, it continued to flourish in Byzantium, where a variety of hospitals had staff who provided care for the sick.[20-22] Around the 11th century, monasteries operated hostel-type hospitals, and the Pantocrator Xenon Monastery Hospital was formed.[21] A service book published by the monastery called Typikon preserved details of the hospital's activities, and this is where the term *nurse* was likely first used to describe paid staff who worked there.[9,21]

Later, during the Renaissance, hospitals began to be opened in Europe for the poor by agencies associated with local provinces and governments as well as volunteer organizations.[12] Most of those who provided the care were lower-class women who only had childrearing as experience.[9] Wars throughout this time also served as opportunities for women to care for injured soldiers and were instrumental in the development of modern nursing. The contributions of Florence Nightingale inspired other women to be trained as nurses, focusing on the art and science of nursing.[23] Revitalization of an interest in scientific knowledge enabled nursing to grow into its own discipline through organized nursing education and practice. During the 1970s, nurses began to focus on original nursing knowledge, describing how one knows in nursing and how the art and caring aspects of nursing relate to the overall discipline.[8,24,25]

Today, caring is a core component of nursing, thus differentiating nurses from other health care providers. Caring is also a core component of telehealth nursing, and nurses are challenged as to how to translate caring in nursing to the virtual environment without the patient being physically present. As more nurses use telehealth in their practice, more inquiry, study, and research should be conducted to clarify the relationship of caring in nursing telehealth practice.

With the ever-increasing ability to provide caring remotely, there are fundamental and aesthetic issues that arise related to transmitting a caring presence in the virtual visit. A 2009 qualitative study was conducted on APRN perceptions of conveying caring during a primary care visit via telehealth.[26] Results revealed that APRNs conveyed nursing qualities and skills of caring using the technology by a process described by the authors as being with the patient, listening, communicating, and staying connected. They reported that being with the patient involved an initiation process where the APRN prepared for the patient's visit by contacting the patient and by reviewing their clinical information. This early contact with the patient conveyed interest and preparation for the visit. The study found active listening and meaningful communications were determined to be especially important when using telehealth because the remote nature of the virtual visit excludes the possibility of using therapeutic touch. Additionally, improved expressions of listening and communicating caring can supplement the encounter in the absence of proximity, as can staying connected after the visit. Virtual visits often use audiovisual technologies such that the images on the screen enable live interaction. Personification of the patient and provider image is heightened on the screen, and attention to details, such as appearance; volume, tempo, and content of speech; and body language send messages that can influence the encounter.[26] Awareness of the importance of these factors can improve the ability to convey caring using technology.

Finally, attributes of the caregiver that were found to heighten the experience of caring in the telehealth encounter included the ability to form a trusting relationship with the patient through honest engagement, showing that decisions made in the telehealth encounter are dependable and will be carried out, and showing competence by empowering patients to make changes or to take health-related actions.[26] The final quality that was found was intentionality. Intentionality was pervasive in all actions the APRNs took to conduct the encounter such that it enabled the APRNs to focus more on the strategies and meaning of those actions to convey caring, connecting with the patient. These are some of the ways nursing can promote and convey caring at a distance in the virtual environment. Additional study is needed regarding how nurses actualize caring in the virtual environment so that evidence for how caring can be enhanced and translated into telehealth practice can be further explored.

FOR REFLECTION 1:

What About Caring in the Virtual Environment?

 Consider how you define caring in nursing and what aspects are most important to achieving a caring presence. What do you think the challenges will be when transferring caring presence to the patient through the videoconferencing experience in the virtual environment?

Distance Communications

Changes in how humans communicate over time are part of the story of telehealth. When thinking about the origins of telehealth, consideration must be given to the history of communicating at a distance. Some of the first distance communications were via runners carrying messages to others to impart important information.[27] Additionally, sound was used to transcend the geographical barriers to communication in early cultures by way of drums and horns.[28] Visual methods such as fire, smoke signals, and flag semaphore were also used in early civilizations to convey distant messages.[29] Another visual method was the heliograph, which was used by the Greek soldiers to convey messages to companion soldiers by reflecting sun from their shields.[30] Written correspondence was also used for communicating at a distance, at times for obtaining medical advice and care. Subsequently, in the 1800s, with the development of the heliotrope for land surveys and the optical telegraph, a new era in communications arrived.[29,31] The modern electronic era of distance communications began with developments such as the telegraph, telephone, radio, and television as they heralded a new age of electrical communication. In the present day, digital data are the norm and are transmitted using wireless forms of communication, as advanced telecommunications technology, wireless transmission, wearables, and IoT are revolutionizing heath care and health care delivery.

Telehealth History: Combining Caring, Distance Communications, Technology, and Health Care Needs

The history of telehealth can be viewed in the context of caring, communications, and application of these advanced communication technologies to demonstrated health care needs. Modern telemedicine development is based on electronic telecommunications technology, including development of the telegraph, radio, telephone, and television. The earliest contemporary application of telemedicine began in the Netherlands in the early 1900s, with transmission of cardiac rhythms through the telephone lines.[29] The first innovators of telemedicine used their insight into what technology could offer to improve medical care by reaching remotely located patients and clinicians and transferring diagnostic and clinical data between the remote site and the physician.[29] During these early years, research focused on relevance, technologic functionality, capabilities and design of systems, and evidence to support its use.[32]

From around 1958, the National Aeronautics and Space Administration (NASA) was instrumental in research and development of technology to monitor astronaut biometric data as well as to provide remote medical care during manned space flights.[33] Otherwise, during these formative years of telehealth development, there was little public or private funding for telemedicine programs. Most programs during this time were developed due to the creative drive of just a few individuals who were determined to solve identified health care problems using distance communications, developing programs such as the Royal Flying Doctors of Australia, and the Boston-Logan Airport Telemedicine Program, in response to aviation accidents.[29,32,34] Closed-circuit television at Nebraska Psychiatric Institute (NPI) in 1959 and 1960 provided the first opportunity to establish a 2-way video and audio link for professional health care provider education between NPI and the University of Nebraska Medical School.[35] Their main goal was to test which clinical functions and physiologic data could be transmitted via technology.[35] Early programs showed that the technology was useful to clinical care, but this was constrained by the technology, costs, and reliability.[29] Results showed both advantages and disadvantages because the technology itself was not consistent and reliable enough for everyday use.[29]

By 1968, 3 major telemedicine programs were developed that moved telemedicine to the point of care: the NPI Telemedicine Program, the Massachusetts General Hospital to Boston-Logan Airport Telemedicine Program, and the Dartmouth Medical Center-Claremont General Hospital Telemedicine Program.[29,32] These programs were successful in providing data on telehealth programs and use of telehealth in health care.[36] All 3 programs were expanded in 1969 and 1970, resulting in the NPI to Nebraska Veterans Administration Network, the Massachusetts General to Bedford Veterans Administration Hospital Program, and the New Hampshire/Vermont Medical Interactive Television Network.[29] The pioneering programs of the early 1960s and the early telemedicine programs of the 1970s focused mainly on research and development.[29] During this time, there was limited federal funding for program development and testing, and, due to the high costs, only projects with federal funding could be developed. Research outcomes provided data on how systems of telehealth could be applied to meet and resolve health care problems, on whether these systems and models were effective at meeting defined outcomes, and on whether telemedicine could improve efficiency of providing care at a distance.[36] Many of these goals were not realized due to the exorbitant costs and technical difficulties.[29] However, telemedicine projects in the 1970s produced an abundance of worthwhile research on telehealth. Unfortunately, these programs were rarely sustainable; therefore, they were not able to adequately address problems of provider shortages, decreasing care disparities, and equitable access to care.[39] The ever-present issues of provider shortages, care disparities in rural and underserved regions, and cost barriers to access continue to plague the health care system and are reasons for the continued interest in telehealth over the decades.

The US federal government provided funding for telemedicine program development and testing between 1972 and 1974 with support for multiple projects.[36] These programs involved interdisciplinary teams and were the first important alignment of the concept of telemedicine and interdisciplinary practice.[29,36] The first national conferences for telemedicine also convened with interdisciplinary participants. Telemedicine grew during this period as several large telemedicine programs for research and development of telehealth programs, processes, and technologies were developed by NASA, including Space Technology Applied to Rural Papago Advanced Health Care, 2 Alaska telemedicine projects, and the Spacebridge programs.[29,36-38] Importantly for nursing, these early programs often involved nurses, and many times APRNs, who collaborated with physicians at the forefront of the care provided in the telemedicine project. A sampling of the nursing involvement in these important programs will be discussed in more detail in the following section.

During the latter 1970s and early 1980s, telemedicine program development was still not robust, due to lack of definitive findings about telemedicine, funding constraints, and growing health care issues restricting expansion.[29] Resurgence of telemedicine programs and technology development in the late 1980s was due to technology advances leading to decreased costs, a renewed focus on the continued deficiencies in our health care system, and the solution that telemedicine offers.[29] Telemedicine was transformed with the digital age, and the technology has picked up speed with

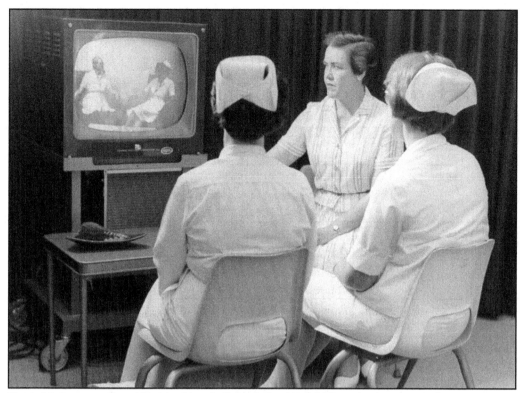

Figure 1-1. Nurses working with telehealth at the Nebraska Psychiatric Institute circa late 1950s/early 1960s. (Courtesy of the University of Nebraska Medical Center's McGoogan Library Special Collections and Archives. A Nebraska Psychiatric Institute Photo.)

each passing year. Today, society is linked by mobile devices, wearables, and wireless technology whose function permeates through all facets of life. Federal and private industry in telecommunications, health care, and health informatics form the basis of the technology for the future development of telehealth.

Telehealth is not only about using technology to deliver care, but the more basic roots relate to where that care is delivered. Delivery of care began in the home in early society, then evolved to centralized delivery in hospitals, clinics, and other facilities, requiring patients to come to the provider where the health care technologies were located. Early telemedicine programs were developed to connect physicians with patients in remote sites because physicians could not always be where they were needed at the moment they were needed. Using APRNs to address this workforce issue was tested in some of the early telemedicine programs. Nurses worked in many associated hospitals and clinics that were part of the first public and private telehealth programs. Nursing was an important component of the early telehealth programs as the nursing role and scope of practice was being explored.

Nursing in Early Telehealth: Projects, Roles, and Nurses

It may surprise some to know that nurses have been working in telehealth for over 60 years (Figure 1-1). It is a recognizable connection because the caring role of the nurse is an essential component of the US health care system. Telehealth nursing has evolved since these early days of telehealth, just as the role, education, and purpose of the nurse has changed over time (Table 1-1). Telehealth nursing can be defined in many ways, but at its core it is the integration of advanced telecommunication technologies in the provision of nursing care and in the practice of nursing.[39]

TABLE 1-1	
THE ROLE OF THE TELEHEALTH NURSE	
EARLY PROGRAM ROLES	**CURRENT AND FUTURE ROLES**
Assists physician	Collaborates with interdisciplinary team
Positions camera	Works with telehealth services industry to develop new technologies
Prepares patients	Educates patients and interdisciplinary team Creates partnerships with patients and provides support in managing the technology
Assists with presenting patient to remote physician	Delivers patient care remotely Consults with specialty providers Provides nursing care of patient at originating site during telehealth visit
Uses physician-developed protocols to deliver care	Provides evidence for practice through conducting and reviewing clinical research
Supervised by physicians through telehealth technology	Has independence of practice and develops innovative programs to provide cost-effective care, increasing access to care, improving satisfaction and the patient care experience, leading to improved patient care outcomes

The role of the nurse in the early telemedicine projects varied from project to project depending upon the purpose, technology, and clinical setting of the program. Additionally, the full scope of the nurse's role in the early telehealth programs was not always clearly discussed in project reports, summaries, and publications. Nurses filled the role of telemedicine coordinator, telepresenter, camera operator, and direct care provider. An exhaustive review of the nursing role and involvement in all telehealth projects is beyond the scope of this book; therefore, a representative sampling of nursing in early telehealth programs related to the projects, the nursing role, and the nurses follows.

Women's Hospital, Birmingham, England

Whether or not Alexander Graham Bell actually used the first transmission of electronic speech in 1876 to summon medical help for a battery acid spill,[29] the telephone quickly became a tool used by medical practitioners to assist in providing health care. Use of the telephone in health care was first mentioned in the *Lancet* on February 9, 1878.[40] A letter to the editor described how the telephone could be used to aid medical diagnoses by transmitting muscle contraction sounds. Another letter described how a physician used the telephone to diagnose a child with a cough and to reduce unnecessary doctor visits. By 1880, the *Lancet* reported that in the Women's Hospital in Birmingham, England, the medical participating staff was using the telephone to connect their facilities located in different geographic areas.[40] It is likely that nurses were some of the users of the telephone in health care within this hospital and the other hospitals that quickly followed.

Nebraska Psychiatric Institute Program, Omaha, Nebraska

Closed-circuit television was an essential design element in the NPI for the purpose of providing exponential education with innovative learning experiences not otherwise available.[41] Using

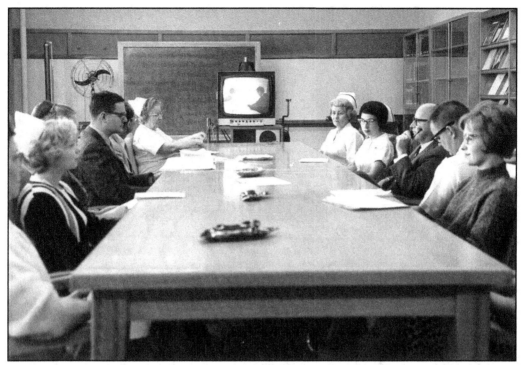

Figure 1-2. Nurses at Norfolk State Hospital working with telehealth. (Courtesy of the University of Nebraska Medical Center's McGoogan Library Special Collections and Archives. A Nebraska Psychiatric Institute Photo.)

closed-circuit television as a tool in nursing education is discussed in a 1956 article that described nurses observing patient activity over the closed-circuit television. The NPI conducted the first systematic study of telemedicine in the United States in 1959.[29] In this study, a control group used standard in-person care and an experimental group used a 2-way television. The purpose of the study was to assess the educational programs and clinical activities such as group psychotherapy sessions using the closed-circuit television to evaluate overall patient and provider acceptance of telemedicine, as well as whether the system was feasible and effective. Additionally, the project provided education and in-service education for staff, including nurses (Figure 1-2). The program was successful, and a fully operational telemedicine program was opened in 1964. The program provided psychiatric, neurologic, and specialty medical consults and medical collaborations between Norfolk State Hospital in Virginia and the NPI (Figure 1-3).

A Survey of Medical Applications of Television

By 1963, the National Naval Medical Center in Bethesda, Maryland, and Walter Reed Medical Center in Washington, DC, were regularly using television as a tool in health care delivery.[32] A survey by Shackel[42] reported that the most widespread use of television in health care was for the purpose of education. However, Shackel also found effective demonstrations of applications of television to aid in remote diagnosis in nursing.

Cook County Hospital Department of Urology Picturephone Project, Chicago, Illinois

Just as a variety of technologies are tested in our current age, so too were they tested in the early period of telemedicine. In 1966, in Cook County Hospital, Chicago, Illinois, the Department of Urology began to use picturephones to improve care and communication between staff and patients.[36] The device was reportedly used to connect clinics and practice sites, including

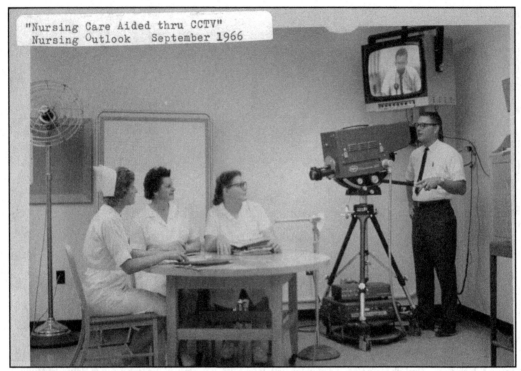

"Nursing Care Aided thru CCTV"
Nursing Outlook   September 1966

Figure 1-3. Nurses at Norfolk State Hospital working with telehealth in 1966. (Courtesy of the University of Nebraska Medical Center's McGoogan Library Special Collections and Archives. A Nebraska Psychiatric Institute Photo.)

radiology, operating rooms, emergency rooms, and exam rooms. Nurses, in addition to physicians, were trained to use the picturephones for care delivery and patient consultations, for education and continuing education, and for patient education.

Alaska Telemedicine Program: Applied Technology Satellites 1 and 6

On August 31, 1933, an amateur radio station operator in Alaska received a call for help.[43] He connected the call to a physician 1,000 miles away who diagnosed a 5-year-old boy with appendicitis. The call was relayed to the US Army Alaska Telegraph, which arranged for a seaplane to take the doctor to the child, saving his life. By the 1950s, an Alaskan communication network was established for access to medical care.[29] Although the radio was used for medical care, successfully improving the ability to provide care in these polar regions, atmospheric ionization caused much interference with transmissions.[43] On July 12, 1966, a satellite station was launched in Alaska, creating NASA's Applied Technology Satellite-1 (ATS-1) program.[29,43] The first uses were for distance education of health care providers. In 1971, the Bureau of Indian Affairs began a health care system for settlements in Alaska, enabling telemedicine consults in the ATS-1 system by using shortwave radio devices in the clinics.[43]

On May 30, 1974, the ATS-6 satellite was launched, enabling initiation of the Alaska ATS-6 Washington-Alaska-Montana-Idaho Telemedicine/Education Program.[28,43] The reported goal was to assess the technology for clinical purposes, and the upgraded equipment enabled better communications among hospitals and nurse outpatient clinics in the extremely remote areas. All clinics and consultant links in this program used live videoconferencing, and tele-auscultation equipment, including tele-electrocardiograms (ECGs) and medical information systems, began to be used. Nurses worked in the remote clinics. For example, Yukon clinic nurses frequently used interactive video transmissions for patient consultations to Tanana Hospital, enabling patients to see the field doctor or medical consultant. Results were reported to be successful, and the Alaska Telemedicine Network provided evidence that the technical quality of the equipment provided satisfactory diagnostic quality for clinical care and that telemedicine was efficient.

Massachusetts General Hospital Telemedicine Program, Boston, Massachusetts

During the late 1960s, health care was experiencing primary care workforce shortages and misdistribution of health care providers and services. Much discussion ensued about innovative ways to provide rural and underserved patients access to care outside of large medical centers. Additionally, the role of the nurse practitioner was evolving, and interest in using nurses in primary care was growing. In this changing environment, a stimulus to the development of telemedicine occurred in response to 2 separate incidents at Boston's Logan International Airport. In 1962, a plane crashed upon takeoff at Logan, causing many deaths, and inefficiencies in medical and emergency management systems were identified.[29] Subsequently, a medical station was established at the airport in collaboration with Massachusetts General Hospital.[29] Shortly after the opening of the medical station, an incident occurred at the airport where a woman suffered a complex fracture.[29,36] It is reported that the nurse practitioner staffing the clinic assessed the severity of the fracture and determined that the physician should evaluate the patient before she was moved. The physician contacted was Dr. Kenneth Bird, and it was at this time that he realized that live television capability between the patient and the physician and the ability to see the radiology imaging remotely would enable more efficient care.[29] Therefore, in 1968, the Massachusetts General Hospital telemedicine program established a connection to Logan International Airport for provision of telemedicine services.[29] At the airport clinic, it is reported that employees and travelers could receive medical care from Massachusetts General Hospital providers via 2-way audiovisual microwave circuit. The medical station was staffed with nurses and physicians. Nurse practitioners staffed the medical station 24/7 and were responsible for triaging, evaluating, and treating patients and using the technology to obtain physician consults. When physicians were not present, they would connect as needed using telephone and/or 2-way radio using microwave transmission for communications and for transmission of radiology images.[29,36] The program was reported to be successful, and a second link was established in 1970 to the Veterans Administration in Bedford, Massachusetts. Initially set up for psychiatric and neurologic consultations, soon other medical consultation ensued, such as cardiology consults at Massachusetts General Hospital. By 1974, nurses such as Elizabeth Quinn and Gertrude B. Nolan were using teleconsultation in nursing practice and incorporating telehealth into the role of the nurse.[29,44]

New Hampshire-Vermont Medical Interactive Television Network, Hanover, New Hampshire

Dartmouth Medical Center in Hanover, New Hampshire, developed an interactive 2-way closed-circuit television network connecting multiple health clinics, correctional facilities, and academic institutions from Dartmouth Medical School and the University of Vermont in 1968.[36] The reported objectives included provision of specialty medical consultations, patient care delivery, and continuing education in a sharing network in New England. The network connected facilities in these institutions using microwave transmissions via mobile carts. Approximately one quarter of the use was for continuing education, including pharmacology courses for Licensed Practical Nurses (LPNs) and student nurses and education for surgical and coronary care nurses. Health care faculty and staff, including nurses, were also involved in the telemedicine care delivery. Although the program was mainly focused on health care education, improved access to medical specialty consultations were provided to patients living in remote areas using telehealth.

Rural Health Associates, Farmington, Maine

The Rural Health Associated Program was located in Farmington, Maine, and was developed for the purpose of providing access to care in west central Maine in 1971.[36] This private health care facility is reported to have used telemedicine as a clinical support service for supervision of nurse clinicians by primary care physicians in the geographically remote areas of Maine using interactive television. Family nurse associates and pediatric nurse associates assisted with general medicine and specialty consultations in this program. The system was used for administration, education, consultation, and direct patient care. The project was successful in showing effectiveness of using nurse practitioners to deliver primary care using telehealth and having physicians supervise nurse practitioners using technology. Widespread patient and provider satisfaction were also reported.

Evaluation of the Impact of Communications Technology and Improved Medical Protocol on Health Care Delivery in Penal Institutions, Miami, Florida

An innovative program was conducted in 1973 at the Dade County, Florida, penal institution targeting inmates in the main jail and the women's detention center.[36] The purpose of this project was to support 6 primary care nurse practitioner students in nurse practitioner training and in jailhouse medical protocols in order to deliver primary care to inmates using telehealth as compared with the traditional in-person delivery of primary care by medical doctors.[45] Wide-band black-and-white audiovisual communications connected Dade County prison and penal health services to Jackson Memorial Hospital. Program results found that the quality of care provided by the nurse practitioners using telehealth was equal to that of the in-person care delivered by medical doctors. In addition to the nurse practitioners, there were registered nurses working in the program to deliver primary care and specialty care at Jackson Memorial Hospital.

Illinois State Psychiatric Institute Picturephone Program, Chicago, Illinois

A telepsychiatry program was developed in 1973 at the Illinois State Psychiatric Institute using picturephone technology, connecting the institute with 4 facilities for the purpose of providing psychiatric care, as well as to evaluate the usefulness of telemedicine for access to crisis care and to assist in coordination of care for patients treated at multiple facilities.[29] Staff at 2 of the linked facilities (psychiatric and pediatric institutes) included registered nurses. Overall results showed that the volume of patients seen increased and the technology was useful in enabling remote care and attendance of educational conferences.

Case Western Reserve University Telemedicine Program, Cleveland, Ohio

At Case Western Reserve University in 1972, a 2-way audiovisual communication system was established between the Cleveland Veterans Administration Hospital and Case Western Reserve University Hospital for the purpose of establishing a consultation portal between the hospital and nurse-anesthetists at the Veterans Administration.[36] The program is reported to have enabled anesthesiologists to consult and supervise an anesthetist remotely. The project's audiovisual capabilities enabled visualization of the patient and nurse as well as the ability to use an electronic stethoscope to hear heart and Korotkoff sounds. The technology also incorporated teletransmission of electrocardiography recordings. The practitioners and administrators using the system reported that the system improved patient care by way of the ease of consultation and supervision.

Nursing Home Telemedicine Project, Boston, Massachusetts

In an effort to address quality-of-care issues and accessibility of primary care, the Boston Nursing Home Project at the Boston City Hospital, Massachusetts, was developed in 1972.[36] The stated goal was to provide more consistent and available care to patients discharged from hospitals to nursing homes. The program is reported to have used an internist and 4 specially trained nurse practitioners, serving 250 patients in 10 nursing homes. The nurse practitioner completed initial evaluations on patients after admission to the nursing home and then met with the physician either in person or via a narrow-band telecommunications system; telephone, facsimile, and instant camera were also used for consultation and communication of findings.[36] Two of the nurse practitioners in the program were trained at Boston City Hospital in a special 12-week course in adult medicine, and all 4 nurse practitioners spent about 80% of their time providing care in the nursing home supervised by the internist. This program had several targeted outcomes, including assessing costs and benefits related to systems operations and the role of the nurse practitioner in telehealth in using advanced communication technology in practice.[29] Results were positive, showing cost-effectiveness and improved outcomes as nurse practitioners contributed to improved quality and access to care.

Blue Hill Interactive Television Project, Deer Isle, Maine

The Blue Hill Interactive Television Project was formed to provide medical care to a remote area of Maine in 1972.[36] The technology used in the program included interactive television using microwave transmission from Blue Hill Memorial Hospital to Deer Island Medical Center. The family nurse practitioner staffing Deer Isle is reported to have connected to 4 physicians at the hospital for consultations as needed. The primary uses of the system included teaching, primary care, and medical and surgery consultations. Nurse practitioners, including Elaine McCarty, used the telemedicine system for approximately 40 patients each month.[36] Results showed the practitioners using this system had increased satisfaction as their experience using the technology increased.[29] A survey asked whether patients were willing to receive care from nurse practitioners if they were able to consult with a physician using telemedicine.[36] Results revealed patient comfort with seeing a nurse practitioner when a consult with a physician was available via telemedicine when needed. This survey was the first to use objective data from a community to support use of telemedicine systems of care.

Telecommunications System Project, Cambridge, Massachusetts

The Cambridge Massachusetts Telemedicine Project was formed in 1972 to provide nurse practitioner–delivered primary care and adult internal medicine consultation services, linking 3 Cambridge Health clinics to Cambridge Hospital.[36] The clinic services were free of charge to anyone within the area, and each clinic is reported to have had one nurse. The goal of this demonstration program was to assess the effectiveness and efficiency of primary care nurse practitioner care delivery.[36] The project used a control group and an experimental group, with the control group using telephone consultation and the experimental group using telehealth consultations. Each nurse practitioner attended a 6-week course at Massachusetts General Hospital. Protocols included standardization of care and when to consult a physician using the telemedicine system. There were at least 220 patients seen at all clinics, resulting in around 55 consults per month, of which approximately half were telehealth consultations. Due to the randomization, some patents required telehealth consults when a simple telephone call would have sufficed, and the nurse practitioners and physicians felt this was inefficient. Overall, both practitioners were satisfied with the program. Physicians enjoyed the ability to see and hear the patient and the nurse practitioner because this also allowed them to elicit patient histories themselves. Patents also reported equivalent satisfaction with the program, and having access to the physician at the hospital when needed comforted them.

Experiment in a Bidirectional Cable Television System to Support a Rural Practice, Waconia, Minnesota

A novel program to address rural health care was developed in 1973 at the Lakeview Clinics in Minnesota.[36] This project used a 2-directional television system to aid communication between physicians, patients, and allied health personnel (including nurses), connecting clinics in Waconia and Jonathan, Minnesota, to a hospital in Waconia. One of the main objectives of the program was to evaluate the effect of telemedicine on allied health personnel participation in patient care and patient management decisions. Both nurses and physicians reported satisfaction with the service. It was reported that the nurses found it useful to have more physician availability using telemedicine than in the traditional in-person setting.

Wagner Bidirectional Cable Link Program, Mount Sinai School of Medicine, New York, New York

The Wagner Bidirectional Cable Link Project in 1973 was a collaboration of the Mount Sinai School of Medicine Pediatric Office and Wagner Child Health Station, a pediatric outreach clinic in East Harlem, New York.[36] The objective of the program was to evaluate whether this technology could be used to replace in-person patient care visits while maintaining quality and decreasing physician time. The codirector of the Wagner Child Health Station was Beatrice E. Thomstad, RN, MPH.[36,43] Four nurse practitioners rotated between the clinic and the pediatric offices. They received training in medical protocols that were used to guide the primary care provided in the clinics. Specialty consults were also enabled by use of the telemedicine system. Both physicians and nurse practitioners were reportedly satisfied using the technology, and patients found it satisfying to save travel time while being cared for by their own providers, with whom they already had a connection.

Space Technology Applied to Rural Papago Advanced Health Care, Indian Health Service, Arizona

Space Technology Applied to Rural Papago Advanced Health Care (STARPAHC) was a NASA telehealth program in collaboration with the Papago Tribe (now the Tohono O'odham Nation), the Lockheed Missile and Space Company, the Indian Health Service (IHS), and the Department of Health, Education, and Welfare.[29,43] The project was an early attempt at using telemedicine to remote populations and focused on exploring possibilities of using technology to provide clinical care and consults in a remote population in southern Arizona in 1973.[37,38] The project used physicians, physician assistants, and nurses in the remote clinics. The project trained staff and reportedly included a course in public nursing. Additionally, the Papago Psychological Service Program was asked by the Australian Ministry of Health for advice as to how to provide psychological services to Aboriginal Australians.[37] Toward this effort, an Aboriginal Australian who was a public health nurse went to the reservation for training for the STARPAHC program. The project was successful and demonstrated the feasibility of public and private partnerships using telehealth in rural populations.[29] The main health care facility in the project was Sells Hospital, where 2 administrative registered nurses, 10 registered nurses (RNs), 7 LPNs, and 6 nurse assistants participated.[37] The Santa Rosa Clinic had one clinical nurse and one public health nurse (PHRN), and the San Xavier Clinic had one PHRN, one RN, and one LPN. There was also a referral center at the IHS hospital in Phoenix with access to medical specialists. Technology included a 2-way video, audio, and data communications link between the facilities, for which clinical care was the primary use. The program identified many salient points for considering when implementing projects of this scale, including the difficulty in managing and sustaining a large-scale project.[29] The project did not show cost-effectiveness, likely due to the increased need for access to care and the many health care problems that were identified.

Puerto Rico Telemedicine Program, Ponce District, Puerto Rico

One strategy to address physician shortages and hospital overcrowding in Puerto Rico was to connect regional hospitals to smaller facilities on the island.[29] In 1974, a telemedicine system using microwave technology was initiated to connect the Ponce District Hospital to a smaller distant facility in Guyama.[36] The population served was approximately 1.8 million low-income patients.[36] The stated purpose of the program was to establish a telehealth model for the island to provide primary, emergency, and medical care as well as medical graduate and continuing education opportunities.[29] Staff at Ponce District Hospital and Guyama Hospital used telehealth in their usual routine of care, also using the technology to transmit diagnostic data and imaging, which improved diagnoses.[36] Nurses from both facilities were reportedly part of the telemedicine project committee. Results revealed that stakeholder involvement affected acceptance, and those involved in the planning of the project rated effectiveness and acceptance higher than those with less involvement or interest in the telemedicine program.

Comparison of Television and Telephone for Remote Medical Consultation, Cambridge, Massachusetts

Advanced practice nursing was at the forefront of this early comparison of television and telephone for remote consultation program. In 1973, a study to assess the clinical application and usefulness of television and telephone consultations was conducted by connecting Cambridge Hospital physicians to remote primary care neighborhood clinics' nurse practitioners.[46] The project focused on whether the efficiency of the nurse practitioner would increase and whether patient referrals to a physician would decrease. Satisfaction was also measured. Standardized protocols guided the 3 participating nurse practitioners' practice and decision making as they saw more than 1400 patients over a 6-month period at 3 separate sites.[46] Project results endorsed longer times for television consultations, causing prolonged times in pre- and post-consultation care and longer scheduling times. However, consultations by television decreased referrals of patients to hospital physicians as compared with telephone consults. Participants reported equivalent satisfaction, although they reported better clinical decision making with the television and more satisfaction with the ability to decrease provider isolation.

Evaluation of Television Consultations Between a Large Neonatal Care Hospital and a Community Hospital, Case Western Reserve University, Cleveland, Ohio

This 1974 telemedicine project used a 2-way television link to connect nurses at a small inner-city hospital with neonatologists at a large university medical center for the purpose of screening for problems in high-risk neonates.[47] Stated goals were to develop a prenatal guideline for screening high-risk mothers and to screen the infants born to these high-risk mothers for illnesses. The technology is reported to have enabled neonatologists and the community nurses to consult daily regarding assessment and management plans for the neonates, as the neonatologists advised nurses in the care of these high-risk infants and recommended transfer to the university hospital when necessary. The program outcome measured transfers from the community hospitals to the university hospitals, and results showed an increase in the transfer rate when patients were assessed with the television. Project researchers reported that the direct visual screening of neonates increased recognition of possible neonatal morbidity and was a positive result. Additionally, guidelines with criteria for transfer and high-risk screening were also more consistent.

Sioux Lookout Program, Ontario, Canada

A systematic study focused on provider and patient satisfaction with telemedicine was conducted in 1977 at the Sioux Lookout Program.[29] This telehealth system used slow-scan video technology to deliver care, and providers were surveyed to assess their attitudes about the system.[48] The survey found that the 34 nurses and 4 physicians participating in the survey were positive about telemedicine, whereas 2 physicians were neutral. The neutral responses indicated that these physicians did not need to use telemedicine for support, but the positive responses indicated recognition of the possibility for increased patient access to care and improved outcomes.

Spacebridge Programs, United States and Russia

A program between the United States and Russia was developed in the early 1980s to provide international broadcast of public programs between the 2 countries using live audiovisual telecommunications.[29] The purpose was to enable engagement and communication, including sharing music, on a variety of subjects. The launch of this endeavor, the US Festival, was held in 1982, and an effort between the Russian radio system, Gosteleradio, and the computer pioneer, Steve Wozniak, through his company at the time, Unison.[49] Subsequent programs were held through 1988. Then, on December 7, 1988, the Spitak earthquake occurred in Armenia, killing 50,000 people, injuring over 100,000, and destroying most of the medical infrastructure and vital services.[50] When the earthquake struck, then-president Mikhail Gorbachev was in the United States visiting with President Ronald Reagan, and Gorbachev asked the United States for help with this disaster.[51] Coincidentally, also at this time, Dr. Nicogossian from NASA and Dr. Gazenko from Russia were at the American Medical Association/Russian Academy of Sciences meeting in California.[51] Through Dr. Nicogossian, NASA agreed to use and upgrade the existing telecommunications infrastructure from the US Festival Programs to provide aid to Armenia.[50] Within 2 weeks, the United States and Russia established connections to Armenia to provide telemedicine support to the people injured in this disaster.[43] The Spacebridge was reportedly fully operational 5 months after the disaster struck, enabling this joint program to establish telemedicine consultations and provision of care from 4 medical centers in the United States to the Russian center in Yerevan. Satellite communications using 2-way audio and 1-way video enabled support for postdisaster recovery. A project of this size took months to set up logistically, and bureaucratic issues had to be overcome.[51] The Spacebridge provided telemedicine consultations for almost 2 months for 209 patients, significantly improving their care.[51] This project demonstrated success in deploying telecommunications across vast geographic distances, cultures, and countries for the purpose of providing medical care during disaster relief efforts.

During the operation of Spacebridge, another disaster occurred in Russia. On June 4, 1989, 2 passenger trains collided in Ulfa, in the Ash-Ulu-Telyak region.[51] This accident caused an explosion of oil pipelines through the leaking of flammable gases. Five hundred seventy-five people were killed and over 600 were injured.[51] This time, Spacebridge set up a telecommunications link with the area to provide real-time telemedicine between Ula and selected US medical centers. This project lasted 3 months, completing 51 consultations for 253 patients and using 400 physicians and nurses from both US sites and the Ulfa site.[51] The project demonstrated the feasibility of mobilizing an existing network for disaster relief operations.

In 1991, NASA and the Uniformed Services University for the Health Sciences in Bethesda, Maryland, held the first international conference on telemedicine and disaster medicine, which led to development of follow-up Spacebridge projects: the Spacebridge to Moscow Project (1993) and the Spacebridge to Russia Project (1994), both at the Clinical Hospital in Moscow.[51] These projects also showed that it was feasible for telemedicine programs to be used to provide health care at a distance. Nurses participated in these programs, although their involvement was limited. Nursing involvement included helping to coordinate activities related to live events between the hospital in Moscow and participating sites in the United States and Russia. The Spacebridge project was an important contribution to telemedicine because it helped to provide a foundation for continued growth of telemedicine by using the established models and examples, by reviewing successes and factors creating barriers to care, and by developing services and technologies. It allowed NASA to use the internet in telemedicine and enabled use of the internet for electronic health records.[50]

"The Wired Prairie" and the Health Information and Technology Scholars Program, Kansas

One of the first distance-learning programs specifically for nurses in a school of nursing was developed in the 1990s at the University of Kansas School of Nursing.[52] Dr. Helen Connors began to work with the established University of Kansas telemedicine program to use technology to expand educational opportunities to student nurses in rural communities.[53] Starting with connections to rural Kansas hospitals and clinics and then transforming the program to become available to nurses worldwide, this successful distance-learning program was developed to provide nursing education to students to whom it would otherwise be unavailable. The program was honored in a *Time* magazine Heroes of Medicine article titled "The Wired Prairie."[52] Additionally, in an effort to empower nursing faculty educators to integrate technology into their courses, Dr. Connors and colleagues developed the Health Information and Technology Scholars collaborative program with 3 US universities and the National League for Nursing.[53] This program focused on teaching faculty about telehealth and health information technologies and how to incorporate them into their student education.

Telemedicine in Critical Care: An Experiment in Health Care Delivery, Cleveland, Ohio

Interactive television was used in 1977 to connect critical care medicine physician experts at the University of Cleveland with a smaller, private, inner-city hospital intensive care unit (ICU) in Cleveland.[50] Nurses participated in the daily consultations and assumed the role of telepresenter: positioning the camera, preparing the patient, presenting the patient to the physician, and implementing recommendations of care as ordered by the remote-site physicians. Results supported using telemedicine to provide critical care consultations to facilities without critical care experts because patient outcomes were improved when consultants' recommendations were followed. Organizational problems and other barriers, such as site selection, were also identified.

The teleICU model has been further studied and developed and, by 2014, 11% of public and private ICUs use the teleICU model.[54] RNs and APRNs are essential to providing care for critical care patients, and they have an important role in teleICUs. ICU nurses use advanced technologies and medical peripherals to monitor patients and clinicians for best practices, which improves outcomes through the provision of this higher level of care.[55] In 2010, the American Association for Critical Nurses formed a task force to study and develop the teleICU nursing role and created guidelines for nursing practice. In 2014, the American Association for Critical Nurses published a consensus statement for teleICU nursing practice.[56]

FOR REFLECTION 2:

What Is My Role as a Telehealth Nurse?

 Now that you have reviewed some of the early telehealth nursing roles, think about the roles and responsibilities of nurses, including APRNs. What were some of the most interesting aspects of the nursing involvement in these early programs? What are your thoughts about the similarities and differences between the early telehealth nursing role and what your role might be today?

Telehealth Nursing Practice in the New Millennium

Telehealth has application to all areas of health care, and nursing has opportunities to embrace the infusion of telehealth technologies into everyday practice. To continue leadership and be at the forefront of care delivery, nurses need to be well-versed in the technology and how to leverage it to improve nursing care and health care outcomes. Just as nurses are advocates for patients and practice in the traditional setting, so too must they be advocates in the expansion and transition to this new way of practicing. Acceptance of the conceptual constructs and actualities of telehealth use is necessary for providers and patients, and in addition to fiscal, legal, and regulatory barriers, this surfaces as an important issue for transition to telehealth practice.[57] In order for transition to happen, nursing should take steps to build acceptance through informing nurses through substantial knowledge and skill development so that they can develop confidence using telehealth to deliver nursing care. Nurses as patient advocates will also be relied upon to introduce and educate patients regarding telehealth, just as nurses provide patient education in traditional nursing practice:

> As one of the most widespread professions with high-level skills, nurses across America are called to action to determine how to leverage informatics and technology in the transformation of care delivery to improve the nation's health with high-quality, cost-efficient, and convenient care.[54]

For nursing to be an essential partner in the remodeling of health care, promotion of an agenda that supports adoption of technology has implications for nursing practice. Nurses could therefore have valuable input in the political arena and influence agendas, as well as work directly with technology companies to develop cost-effective solutions that address needs as viewed through the eyes of the nurse. Nursing can also work to develop telehealth networks for education and patient care, becoming experts in matching the correct telehealth solution to the patient care need.[57] This can result in nursing remaining significant as traditional health care and telehealth merge into a collaborative and cohesive partnership.

Nursing as an Essential Interdisciplinary Team Partner in Telehealth

Just as nursing and nurses were important team members in the early telehealth programs, they are important interdisciplinary partners in the new generation of technology-enhanced delivery and integration of care. "Progressive development and sophistication of communication and technology, coupled with demand for novel approaches to care, positions nurses to collaborate and address health disparities in these communities through deployment of telehealth technology."[54] The majority of health care involves nurses, who are the largest and most trusted health care workforce in the United States.[58,59] Nursing has always held a significant role in health care, and as an essential partner, nursing should work to promote engagement with the patient as well as the interdisciplinary team when using telehealth (see Chapter 9).

GROUP EXERCISE

What About Attitudes?

Supporting adoption of telehealth in nursing practice can be influenced by the attitudes of the nurse and the patient regarding the technology. Consider that nurses have long introduced new technologies to patients, from the stethoscope, to cardiac monitors, to automatic blood pressure machines, to electronic intravenous pumps. Now, nurses will play a major role in introducing patients to telehealth. How can a nurse's personal knowledge, skills, and attitudes about telehealth affect how he or she will teach and inform patients about telehealth? How can this influence patient attitudes and willingness to use telehealth?

CONCLUSION

Nurses have long been essential providers of care, responding to the needs of family, friends, community, and society as a whole through the art and science of nursing practice. Advanced technologic capabilities for health care has roots in distance communication, evolving from simple visual methods such as fires and flags to our present-day highly technological capabilities. The role of the nurse has been transformed over time, responding to societal norms, environment, available evidence, and technological capabilities. As technology converges with health care, nurses have the opportunity to provide an essential link in telehealth care. Successful telehealth nursing practice in the new millennium will leverage technology to improve health care outcomes. Substantive nursing telehealth knowledge and skill acquisition can build confidence and acceptance in nurses to use telehealth in nursing practice. The partnership of nursing and the patient care team, as demonstrated in the early telehealth programs, as well as in nursing practice today, is also an important element of current and future nursing telehealth practice. As these factors coalesce, at some point in the future, nursing will be able to say that we are able to provide the right care, in the right place, and at the right time.

THOUGHTFUL QUESTIONS

1. What questions do you have when considering how to bring the art of nursing into the virtual environment?
2. How does the connected consumer influence the acquisition of telehealth?
3. How can telehealth aid the personalization of health care? What strengths and alignments does nursing offer?
4. How do you envision your role as a telehealth nurse? What is one strength you bring when considering the changes in practice going forward?

CASE STUDY

A small, rural primary care clinic has a high rate of patients with heart failure with a higher than national rate of being readmitted within 30 days of hospitalization for a heart failure exacerbation. The clinic has 2 physicians and 4 APRNs serving a large, underserved population. In the recent past, a distant university medical center has provided remote patient monitoring services for the clinic's patients with strokes who were discharged from the medical center, and the clinic providers were involved with the collection and assessment of the remote data as well as with providing follow-up for any patient data outliers. This program worked well to provide better access to care for these patients and decreased their readmission rates substantially through the timely management of problems. The medical center has recently contacted the clinic and offered to partner with them to develop a pilot remote patient monitoring program to address their high heart failure readmission rates. Several of the APRNs are excited for the possibility of improving the health outcomes in their heart failure population and begin to work with the medical center to develop the program.

Questions

1. If you were one of the involved practitioners, what roles could you play in the development of this telehealth program?
2. Who would you partner with to implement the program?
3. What would you need to teach the patients about telehealth to build their confidence with the technology, enabling them to see how it can personally benefit their health?

REFERENCES

1. Health IT.gov. What is telehealth? How is telehealth different from telemedicine? https://www.healthit.gov/faq/what-telehealth-how-telehealth-different-telemedicine. Accessed December 21, 2019.
2. Bashshur RL, Krupinski EA, Doarn CR, Merrell RC, Woolliscroft JO, Frenk J. Telemedicine across time: integrated health system of the future–a prelude [published online ahead of print March 11, 2019]. *Telemed J E Health*. doi:10.1089/tmj.2019.0025.
3. Schlachta-Fairchild LM. Description of the professional role and predictors of role stress, role ambiguity and role conflict. *Augusta University Thesis and Dissertations*. 2000. https://augusta.openrepository.com/handle/10675.2/575461. Accessed February 12, 2020.
4. Grady JL, Schlachta-Fairchild L. Report of the 2004-2005 International Telenursing Survey. *Comput Inform Nurs*. 2007;25(5):266-272.
5. Adams LY. The conundrum of caring in nursing. *International Journal of Caring Sciences*. 2016;9(1):1-8.
6. Lordkipanidze D, Vekua A, Ferring R, et al. Anthropology: the earliest toothless hominin skull. *Nature*. 2005;4(7034):717-718.
7. Leininger MM. The culture care concept and its relevance to nursing. *J Nurs Educ*. 1967;6:27-37.
8. Watson J. *Nursing: The Philosophy and Science of Caring*. Boulder, CO: University Press of Colorado; 2008.
9. Theofanidis D, Sapountzi-Krepia D. Nursing and caring: an historical overview from ancient Greek tradition to modern times. *International Journal of Caring Sciences*. 2015;8(3):791-800.
10. Stewart IM, Austin AL. *History of Nursing: From Ancient to Modern Times: A World View*. New York: G. P. Putnam's Sons; 1962.
11. Risse G. *Mending Bodies, Saving Souls: A History of Hospitals*. Oxford, UK: Oxford University Press; 1999.
12. King H. *Hippocrates' Woman: Reading the Female Body in Ancient Greece*. London: Routledge; 1998.
13. Blainey G. *A Short History of Christianity*. Lanham, MD: Rowman & Littlefield; 2011.
14. Callahan J. 7 Bible verses that illustrate the importance of caring for others. *The Christian Post*. http://www.christianpost.com/buzzvine/7bible-verses-that-illustrate-the-importance-of-caring-for-others-125056/. Accessed February 12, 2020.

15. Osiek C. Diakonos and prostatis: women's patronage in early Christianity. *HTS Theological Studies.* 2005;61(1&2):347-370.

16. Ogilive MB. *Women in Science: Antiquity Through Nineteenth Century.* Cambridge, MA: MIT Press; 1986.

17. Cilliers L, Retief F. The evolution of the hospital from antiquity to the end of the middle ages. *Curationis.* 2002;25:60-66.

18. Nutting M, Dock L. *History of Nursing (Vol I).* New York: Putman & Sons; 1907.

19. Benedictow OJ. *The Black Death 1346-1353: The Complete History.* Trowbridge, UK: Cromwell Press; 2004.

20. Kourkouta L, Lanara V. Terms used in Byzantium for nursing personnel. *Int Hist Nurs J.* 1996;2(1):46-57.

21. Miller T. *The Birth of the Hospital in the Byzantine Empire.* Baltimore, MD: Johns Hopkins University Press; 1997.

22. Abel-Smith B. *A History of the Nursing Profession.* London: Heinemann-Kingswood; 1960.

23. Nightingale, F. *Notes on Nursing: What It Is, and What It Is Not.* New York: Appleton-Century; 1946.

24. Carper BA. Fundamental patterns of knowing in nursing. *Adv Nurs Sci.* 1978;1(1).

25. Leininger, M. Leininger's theory of nursing: cultural care diversity and universality. *Nurs Sci Q.* 1988;1(4):152-160.

26. Varghese SB, Phillips CA. Caring in telehealth. *Telemedicine and e-Health.* 2009;15(10):1005-1009.

27. Rheuban KS, Krupinski EA. *Understanding Telehealth.* New York: McGraw Hill; 2018.

28. Martin S. *A Short History of Disease: From the Black Death to Ebola.* Harpenden, UK: Oldcastle Books; 2015.

29. Bashshur RL, Shannon GW. History of telemedicine: evolution, context, and transformation. *Healthc Inform Res.* 2010;16(1):65-66.

30. Dakyns H. *Hellenica by Xenophon.* 1998. https://www.gutenberg.org/etext/1174. Accessed February 10, 2020.

31. Dilhac JM. The telegraph of Claude Chappe: an optical telecommunications network for the XVIIIth century. 2001. https://ethw.org/w/images/1/17/Dilhac.pdf. Accessed February 10, 2020.

32. Park B. *An Introduction to Telemedicine: Interactive Television for Delivery of Health Services.* New York: Rockefeller Foundation; 1974.

33. National Aeronautics Space Administration. A brief history of NASA's contributions to telemedicine. 2013. https://www.nasa.gov/content/a-brief-history-of-nasa-s-contributions-to-telemedicine/. Accessed May 11, 2019.

34. Eikelboom RH. The telegraph and the beginnings of telemedicine in Australia. *Global Telehealth 2012.* 2012;182:67-72.

35. Grigsby J, Kaehny MM, Sandberg EJ, Schlenker RE, Shaughnessy PW. Effects and effectiveness of telemedicine. *Health Care Financ Rev.* 1995;17(1):115-131.

36. Bashshur RL, Armstrong PA, Youssef ZI. *Telemedicine: Explorations in the Use of Telecommunications in Health Care.* Springfield, IL: Charles C. Thomas; 1975.

37. Freiburger G, Holcomb M, Piper D. The STARPAHC collection: part of an archive of the history of telemedicine. *J Telemed Telecare.* 2007;13:221-223.

38. Fuchs M. Provider attitudes toward STARPAHC: a telemedicine project on the Papago reservation. *Med Care.* 1979;1:59-68.

39. Schlachta-Fairchild L, Varghese SB, Deickman A, Castelli D. Telehealth and telenursing are live: APN policy and practice implications. *J Nurse Pract.* 2010;6(2):98-106.

40. Aronson S. The *Lancet* on the telephone 1876-1975. *Med Hist.* 1977;21(1):69-87.

41. Wittson C, Dutton R. A new tool in psychiatric education. *Psych Serv.* 1956;7(9):11-14.

42. Shackel B. Medical applications of television: a survey. *Med Biol Eng.* 1963;1:35-50.

43. Vladzymyrskyy A, Jordanova M, Lievens F. *A century of telemedicine: curatio sine distantia et tempora.* International Society for Telemedicine and eHealth. https://www.isfteh.org/files/media/Telemedicine_history_CD.pdf. Accessed February 12, 2020.

44. Quinn EE. Teleconsultation: exciting new dimension for nurses. *RN.* 1974;37(2):36-42.

45. Hastings GE, Vick L, Lee G, Sasmor L, Natiello TA, Sanders JH. Nurse practitioners in a jailhouse clinic. *Med Care.* 1980;15(7):730-744.

46. Moore GT, Willemain TR, Bonanno R, Clark WD, Martin AR, Mogielnicki RP. Comparison of television and telephone for remote medical consultation. *N Engl J Med.* 1975;292:729-732.

47. Jones PK, Jones SL, Halliday HL. Evaluation of television consultation between a large neonatal care hospital and a community hospital. *Med Care.* 1980;18(1):110-116.

48. Higgins CA, Conrath DW, Dunn EV. Provider acceptance of telemedicine systems in remote areas of Ontario. *J Fam Pract.* 1984;18(2):285-289.

49. Himmesbach-Winestein E. The music festival that time forgot: inside Steve Wozniac's US Fest. *Los Angeles Magazine.* June 28, 2017. https://www.lamag.com/mag-fetures/steve-wozniak-us-fest/. Accessed February 12, 2020.

50. Grundy BL, Jones PK, Lovitt A. Telemedicine in critical care: problems in design, implementation, and assessment. *Crit Care Med.* 1982;10(7):471-475.

51. Doarn CR, Merrell RC. Spacebridge to Armenia: a look back at its impact on telemedicine in disaster response. *Telemed J E Health.* 2011;17(7):546-552.

52. Gorman C. The wired prairie. *Time.* October 1, 1997. http://content.time.com/time/magazine/article/0,9171,987110,00.html. Accessed February 12, 2020.

53. Connors HB, Skiba DJ, Jeffries PR, Rizzolo MA, Billings DM. Health information technology scholars program: from implementation to outcomes. *Nurs Educ Perspect.* 2017;38(1):3-8.

54. Lilly CM, Zubrow MT, Kempner KM, et al. Society of Critical Care Medicine Tele-ICU Committee Critical care telemedicine: evolution and state of the art. *Crit Care Med.* 2014. November; 42 11: 2429– 36.

55. Udeh C, Udeh B, Rahman N, Canfield C, Campbell J, Hata JS. Telemedicine/virtual ICU: where are we and where are we going? *Methodist Debakey Cardiovasc J.* 2018;14(2):126-133.

56. American Association of Critical Care Nurses. TeleICU nursing practice: an expert consensus statement supporting high acuity, progressive, and critical care. *Crit Care Nurse.* 2018;38:77-78.

57. Dineson B, Nonnecke B, Lindemen D, et al. Personalized telehealth in the future: a global research agenda. *J Med Internet Res.* 2016;18(3);e53.

58. American Association of Critical-Care Nurses. https://www.aacn.org/. Accessed February 12, 2020.

59. American Hospital Association. For the 17th year in a row, nurses top Gallup's poll of most trusted profession. January 9, 2019. https://www.aha.org/news/insights-and-analysis/2019-01-09-17th-year-row-nurses-top-gallups-poll-most-trusted-profession. Accessed February 12, 2020.

Telehealth Basics

Rebecca A. Bates, DNP, FNP-C
Kristi Henderson, DNP, FNP-BC, FAAN, FAEN
Carolyn M. Rutledge, PhD, FNP-BC

CHAPTER OBJECTIVES

Upon review of this chapter, the reader will be able to:
1. Describe telehealth and how it impacts and benefits health care.
2. Discuss the changes that have occurred in health care that are allowing for better incorporation of telehealth.
3. Outline types of telehealth and their application to use cases.
4. Summarize steps needed to implement telehealth within practice.

Twenty-first–century telecommunications technology permeates virtually all aspects of life and is becoming immersed in present-day health care. These advanced technologies provide a unique opportunity for patients to receive care remotely, presenting real options to improve the health of rural, economically and educationally disadvantaged, and underserved populations. The application of technology within health care is so diverse that it is not surprising that many are confused regarding differences in terms such as *telemedicine*, *telehealth*, and *connected health* and how they can be applied to health care. In fact, there have been over 100 definitions found in the literature.[1,2] Practitioners and professional organizations define terms such as *telemedicine* and *telehealth* with variations; thus, a clear conceptual understanding of telehealth and telemedicine is needed. The World Health Organization (WHO) defines *telemedicine* as the following:

> The delivery of health care services, where distance is a critical factor, by all health care professionals using information and communication technologies for the exchange of valid information, for diagnosis, treatment and prevention of disease and injuries, research and evaluation, and for the continuing education of health care providers, all in the interests of advancing the health of individuals and their communities.[3(p8)]

Schweickert PA, Rutledge CM, eds.
Telehealth Essentials for Advanced Practice Nursing (pp 23-44).
© 2020 Taylor & Francis Group.

Telehealth is defined by the Health Resources and Services Administration (HRSA) as the following:

> The use of electronic information and telecommunications technologies to support and promote long-distance clinical health care, patient and professional health-related education, public health and health administration. Technologies include videoconferencing, the internet, store-and-forward imaging, streaming media, and terrestrial and wireless communications.[4(p1)]

The term *connected health* has been used as a synonym for telehealth because it focuses on placing the patient at the center and connecting him or her to health care and health care resources through technology.

For the purposes of this book, telehealth will be defined using the definition that was developed by the HRSA.[4] This will include virtual visits, remote monitoring, and the transfer of data and diagnostic imaging.

TELEHEALTH IS HEALTH CARE

Telehealth is fully present in the developed world and is rapidly expanding to developing countries. Its presence can be found in all 50 states and a majority of provider environments. Over 50% of all US hospitals have a telehealth program,[5] and 48 states now have some mechanism to pay for telehealth, with Medicaid agencies in the United States covering some forms of telehealth.[6] It is estimated that 7 million people were seen by telehealth in 2018.[7] These facts lead to an inevitable conclusion: telehealth technology is here to stay and will be a force in contemporary health care and advanced practice nursing.

Given the rapid rise of telehealth within health care, it is important to understand what it can do and what it cannot do. Building on the HRSA and WHO definitions to develop a common framework of understanding, telehealth can be understood to include the use of digital information and communication technologies, such as computers and mobile devices, to access health care services remotely to manage care. These may be technologies originating from a home or one that a provider uses to improve or support health care services. Telehealth is increasing as a tool used by nursing, particularly advanced practice nursing, to provide virtual clinic visits and virtual consultation.[1] Consider, for example, the ways telehealth or virtual care could help a provider if his or her patient is at risk for hypertension. Telehealth could be a valuable resource for the following:

- Employing a smart device to upload blood pressure, medications, and exercise
- Watching a video on a heart-healthy diet and downloading an app for it to the smartphone
- Connecting through a secure online patient portal to see test results, schedule appointments, request prescription refills, or access email
- Having a video appointment with a provider to discuss follow-up, medication changes, and ongoing care

Telehealth is at a tipping point that is changing the face of health care. Indeed, it is putting a face, rather than a phone call, at the heart of advanced practice nursing. Telehealth holds the promise to significantly impact some of the most challenging problems of our current health care system: access to care, cost-effective delivery, and workforce shortages. The application of digital technology is moving to improve community and population health, expand the patient experience, reduce costs, and increase provider satisfaction. Therefore, advanced practice registered nurses and other health professionals, administrators, payers, and government entities all stand at a crossroads: do we move to apply telehealth? Or do we continue on the uncertain and expensive course the nation is on?

FOR REFLECTION 1:

Benefits of Telehealth

Think about a patient you have cared for that has an unmet health care need. Consider how telehealth could assist in addressing this unmet health care need using common technologies including apps, smartphones, or the internet. What is the potential to improve the health of this population of patients addressing unmet needs via telehealth?

A FRAMEWORK FOR UNDERSTANDING TELEHEALTH

The term *telehealth* is the overriding term that addresses all uses for technology in the health care arena. Telehealth can be described as synchronous or asynchronous. Synchronous applications consist of real-time encounters where 2 or more people are connected via technology at the same time. This occurs primarily through videoconferencing or live interaction with peripherals such as a blood pressure cuff, otoscope, or stethoscope. Synchronous encounters are frequently used for mental health care where the provider is connected to the patient via a videoconferencing platform allowing for real-time counseling at a distance. Synchronous encounters can enable the provider to observe and/or participate in an assessment, treatment, or surgery at a distance using videoconferencing platforms and/or peripherals. This approach also works well for the assessment of student performance at a distance.

Asynchronous applications of telehealth occur when data and information are transferred via technology and stored for later viewing. This allows data to be obtained and reviewed at a time that is convenient to the provider. There is no need for the person sending or receiving the data to be present for its review. Examples of this include store-and-forward technologies that allow for the transfer of physiologic and diagnostic data from the patient site to another site for review.[3] The data or patient information are stored at a intermediary site (ie node), often on a server, until it is forwarded to a recipient.[8] Store-and-forward applications are often used to obtain expert advice on radiographs and medical images, physiologic data (vital signs, weight, blood glucose levels, oxygen saturation levels), electrocardiograms (ECGs), and images of skin conditions.[1,9] They can also be used to provide patient or provider education.

In order to help the reader better understand telehealth, there is a need for clarification of each of the delivery methods, as well as the purpose of using the method. Figure 2-1 provides a detailed outline of telehealth and its connection to telemedicine. Further understanding of telehealth can be gained by clarification of telehealth nomenclature related to the technology, enabling readers to layer this knowledge into the application of care and telehealth program development. Many sources for definitions are present through the literature and professional organizations. A working knowledge of telehealth nomenclature can deepen the reader's understanding of telehealth technologies, allowing for assimilation of telehealth knowledge into existing knowledge.

This section will provide a detailed explanation of each component identified in the model related to telehealth (see Figure 2-1). This includes telemedicine, remote home monitoring/remote patient monitoring, videoconferencing, mHealth, eConsults, patient education, and continuing education for the provider.

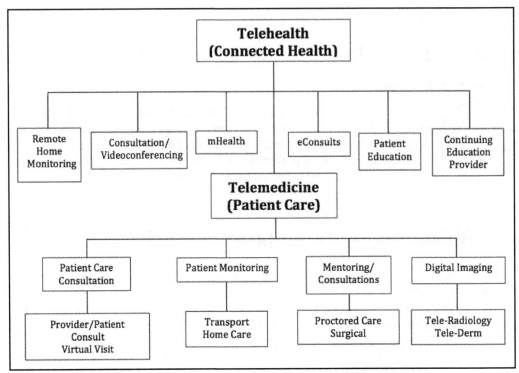

Figure 2-1. Diagram of telehealth/connected health and telemedicine.

Telemedicine

Telemedicine, a fundamental component of telehealth, is used to describe the actual care provided to the patient and is just one component of telehealth.[1] It uses both synchronous and asynchronous applications to provide virtual medical consultations between patients and providers or between providers, virtual clinic visits, remote patient monitoring, mentoring, and teletransfer of diagnostic imaging.[10] In essence, it is the delivery of patient care using technology. It is a key strategy to maximize efficiency and resource use among hospitals and clinics and with partner locations. Sharing health care resources across various locations allows for improvement in the delivery system in a financially responsible way that improves timely access to health resources. Many providers take calls at more than one hospital and in rural areas providers are often doing this while covering a busy clinic. Using telemedicine as a triaging tool can help providers determine where they are physically needed, such as for a procedure, vs being able to deliver the same services through telemedicine. It allows providers to use their time in the most efficient way and reach more people than they could in the traditional model of care without telemedicine.

In addition to the improved efficiency of existing resources, telemedicine allows for access to high-need, low-availability services such as neurology, rheumatology, and other specialty care. When a community does not have access to specialists, either the patient or the provider must travel for the needed services. Telemedicine offers an alternative approach to solving this gap in care. Telemedicine allows the distribution of services to varying locations based on need and removes many geographic barriers. However, this does not remove the requirement to obtain the appropriate provider licensure in the location where the patient is located.

Telemedicine can fill gaps in services and provide alternative options when clinicians need to cover lower-volume hospitals or outreach clinics that require travel. Sharing health care resources across various locations provides a highly efficient delivery system operating in the most financially responsible way while improving timely access to health services. The integration and coordination of telemedicine into the system of care unleashes a much bigger opportunity than treating each modality individually.

Patient Care/Consultation (Virtual Visits)

Virtual clinical visits, a form of telemedicine, can be used as an extension of a provider's brick-and-mortar practice using technology to assess, diagnose, and treat patients. Clinical algorithms can be used to determine when the patient should be seen in a standing clinic space vs through a virtual clinic visit. The uses of virtual visits in health care are as numerous as the number of different clinics and specialties. The following are 3 primary models:

- Multi-specialty virtual clinics are for all specialties and allow any health care provider to improve access and follow-up for their existing patients as well provide intake assessments for referred patients.
- Primary care virtual clinics provide episodic care via telehealth technology for new and established patients. This service can be for a practice's established patients, can be open to the public, or can be provided as employee health services to businesses.
- Virtual school clinics provide care to children in the schools. This allows children to receive access to a primary care provider such as a nurse practitioner when they are seen by the school nurse.

Each of the virtual clinics allows for the patient to be assessed using videoconferencing equipment such as smart tablets, telehealth carts, and computers that are often equipped with peripherals such as a stethoscope, otoscope, ophthalmoscope, and skin cameras. An example of a virtual visit is when a school nurse needs to consult with a primary care provider/nurse practitioner on a student that has come to the school clinic feeling ill. For children who have signed up for the virtual school health program and thus have an electronic health record established, the school nurse can connect with the nurse practitioner on call for the school. The nurse practitioner can observe the patient and participate in the physical exam while the school nurse uses the otoscope to check the ears and the stethoscope to listen to the heart and lungs. Through videoconferencing, the nurse practitioner can ask the patient and school nurse questions. Many of these programs are also set up so that the school nurse can do testing such as for strep throat. If the patient is deemed to have a contagious illness like strep throat, the nurse practitioner can send in a prescription to the child's pharmacy and document the visit using the established electronic health record. Programs such as this have been monumental in keeping children in school and their patients at work. This is an example of how both the registered nurse that is with the patient and the advanced practice registered nurse at a distance can provide care at the highest level of their license and scope of practice.

Patient Monitoring

At times, it is important for a provider to monitor a patient at a distance. This can be used to assess a patient's health status and provide guidance on patient care. For instance, there are programs such as the tele-intensive care unit (teleICU), where providers at one location monitor patients who are in the ICU at another site. This has been beneficial in enabling critical access hospitals to stay open and keep patients they would have had to transfer before the advent of telehealth. Patient monitoring is also seen during transport, enabling providers to assess a patient's condition from one site while the patient is in a medical transport vehicle. This enables the provider to conduct assessment and develop treatment plans in order to best stabilize the patient until he or she gets to the health care facility.

Mentoring

Telehealth has become a venue for mentoring other providers at a distance. Two increasingly accepted uses have been in mentoring students in ambulatory care settings at a distance and assisting surgeons using robotic surgery. Both videoconferencing and peripherals can be used to assess the performance of students at a distance. For example, rather than having a faculty member travel distances in order to conduct a site visit on a nurse practitioner student, the site visit can be conducted using telehealth equipment. The student can conduct his or her assessment using the videoconferencing equipment and the peripherals. This would allow the faculty member to determine if the student is able to properly conduct a physical assessment, diagnose, and develop a treatment plan. One great advantage to using the peripherals is that the faculty can hear the heart and lung sounds and see the results of the fundoscopic exam or the otoscopic exam at the same time the student is assessing them. The student can then describe the findings. This approach can actually result in a more thorough assessment of the student's knowledge and skills.

Digital Imaging

Digital imaging uses store-and-forward technology where data are collected at the patient site and sent to a node, or server, where they stay until they can be reviewed at the receiving site. Digital images include radiographs, photographs of skin conditions, ECG strips, views of both eye and ear exams, and even pictures taken of findings in surgery. Many of these images can readily be incorporated into the electronic health record. One of the most noted uses of digital imaging is in the assessment and management of stroke patients seen in critical access hospitals. In order to save many critical access hospitals, they are now connecting with larger health centers. When a patient is suspected of having a stroke, computed tomography imaging can be obtained and forwarded to the neurologist for review. Based on the review, the neurologist can determine whether the patient is having a hemorrhagic or ischemic stroke and thus prescribe appropriate treatment. This is allowing critical access hospitals to continue treating many of their patients rather than referring them. This is also resulting in better outcomes as patients receive appropriate treatment in a timely manner.

Remote Patient Monitoring

Remote patient monitoring (RPM) is a form of telehealth that is used for chronic disease management and postoperative follow-up to achieve individual and population health. RPM is rapidly evolving as technology advances and as smart home devices and wearable devices become more mainstream. In the earliest days of remote monitoring, equipment and devices had to be provided to a patient, were limited by wireless internet connectivity at the patient's home, and were not reimbursed by insurance companies. Due to these barriers, remote monitoring adoption was slow and often dependent on grant funding. Today, barriers to RPM are fading. Insurance reimbursement is available, cellular and broadband connectivity has improved, and personal devices or smartphones can be used instead of having to use a special piece of equipment for RPM. All these advances have led to increased use of RPM. However, an understanding of the best use, the right duration, and the effectiveness of RPM is still in its infancy. Additional research is needed to understand how, when, and where to use RPM in care pathways and care management plans.

RPM should be viewed as a tiered health information technology (IT) solution that connects patients to their health care team when they are outside of a health care facility. It is typically used for conditions such as congestive heart failure, diabetes mellitus, and chronic obstructive pulmonary disease, where daily control of the condition is important and is often used for the most costly and vulnerable patients. For example, RPM has been very effective in the management of patients with congestive health failure. By providing the patient with peripherals such as scales, pulse oximeters, and blood pressure cuffs, patients can obtain their levels daily and have them transmitted to the provider through a store-and-forward process. The provider or medical staff can review the readings and determine if the patient's health status is decompensating. This allows the provider to alter medications as needed to address the condition before emergency care or hospitalization is needed.

Risk stratification and segmentation of the population will ensure the right patients are selected for RPM services. This service is typically led by nurses and may include a remote care team of other health professionals such as health coaches, dieticians, pharmacists, social workers, and diabetes educators. The service includes education, behavior modification, medication reminders/adherence monitoring, biometric monitoring, and motivation using technology in the home setting. This service can be implemented in various populations but has increased use in the following:

- Managed care organizations/accountable care organizations
- Care management programs
- Home health
- Hospitals for readmission prevention
- Optimization for surgical patients

Videoconferencing

When people think of telehealth, many times their perspective is that of videoconferencing. Videoconferencing is the synchronous or live 2-way exchange of both audio and visual data. Many individuals have become accustomed to using videoconferencing technologies through routine encounters such as FaceTime (Apple), WebEx (Cisco), Zoom, or Skype (Microsoft). This enables an individual to see the person he or she is communicating with in real time. This is one of the most widely used types of telehealth in mental health counseling because it allows the provider to not only hear the patient but observe his or her facial expressions and body language. It also allows the patient to observe the mental health provider, thus enhancing the ability of the patient to portray empathy. Videoconferencing has also been found beneficial when providing education, conducting history and physical exams, providing preoperative counseling, and consulting between providers. Although there are many benefits to videoconferencing, the user must realize that not all platforms are secure or Health Insurance Portability and Accountability Act (HIPAA) compliant. They must choose the platform used for health care carefully. The fact that many individuals use videoconferencing for social interactions may seem to be an advantage. However, it may actually be detrimental in that the users may become too casual, thus creating an encounter that interferes with the professional approach needed in health care. Chapter 8 describes human factor issues such as telehealth etiquette that must be addressed in order to optimize videoconferencing as a form of telehealth.

mHealth

Mobile health, also known as mHealth, is one of the fastest growing areas of telehealth. mHealth is the use of mobile technology such as the smartphone, smart tablet, smart watch, or activity tracker to optimize health. The use of mHealth is one of the most common forms of telehealth that is originated by the patient. It is not uncommon to find individuals discussing how they are able to track of their exercise level, check their vital signs or blood sugar, or access a mobile app to address health care issues using their mHealth device.

mHealth is also becoming a frequently used means of telehealth for the providers. Many providers now use peripherals attached to their smartphone to obtain an ECG, conduct an ultrasound, or review and transmit views of the retina to an ophthalmologist. The uses of mHealth are increasing daily. mHealth is reviewed in detail in Chapter 4.

eConsults

eConsults are being used as a method for connecting providers to each other for asynchronous consultation. More specifically, eConsults are being used by the following:

- Providers to connect with specialists to obtain their expertise in managing complicated patients
- Specialists to expand their practice
- Retiring providers who want to minimize their practice

eConsults use an asynchronous or store-and-forward platform to conduct a consultation. This allows the provider to send and review information on his or her own time. The provider presents the patient's case along with data/images on a secure online portal. The specialist receives a text message that there is an eConsult to be reviewed. The specialist reviews the case and then sends back information regarding diagnosis or treatment. This form of telehealth is allowing providers to consult without having to find a time to meet synchronously. It allows for a timely consultation to occur. More details on the eConsult can be found in Chapter 4.

Patient Education/Coaching

Telehealth is being used as a means for educating, coaching, and empowering patients regarding health promotion/prevention, as well as for management of medical conditions. The platform used can vary tremendously. Common platforms for patient education/coaching can be synchronous or asynchronous. Common asynchronous platforms include smartphones with apps and other mHealth devices.

Videoconferencing sessions with providers/educators are often used to provide synchronous educational/coaching sessions. These sessions can be provided individually or in groups. For example, videoconferencing can be used to provide diabetes education to groups of patients with diabetes. This can be provided via platforms such as WebEx or Zoom and allows for all participants to be seen and to ask and answer questions in real time.

Continuing Education for the Provider

Telehealth is also becoming an important mechanism for providing provider education. One of the most commonly used telehealth programs for provider education is Project ECHO (Extension for Community Healthcare Outcomes). Project ECHO is similar to virtual grand rounds. A provider can submit a case for review. During a Project ECHO session, providers interested in the topic can connect to the videoconferencing platform where a team of experts present the case. The experts discuss how the case should be approached from the perspective of each expert on the team. This allows the participating providers to gain knowledge and a plan for addressing patients like the one presented.

FOR REFLECTION 2:

Selecting a Telehealth Methodology

 Reflect on a patient that you have worked with who has had a chronic disease. Select 3 telehealth approaches that would work well in optimizing the patient's health. How would the approaches be used with the patient? What benefit would they provide?

THE CASE FOR TELEHEALTH: HEALTH CARE NEEDS AND THE CHANGING ENVIRONMENT

Telehealth was born out of necessity. Patients living in rural, remote areas have always lacked access to health care. Those with the means to travel great distances were able to access care. However, those who were not able to travel often received inadequate care or no care at all. Now, even in the 21st century, many patients are still not able to see a specialist or get the treatment they need without traveling long distances or waiting extended periods of time for an appointment. The health care provider shortage is partially to blame, but a more crucial factor is the inefficient use of our existing health care workforce. The number of health care providers needed would change if schedules were optimized, the system were efficient, travel time were reduced, and the patient volume were shared across the entire health care providers/staff regardless of location. Telehealth can have an impact on the health care workforce and physical space needs. Telehealth extends the walls of clinics and hospitals to places such as the workplace, schools, homes, and to people on the go through their smartphones, laptops, and tablets. Much of the nonemergency patient volume in emergency rooms can be shifted to virtual clinics where the expense of a hospital and its associated staff is reduced or eliminated. Workforce and space requirements for health care are decreased, and secondary gains come from having the ability to be more connected to patients. Over time, the health of the population could improve because the population would gain convenient and afford-able health care services. Large health systems that have embedded telehealth into their operations are projecting the need for fewer hospital beds and less clinic space. Telehealth services can be highly impactful if deployed through a systemic and comprehensive approach and if public-private partnerships are secured to achieve this goal.

An effective redesign of the health care delivery system requires a change in how we reach and engage with individuals. The delivery of health care services through telehealth technologies allows care to be delivered when and where it is needed with a convenience and accessibility that people expect in every other aspect of their lives. When telehealth services are integrated into a system of care in a coordinated manner, it has the potential to revolutionize the US health care delivery system and achieve the quadruple aim of improved health outcomes, an improved individual experience, an improved clinical team experience, and a lower total cost.

Improved Health Outcomes

The American Telemedicine Association's (ATA's) 2015 paper entitled "Telemedicine's Impact on Healthcare Cost and Quality" reveals over 12,000 citations within PubMed on telemedicine/telehealth, including greater than 2,000 evaluative studies on telehealth.[10] The evidence continues to grow to support telehealth in all types of settings and within all types of specialties. The evidence has been demonstrated in areas such as improved access to care, improved coordination and collaboration, and improved chronic disease management.

Chronic disease is a major issue contributing to the US health crisis, particularly for the uninsured and underinsured. A review of data provided by the Centers for Disease Control (CDC) on chronic disease reveals that approximately 60% of all adults in the United States live with one or more chronic health conditions. More than 75% of health care costs are due to chronic conditions—nearly $7900 for every American with a chronic disease.[11] One in 5, or 2.6 million, Medicare patients are readmitted to the hospital within 30 days of discharge, which generates costs of over $26 billion each year.[12] High hospitalization rates are indicative of many negative factors influencing a population's health status, including low socioeconomic status, educational level, and access to primary health care and inpatient hospital services.[13] Due to limited physical mobility and lack of transportation, patients often lack access to vital primary care health services that focus on prevention and management of chronic illnesses, leading to inadequate continuity, poor coordination of care, and fragmentation of care. Therefore, postdischarge transitional care interventions can be extremely beneficial in reducing hospital readmissions.[14,15] Telehealth services used in the home can bridge care from the hospital to the home through RPM where video chats with a personalized health care team, biometric monitoring, video-based education, postdischarge instructions, and behavior modification interventions support patients during their most vulnerable time.

Management of chronic diseases and population health are the areas of greatest need and greatest potential. Accountable care organizations, care coordination programs, and readmission prevention programs are a few examples of how health systems are attempting to curtail costs and improve the quality and impact of chronic disease management and population health. Unmanageable cost is one major barrier to the success of these types of programs that are often resource intensive and lack scalability. This is where telehealth services can have a major impact.

RPM is being used to address chronic disease management and can help achieve improved population health. To deliver personalized care and reach a person wherever he or she falls on his or her continuum of health can only be achieved through a tiered health IT approach connecting with patients outside of our health care facilities.

St. Vincent Health, an Ascension Health system in Indiana, had remarkable success from a pilot project using home monitoring technology. The study suggests a 75% reduction in hospital admissions to a 5% readmission rate compared with the national average of 20%.[16] There are numerous other examples, with some of the largest studies found within the Veterans Administration (VA). The VA implemented a national home telehealth program, Care Coordination/Home Telehealth (CCHT), in 2003. This program resulted in a 25% reduction in numbers of bed-days of care, a 19% reduction in number of hospital readmissions, and a mean satisfaction score rating of 86% after enrollment in the program. These results demonstrate a dramatic reduction in costs and an equally dramatic increase in quality.[17] From this initial study, the VA has expanded their RPM program, with $1.2 billion of their $68.6-billion-dollar budget being earmarked to fund telehealth. In 2015, the VA provided 677,000 veterans with telemedicine services, which they planned to grow to 765,000 veterans in 2017.[18]

Another project demonstrating the benefits of telehealth is a study of discharged heart failure patients who were monitored remotely.[19] It demonstrated that telemonitoring is a promising strategy for reducing hospital readmissions. This retrospective cohort study of a hospital-to-home model targeting 759 heart failure patients recently discharged from the hospital revealed a decrease in 30-day mortality along with a 24% decreased 30-day readmission rate compared with the group that did not receive telemonitoring services. In addition to preventing costly readmissions, telemonitoring has the added benefit of being cost-effective, helping patients comply with their medication instructions, and improving patients' quality of life.

A study of the Health Buddy Program implemented by the Center for Medicare and Medicare and Medicaid Services (CMS), which integrated content-based telehealth with care management to risk, stratify, and improve care processes for beneficiaries with congestive heart failure, diabetes mellitus, and chronic obstructive pulmonary disease (COPD), revealed that the intervention reduced spending by approximately 7.7% to 13.3% over 2 years compared with a control group. Overall findings on reductions in spending indicated a reduction of $312 to $542 per patient per quarter, totaling approximately $1248 to $2168 per year.[20]

A 4-month study at a Cox Health Systems hospital in Springfield, Missouri, demonstrated that follow-up phone calls to patients are an effective way to reduce hospital readmissions. Patients who received 5 calls over a 30-day period were less likely to be readmitted within 30 days after they were discharged. Hospital officials were so encouraged by the findings they greatly increased the study's scope. Today, all medical surgery patients discharged from Cox South and 2 other Cox hospitals, a total of 400 to 450 patients, are receiving follow-up calls.[21]

The North Carolina–based Patient Provider Telehealth Network used RPM for high-risk chronic disease patients living in rural areas. Providers who participated in the program noted that telehealth helped inform their decision making and improved efficiency and quality of care. Telehealth helped the providers understand what challenges their patients were dealing with daily and allowed for quick resolution of issues that arose. Telehealth also helped patients take a more active role in their own care. Patients reported feeling empowered to make healthier decisions because their providers were paying attention to their behaviors. Telehealth increased access to services for these patients as well. Evaluations of the project revealed a 50% reduction in hospital bed-days and an 81% reduction in emergency department visits. These outcomes resulted in a 72% reduction in hospital costs during the telehealth intervention and a 64% reduction postintervention.[22]

Telehealth provides a method to address chronic disease prevalence, the social determinants of health, and an aging population, in new ways that the traditional face-to-face visit has been unable to provide. Building a new model that extends the system's reach to deliver personalized care when and where an individual has needs can have a profound impact on the health ecosystem, both in quality and cost. Telehealth technology that powers remote care models will play an increasingly significant role in allowing health care providers to extend the reach of scarce or expensive expertise. Telehealth technology allows the principles of supply chain logistics to be applied to health care. When health resources can be pooled and then distributed based on demand and need, the limitations and barriers from geography are lifted.

Another area where telehealth has demonstrated improved quality and lower costs is in nursing homes. From a baseline of 2.7 million transports made annually from nursing home facilities to emergency departments at a cost of $3.62 billion in current transportation and emergency department visit costs, hybrid technologies could avoid 387,000 transports, with a cost savings of $327 million. In addition, of the 10.1 million physician office visits made annually from nursing facilities at a cost of $1.29 billion for in-person physician office visits and transportation, hybrid telehealth technologies could avoid 6.87 million transports with a cost savings of $479 million.[23]

FOR REFLECTION 3:

Telehealth Care Models

Think about your patient population and the challenges your patients face accessing health care services to improve health outcomes. What care models could you consider in your practice to provide cost-effective care that improves patient health outcomes?

Improved Patient Experience

Patients have greater expectations from the health care delivery system as technology advancements have made people intolerant of a system that does not meet their needs when and where they want it. The digitization of every aspect of a person's life, as in retail, travel, shopping, and banking, has led a shift to a consumerization of health care. The technological capabilities have been present for numerous years, but only now is the United States beginning to see significant adoption and use of telehealth. A tipping point has been reached now that the demand has put pressure on the needed policy, regulatory, and stakeholder groups to clear barriers for widespread integration of telehealth services. Compounding the changing landscape are the new entrants into health care, such as organizations providing retail health care, including Amazon, Walmart, CVS

Pharmacy, Walgreens, and many others, joining the health care delivery space. Some of these new entrants are best known for their consumer experience, which will put increased pressure on the traditional health care provider organizations to rethink how they deliver a customer-friendly product or service.

A patient's experience is about more than the treatment provided. It is about a seamless, intuitive, on-demand, and personalized experience. Health care is challenged to meet these expectations, and telehealth will be an essential component to achieving it. Telehealth will not be the only lever that health care organizations will need to pull to meet patient/customer expectations, but it should be thought of as more than just untethering a patient or provider from a site of service. Telehealth can extend services to new locations, but it can also connect multidisciplinary teams, facilitate second opinions, monitor ongoing health status, and help coordinate a multitude of services and appointments.

Improved Clinician/Clinical Team Experience

The burnout rate (>50% of physicians) within the health care workforce is high, with satisfaction on the decline (5% decrease in 5 years).[7] The provider workforce shortage continues to increase each year.[7] With this ongoing deficit, the key to resolving the US health care system's challenges are far more than just an issue of access or even health outcomes. There is a need to focus on our health care workforce to ensure a healthy work environment, so providers can be recruited and retained into the field. Telehealth can be part of the solution. Telehealth can positively impact areas such as capacity management, collaboration, health education/training, comanagement, access to specialists, and second opinions. All of these are key areas of opportunity for improved satisfaction and experience for the health care workforce.

When telehealth is viewed as a modality to deliver health care services in new ways and in new locations, the value can be better understood and the possibilities imagined. Telehealth brings far more benefits than just untethering a provider and patient from a specific site or location for care. It also unlocks new opportunities to redesign the consumer/patients and clinicians experience with the health care ecosystem.

Lower Cost of Care

Much debate exists on whether telehealth lowers the cost of care. A comprehensive analysis and understanding of health care cost is necessary when evaluating the impact of telehealth on the total cost of care. If telehealth is integrated into a system of care, duplication or additive cost can be avoided. In many cases, telehealth provides access to a service that may avoid additional medical expenses, such as the case with an early intervention that prevents a deterioration of a health condition that avoids a hospitalization. In this case, telehealth would not necessarily result in a lower cost of care but over time would demonstrate a lower cost from what was projected for an individual. Another example is in a patient with hypertension and diabetes who receives remote monitoring that assists him or her to better manage and control his or her chronic disease. Without disease control, the individual may have had a future of dialysis and even amputations. With remote monitoring and disease control, the patient could avoid both devastating and expensive complications of chronic disease.

TABLE 2-1

SAMPLE METRICS TO DETERMINE IMPACT ON TOTAL COST OF CARE

HEALTH OUTCOMES	FINANCIAL OUTCOMES	OPERATIONAL EFFICIENCY	EXPERIENCE AND SATISFACTION
Emergency department use Hospital admission and readmission frequency Specific disease clinical markers (eg, HbA1c, BP, BMI) compared with individual's baseline and control group HCAHPS	Annual insurance and individual health costs Health organization's cost for services and telehealth equipment Clinician cost Revenue from services (reimbursement, contracted fees for service, and self-pay)	Travel miles saved for providers and patients Staffing ratios and productivity measures of providers (wRVUs can be used if telehealth visits are given RVU credit) Hospital and emergency department length of stay	HCAHPS/CAHPS and other satisfaction survey measurement tools Clinician/provider satisfaction survey Workforce retention and turnover rates Patient loyalty

BMI, body mass index; BP, blood pressure; CAHPS, Consumer Assessment of Healthcare Providers and Systems; HbA1c, hemoglobin A1c; HCAHPS, Hospital Consumer Assessment of Healthcare Providers and Systems; RVU, relative value unit; wRVU, work relative value unit.

In evaluating the value of telehealth, a comprehensive research approach should be developed and will be discussed in more detail later in the chapter. In determining telehealth's impact on the total cost of care, the following 4 primary categories should be analyzed:

1. Health outcomes
2. Financial outcomes
3. Operational efficiency measures
4. Clinician/patient satisfaction

All 4 categories have an impact on the total cost of care, some directly and others indirectly. These will need to be tracked over time to understand the full value. Table 2-1 reflects examples of metrics for each category that could be assessed at baseline and after the implementation of telehealth services.

It is recommended that the National Quality Forum's (NQF's) conceptual framework for evaluating telehealth be used as the model for evaluation. In August 2017, the NQF released a report entitled "Creating a Framework to Support Measure Development for Telehealth" that detailed a measurement framework for evaluating various forms of telehealth used to provide care.[24] The underlying 4 domains that illustrate the main components of telehealth include access to care, financial impact/cost, experience, and effectiveness. This report also included 6 areas for measurement: travel, timeliness of care, actionable information, added value of telehealth to provide evidence-based best practices, patient empowerment, and care coordination. Additionally, this NQF report provides detailed descriptions of the domains, subdomains, and measures with examples for the researcher to improve the iterative process of quality measurement of various telehealth delivery modalities.

FOR REFLECTION 4:

Benefits of Telehealth

Consider the ways in which enhancing the patient and clinician/team experience through telehealth use can affect the cost of care. Create a chart with at least 3 metrics for each category (see Table 2-1).

PLANNING HOW TO IMPLEMENT TELEHEALTH

A new care model is required to address the everchanging health ecosystem amidst alterations in reimbursement and increasing penalties. Health care reform is forcing new models of care where health systems are now being held responsible for their patients' activities outside of their hospital and clinics. Readmission penalties, bundled payments, Medicare Access and CHIP Reauthorization Act (MACRA), and value-based contracts demand that health systems become more skilled at chronic disease management, prevention, and wellness. Issues such as these require an organized and phased approach that maximizes existing resources, ensures quality and safety, and takes advantage of the latest in technology and scientific advances. Careful sequencing and integration of telehealth services can help health care organizations deliver consumer-friendly health care services that differentiate them from the market, provide tools to achieve desired health outcomes, and increase the organization's reach and impact.

Strategic Planning for the Use of Telehealth

A successful health care delivery model requires a coordinated and systematic approach that connects an integrated system of care in a patient-friendly, convenient, and cost-contained manner. Patients and clinical teams want reliable, dependable, and simple access to the services and resources they need. The use of telehealth can help achieve this model.

Telehealth services can be used in many different settings beyond the traditional hub site (hospital) to spoke site (remote end user) model. Telehealth is a prime opportunity to extend the reach and impact of clinical services without requiring the costly overhead of a physical space. Approaching population health and continuity of care with the traditional approach of building and buying is no longer sustainable. Patients expect quality care and pick a health care provider based on the experience. Individuals intersect with the health care system in a variety of ways as a member of a health plan or managed care organization, as a recipient of services at a hospital/ clinic, as a resident in an assisted living or skilled nursing facility, or as a recipient of home health services. Each of these entry points is a silo of information and services that result in fragmented care instead of achieving integrated population health. Understanding the population's needs, social determinants of health (factors impacting health status such as education, transportation, and socioeconomic status), and individual needs will uncover the information necessary to create a model that delivers high impact while driving down costs. Many have attempted to segment populations to achieve population health, but data were limited and accountability was dispersed.

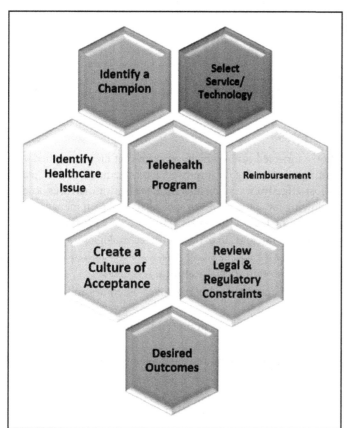

Figure 2-2. Components to establishing a telehealth program.

The health care landscape has changed and now data, accountability, and cost are coming together to create the ideal environment for real change. Telehealth will be an integral part of the redesign of health care. Proactive care delivery in new settings will offer new ways to engage with the population. Employee health, school health, and member health are 3 examples. Support for employee health is in high demand, as evidenced by the recent partnership of Amazon, Berkshire Hathaway, and CVS Pharmacy. Unique partnerships are arising with new entrants into health care with a new perspective and new focus on the patient as a consumer or customer. A strategic plan for the use of telehealth should consider this rapidly changing health care environment, the new players in health care, and the new payment models.

When developing a strategic plan for the use of telehealth, it should be approached as a modality to enhance a system of care vs being deployed as a siloed program or initiative. The strategic aim is to improve health through an efficient and coordinated care delivery system that uses technology while lowering the cost of care.

Priority goals should include the following:

- Optimized patient experience
- Improved system efficiency through resource sharing
- Increased patient engagement
- Improved clinician experience
- Provision of evidence-based, patient-centered, quality care

In order to integrate telehealth into a practice, there are specific issues that must be addressed (Figure 2-2). These include the following:

- Identifying patient/health care issue that you want to address

- Establishing a champion
- Identifying service to deliver/technology
- Figuring out the reimbursement
- Understanding legal and regulatory issues
- Creating a culture where providers and patients accept the telehealth
- Identifying desired outcomes

Patient/Health Care Issue to Address

Telehealth, mobile health, and digital connected care—whichever term that may be applied—is changing the current paradigm of health care, allowing for improved access, reduced costs of travel, and improved health outcomes in cost-effective ways. For instance, telehealth increases access to health care in rural communities, allowing for connections to specialists like pain management or mental health providers who may help in the face of the opiate crisis.

Ultimately, there are several drivers pushing integration of telehealth technologies into provider practices:

- Rural or isolated patients can more easily obtain specialty clinical resources.
- Patients can be diagnosed and treated earlier, often having improved outcomes and less costly treatments.
- Telehealth can support ICU, having substantially reduced mortality rates, reduced complications, and reduced hospital stays.
- Remote monitoring programs can reduce readmissions and emergency rooms visits, reducing high cost hospital visits.
- Workforce shortages can be addressed.
- Providers can have access to educational resources like Project ECHO.
- Telehealth can improve support for patients and families, such as Alzheimer's caregivers.
- Patients can stay in their local communities and, when hospitalized away from home, can keep in contact with family.

Telehealth Champion

In order to have a successful telehealth program, it is important to identify or develop a champion. The champion is invested in seeing that the telehealth program is developed and meets the expectation of the practice. The champion drives the entire process. Specific roles for the champion include the following:

- Overseeing the implementation of the telehealth network
  - Identifying the services needed
  - Selecting a vendor
  - Collecting data regarding legal and regulatory issues and reimbursement
  - Presenting practices/providers with information
  - Developing protocol
  - Identifying patient and understanding how to connect them
  - Marketing program
- Providing training for providers/staff
- Stimulating enthusiasm
- Troubleshooting problems
- Connecting providers, staff, patients, IT, and vendors

Champions can be either providers or administrative staff. However, they must be supported by others in the practice. The champion cannot be successful if there is opposition from the leaders in a practice. Yet, they are often the ones who bring the idea to a practice. They often come convinced that telehealth will benefit the practice by improving patient care, increasing efficiency and effectiveness, connecting providers to specialists or other resources, minimizing patient decline/recidivism to the hospital, and improving cost-effectiveness. They see telehealth as a means for addressing gaps that have been identified in the practice/patient care.

Telehealth programs often fail when there is no one serving as the champion. With the high workload of providers and staff, it is not uncommon for practices to focus on the current crisis, leaving very little time for implementing a telehealth program that in the long run could minimize the crisis approach to care. In order for success to occur, the champion must be empowered to implement change.

Choosing Service/Technology

The advent of telehealth opened opportunities for myriad ways to interact with patients, monitor chronic diseases, consult with specialists, and provide health education that supports patient self-management. These new methods of care delivery are increasingly used in a variety of novel ways to assist with the patient-centered provision of health care services. Care delivery using telehealth involves many types of electronic communication that may be delivered synchronously or asynchronously. For example, an eConsult may be initiated by the primary care provider to receive specialty consultation recommendations (asynchronous), or a virtual consult may be arranged for the patient to see a specialty provider via telehealth (synchronous). Providers may monitor patients remotely using Bluetooth-enabled home monitoring equipment or by receiving mHealth information provided by the patient from a patient's wearables via an application on a mobile device. Health education may be delivered to a patient via secure text messaging services. Chapter 4 will discuss these areas in more detail and provide information on additional ways that telehealth may benefit patient outcomes while improving care delivery.

Reimbursement

Reimbursement remains the single biggest barrier to health system use and expansion of telehealth. There is a lack of understanding and consistency about how payers reimburse for telehealth services. The state specific laws related to telehealth reimbursement vary and are changing annually. The Center for Connected Health Policy (CCHP) is a resource for telehealth laws, regulations, and reimbursement. In a report released by CCHP, "Current State Laws & Reimbursement Policies," as of September 2018, 39 states and the District of Columbia had mandates for commercial reimbursement of telehealth services, with other states considering legislation.[6] Massachusetts was the only state that did not have regulatory language for Medicaid reimbursement. The largest reimbursement barrier is with Medicare, which imposes restrictions based on the patient's location. Currently, the patient must be in a designated rural area within an approved Medicare clinical location for reimbursement to occur. There are several congressional efforts underway that focus on Medicare reform to improve this. Whereas Medicare has these limitations, many Medicare Advantage programs do not impose these geographic restrictions and have embraced telehealth as a viable solution for the aging population. It is imperative that programs review the reimbursement of plans that are frequently seen by the practice. See Chapter 5 for more information on reimbursement.

Regulatory/Statutory

When telehealth is integrated into an existing system of care, existing forms, consents, rules/regulations, and policies must be updated to reflect that care may now be offered via telehealth. There are state and federal laws outlining the requirements related to the use of telehealth, and legal counsel should be consulted to make the appropriate changes in existing documents while adding new forms, consents, and policies when needed. The following are a few examples of areas that will need legal review; they will vary depending on the location, type of service, and governing body:

- Credentialing and licensure of providers and other clinical staff using telehealth
- Hospital bylaws
- Consent forms, privacy notice, assignment of benefits for telehealth visits
- Policies and procedures for telehealth for items such as appropriate patient use, use of telehealth, competency, technology support and maintenance, documentation, data sharing, downtime procedures, and performance improvement
- Data management and security for telehealth data and remote monitoring devices

As the use of telehealth increases, associated litigation will likely increase. To date, most lawsuits have been around patent infringement or for hospitals who had a negative patient outcome when telemedicine was not used for specialist consultation but was available. With the push into mobile solutions, there has been an associated increase in litigation related to patient privacy and data security. This area will need to be monitored, and a skilled legal team should be consulted to gain knowledge and awareness of this area of health law. For more information on addressing regulatory and legal issues, see Chapter 5.

Culture and Attitudes

The bigger risk to the success of telehealth comes from the culture and the attitudes of those working within the existing health system. There must be a culture that is supportive of telehealth and a positive attitude or at least open toward its implementation. Success requires a significant commitment to rethinking and redesigning the system. A system-wide commitment to use telehealth strategies to optimize care delivery is required. Otherwise, the time and cost of implementation will be of little or no value. Leadership will have to ignite excitement and support change and management efforts for adoption of telehealth by the organization. This includes reexamining provider compensation plans, policies, and processes that encourage telemedicine when an in-person visit is not needed for both established patients and new patients. Clinicians will need to develop trust in the telehealth program and be assured that it will be safe for their patients and will not negatively impact their compensation if adoption is to follow. Changing attitudes within an organization takes time and effort but should be part of strategic planning to gain a return on the up-front investment with stakeholders. Understanding stakeholder concerns and perceived barriers will help the leadership team overcome the challenges to implementation by addressing these issues and working together to provide a resolution. It will be imperative to train all participants in using telehealth. This includes the providers, staff, and IT personnel, as well as the patients. Chapter 3 provides strategies for implementing education/training programs.

Expected Outcomes

Planning for evaluation of telehealth services should be in advance of program deployment and should outline how success will be measured. Baseline data, where available, should be determined for comparison across time. Operational metrics, such as telehealth volume, are important to understand the program adoption but are only the first step of analysis that is needed to determine the full value of telehealth.

It is recommended that an outcomes dashboard be created and refined as the program matures and as more data are available. Initially, basic operational metrics and direct financial metrics (cost and revenue) should be monitored monthly. Next, a more robust analysis should include metrics measuring the program against the quadruple aim. The data can be analyzed to answer questions such as the following:

- Did the program improve health outcomes?
- Did the program improve operational efficiency?
- Did the program improve patient experience?

• Did the program improve clinician/clinical team experience?

For patients using telehealth services, whether for an episodic urgent-care telehealth visit or for remote monitoring of a chronic disease, patient activities, health care costs, and overall health over time will begin to reveal the individual and the population health impact attributable, in part, to the telehealth services. When evaluating clinical outcomes, established health metrics for specific conditions can be assessed to determine effectiveness of a specific intervention. Additionally, a comparative effectiveness analysis can be conducted between similar populations with one cohort receiving services via telehealth and the other cohort via in-person care. An alternative analysis can use the patient as the control group looking at health status and expenditure in the years prior to telehealth use and then after use for an appropriate period of time. There are numerous ways to evaluate the effectiveness of telehealth and to account for the multitude of variables impacting health. Ongoing analysis should be a component of the telehealth program.

GROUP EXERCISE

Benefits of Telehealth

Consider how telehealth could be used at a facility you have encountered. Who are the stakeholders, and what outcomes are you trying to effect? How would you explain its benefits to patients, providers, and administration at the site? What barriers would you need to be prepared to address, and how would you address them? What outcomes would you assess to determine the effectiveness of the program?

CONCLUSION

Telehealth can be used in many different settings beyond the traditional hospital or clinic location and is now being used on smartphones and other personal electronic devices, reducing barriers to care due to a physical location. When discussing the various locations for use of telemedicine, it is important to be familiar with the federal, state, and professional board regulations and practice laws related to health care delivery and telemedicine. Technology makes care possible anywhere, but current laws and regulations continue to limit the possibilities. However, each year, policy changes are advancing to unleash its full potential.

Telehealth provides the opportunity to connect with people wherever they live, work, or play and should be viewed as a way to extend the health system and target regions without the requirement of purchasing new health facilities or hiring new providers if existing providers have capacity. This can be done by expanding existing partnerships to include telehealth services or by forging new partnerships to bring needed medical services to a region. Potential telehealth service sites include schools, businesses, correctional facilities, retail pharmacies, nursing homes, critical access hospitals, community hospitals, mental health facilities, and clinics.

Various elements should be considered in selecting strategic locations for deploying telemedicine services, including the following:

• Strategic locations to reach new populations
• Medicare reimbursement implications based on rural locations
• Medically underserved locations across the state as identification of service gaps is critical to getting adoption
• Broadband and cellular network availability
• Telehealth or other policies impacting the use of telehealth in various locations

As Medicare imposes geographic restrictions to telehealth reimbursement, a careful review should be done for each site being considered for telehealth services. The Medicare telehealth payment eligibility analyzer can be found at https://data.hrsa.gov/tools/medicare/telehealth. Maps reflecting current broadband coverage can be found at the Federal Communications Commission (https://broadbandmap.fcc.gov/#/). There are several organizations, such as the CCHP and the ATA, that provide resources of state telehealth reimbursement and other related regulations and policies by state that should be referenced when developing a telehealth strategic plan. In addition to these resources, state medical, nursing, and pharmacy boards; state health and human services departments; and state Medicaid and private insurance companies should be contacted to review any related telehealth rules and regulations.

The strategic plan should also include information related to the resources and budget needed to deploy telehealth services. Resources include workforce, telehealth technology hardware and software, broadband or wireless infrastructure, and support/maintenance services. There can be significant costs associated with initial deployment of telehealth that are often overlooked and not budgeted. These costs are related to staff training, legal needs (eg, credentialing, licensure, bylaws, policies and procedures, consent forms), marketing, and community education. The health care organization needs to complete a program pro forma with the business plan prior to implementing telehealth to help manage expectations and avoid unexpected costs.

Selection of telehealth technology can be overwhelming if an experienced telehealth executive is not involved. The number of vendors providing telehealth technology is extensive and growing. Cost varies dramatically, so a detailed understanding of the clinical requirements is foundational before technology selection should occur. Consideration of the patient's and provider's experience is critical when selecting technology. A strategic plan will help avoid unnecessary technology expenses and a technology architecture that is difficult to incorporate into the clinical team's workflow. Clinicians should work closely with the IT department to select the best technology solution, and patients should be consulted for their feedback in the design and experience to ensure optimal support.

When telehealth technology is selected without a comprehensive plan and done as each specialty or provider decides to use telehealth, a fragmented infrastructure will arise that does not integrate into the clinical team's workflow, leading to limited and temporary adoption. Unfortunately, this approach has been the norm to date because most telehealth initiatives were being tested as pilot studies until a greater confidence was achieved. Today, this approach is not necessary and is harmful to the success and scalability of any telehealth program. A model with multiple devices and telehealth platforms that require different log-ins and modified workflows hamper adoption and create an unpleasant experience for both clinicians and patients.

A comprehensive implementation plan will help ensure the strategic plan moves from a concept to operational success. The plan should include information related to technology installation and testing, provider and staff training, policies and procedures, documentation, site/specialty readiness, revenue cycle, public education/awareness (marketing plan), and performance improvement. Each of these components is a fundamental element of any clinical operation but can get overlooked or skipped with significant consequences to the program's success. The education, training, and change management components of integration of telehealth are frequently underestimated. A realistic timeline should be mapped to an overall roadmap for the telehealth program implementation.

It is important to be aware of threats to the success and sustainability of telehealth. Intentional steps can be taken to minimize the threats. The following are 3 primary threats to telehealth that can be underestimated:

- Reimbursement
- Regulatory/statutory
- Culture and attitudes

Additionally, planning outcomes evaluations is an essential component of telehealth programs because achieving program outcomes determines whether the program is effective and sustainable to meet the needs of the patients and providers.

THOUGHTFUL QUESTIONS

1. What approaches to telehealth do you see as beneficial to the patient population that you serve and why?
2. How can telehealth enhance the care that is provided to patient populations?
3. How can a provider's approach to his or her role in health care be enhanced through the use of telehealth?
4. How can you advocate for the use of telehealth in practice?

CASE STUDY

You have a large panel of patients with type 2 diabetes mellitus who are interested in taking a more active role in managing their illness. They are willing to use technology as a means of improving their health status. You have felt that you have not been as effective as you would like with these patients. They continue to have high hemoglobin A1c levels and gain weight, and you are witnessing more complications such as kidney disease, diabetic retinopathy, and peripheral neuropathy. You are interested in establishing a telehealth program for these patients that would empower them to make behavioral changes, monitor their diabetes, receive prompt responses to their concerns, and provide you with data on their health status so that you can intervene more frequently. You have heard that there are both synchronous and asynchronous telehealth approaches to such care. You are in the planning stage of developing a telehealth program for these patients.

Questions

1. Thinking about strategic planning in your practice, who are the stakeholders that need to be included in designing the telehealth program?
2. What gaps in care are you planning to address?
3. What outcomes are you trying to impact?
4. What steps would you take to implement the program?
5. Whom would you involve?
6. What support staff would you hire, and what role would they take on?
7. What types of telehealth equipment would you incorporate, and why?

REFERENCES

1. Rutledge CM, Kott K, Schweickert PA, Poston R, Fowler C, Haney TS. Telehealth and eHealth in nurse practitioner training: current perspectives. *Adv Med Educ Pract*. 2017;8:399-409.
2. Sood SP, Negash S, Mbarika VWA, Kifle M, Prakash N. Differences in public and private sector adoption of telemedicine: Indian case study for sectoral adoption. *Stud Health Technol Inform*. 2007;130:157-268.

3. World Health Organization. Telemedicine: opportunities and developments in member states. Report on the second global survey on eHealth. Global Observatory for eHealth Series – Volume 2. http://www.who.int/goe /publications/goe_telemedicine_2010.pdf. Accessed February 14, 2020.

4. Health IT.gov. Telemedicine and telehealth. https://www.healthit.gov/topic/health-it-initiatives/telemedicine -and-telehealth. Accessed February 14, 2020.

5. American Telemedicine Association. About telemedicine. http://legacy.americantelemed.org/main/about /telehealth-faqs-. Accessed February 14, 2020.

6. Center for Connected Health Policy. Current state laws & reimbursement policies. https://www.cchpca.org /telehealth-policy/current-state-laws-and-reimbursement-policies?jurisdiction=All&category=All&topic=All. Accessed February 14, 2020.

7. Jackson Healthcare. 2016 physician trends. https://jacksonhealthcare.com/physician-trends/articles/physician -trends-2016-report/. Accessed February 14, 2020.

8. Armstrong A, Sanders C, Farbstein A, et al. Evaluation and comparison of store-and-forward teledermatology applications. *Telemed J E Health.* 2010;16(4):424-438.

9. Rand Corporation. Paul Baran and the origins of the internet. https://www.rand.org/about/history/baran.list .html. Accessed February 14, 2020.

10. American Telemedicine Association. Telemedicine's impact on healthcare cost and quality. https:// higherlogicdownload.s3.amazonaws.com/AMERICANTELEMED/3c09839a-fffd-46f7-916c-692c11d78933 /UploadedImages/Policy/examples-of-research-outcomes---telemedicine%27s-impact-on-healthcare-cost-and -quality.pdf. Published April 2015. Accessed February 14, 2020.

11. Centers for Disease Control and Prevention. Chronic diseases in America. https://www.cdc.gov/chronicdisease /resources/infographic/chronic-diseases.htm. Published January 16, 2019. Accessed February 12, 2019.

12. PerryUndem Research & Communications. *The revolving door.* The Dartmouth Institute for Health Policy and Clinical Practice, Robert Wood Johnson Foundation. https://www.rwjf.org/en/library/research/2013/02 /the-revolving-door--a-report-on-u-s--hospital-readmissions.html. Published February 11, 2013. Accessed February 14, 2020.

13. Mississippi State Department of Health. *Hospital inpatient discharge data: annual report.* https://msdh.ms.gov /msdhsite/_static/resources/5169.pdf. Published 2010. Accessed February 14, 2020.

14. Centers for Medicare & Medicaid Services. Community-based care transitions program. https://innovation.cms .gov/initiatives/CCTP/. Updated December 9, 2019. Accessed February 14, 2020.

15. Agency for Healthcare Research and Quality. Some transitional care interventions reduce 30-day readmissions and emergency department visits. https://archive.ahrq.gov/news/newsletters/research-activities/13sep/0913RA8 .html. Published September 2013. Accessed February 14, 2020.

16. Snell A. The role of remote care management in population health. Health Affairs blog. https://www .healthaffairs.org/do/10.1377/hblog20140404.038196/full/. Published April 4, 2014. Accessed February 14, 2020.

17. Darkins A, Ryan P, Kobb R, et al. Care coordination/home telehealth: the systematic implementation of health informatics, home telehealth, and disease management to support the care of veteran patients with chronic conditions. *Telemed J E Health.* 2008;14(10):1118-1126.

18. Bowman D. VA FY 2017 budget anticipates expansion of telehealth services. FierceHealthcare. https://www .fiercehealthcare.com/it/va-fy-2017-budget-anticipates-expansion-telehealth-services. Published February 10, 2016. Accessed February 9, 2019.

19. Bilchick K, Moss T, Welch T, et al. Improving heart failure readmission costs and outcomes with a hospital-to- home readmission intervention program. *Am J Med Qual.* 2018;34(2):127-135.

20. Baker LC, Johnson SJ, Macaulay D, Birnbaum H. Integrated telehealth and care management program for Medicare beneficiaries with chronic disease linked to savings. *Health Aff Proj Hope.* 2011;30(9):1689-1697.

21. Advanced TeleHealth Solutions/Cox Health Systems. Follow-up call study: whitepaper. https://healthcare.report /Resources/Whitepapers/a5462c23-41bc-4e4d-8d92-594e7d88f3ca_AdvancedTeleHealth-White-Paper-Follow -Up-Call-Study.pdf. Published April 1, 2014. Accessed February 14, 2020.

22. NORC at the University of Chicago. Patient provider telehealth network – using telehealth to improve chronic disease management. https://www.healthit.gov/sites/default/files/pdf/RCCHCandPHS_CaseStudy.pdf. Published June 2012. Accessed February 14, 2020.

23. Schiff M, Bell E, Chao S, Huh K, McGaffey F, McKillop M. State health care spending. A report from The Pew Charitable Trusts and the John D. and Catherine T. MacArthur Foundation. http://www.pewtrusts.org/~/media /assets/2016/05/state-health-care-spending.pdf. Published May 2016. Accessed February 14, 2020.

24. National Quality Forum. Creating a Framework to Support Measure Development for Telehealth. https://www .qualityforum.org/Publications/2017/08/Creating_a_Framework_to_Support_Measure_Development_for _Telehealth.aspx. Published August 2017. Accessed February 14, 2020.

3

Building Blocks of Nursing Telehealth Education
The Multimodal Approach

Carolyn M. Rutledge, PhD, FNP-BC
Katherine E. Chike-Harris, DNP, APRN, CPNP-PC, NE
Susan V. Brammer, PhD, RN, CNE
Patty Alane Schweickert, DNP, FNP-C

CHAPTER OBJECTIVES

Upon review of this chapter, the reader will be able to:
1. Identify components of a comprehensive telehealth educational program.
2. Outline topics that are essential to include within a telehealth educational program.
3. Discuss the steps needed to institute a telehealth educational program within a health care curriculum.
4. Establish telehealth programs that will provide improved faculty oversight during clinical rotations.

As telehealth becomes more commonplace within health care, the need for telehealth education within professional health care programs becomes more imperative. In 2018, the National Organization of Nurse Practitioner Faculties (NONPF)[1] developed one of the first position statements on telehealth education. NONPF came out in support of telehealth education and outlined the competencies needed within the nurse practitioner profession. NONPF stated that nurse practitioners that were educated to use telehealth to deliver care were poised to make great contributions to health care as leaders. Expertise in telehealth would position nurse practitioners to be at the forefront of addressing the challenges in health care through innovative approaches that break down barriers and allow for more immediate access to care. The NONPF statement on telehealth is consistent with the NONPF nurse practitioner core competencies,[2] specifically the technology and information literacy competencies.

The NONPF statement is congruent with previous statements, such as those found in the Institute of Medicine (IOM) report, "The Future of Nursing: Leading Change, Advancing Health."[3] The IOM report called for the advancement of education and the provision of care using

Schweickert PA, Rutledge CM, eds.
Telehealth Essentials for Advanced Practice Nursing (pp 45-70).
© 2020 Taylor & Francis Group.

innovative approaches to health care, including technology, in order to address the inherent challenges. Specific emphasis was on the use of electronic health records (EHRs), remote patient monitoring (RPM), health and information technology (HIT), and other forms of telehealth.

Emphasis on telehealth education is also found in the Master of Science in Nursing (MSN) and the Doctor of Nursing Practice (DNP) essentials for nursing. According to the American Association of Colleges of Nursing 2011 Essentials of Master's Education in Nursing,[4] technology and telehealth education is a requirement of MSN education. In "Essential V: Informatics and Healthcare Technologies," informatics and health care technologies are addressed as they relate to care delivery, communication and care coordination, outcome evaluation, and health education. It is expected that master's-prepared nurses be equipped with the knowledge and skills required to address and use telehealth in health care. They should be prepared to determine how to analyze technologies and best integrate telehealth within practices and health care systems. Master's-prepared nurses should be able to promote policies and address ethical, legal, and regulatory considerations when implementing telehealth. They must be aware of security, privacy, and copyright issues.

According to the Essentials of Doctoral Education for Advanced Nursing Practice published in October 2006,[5] there is specific need for preparing DNP students in the use of technology in health care. Specifically, telehealth is addressed in "Essential IV: Information Systems/Technology and Patient Care Technology for the Improvement and Transformation of Health Care." The expectations of DNP graduates include being equipped to implement and use health care technologies, including telehealth, to address patient needs and improve health care; to provide leadership in its integration within the health care system; and to assess outcomes of use. Specific emphasis of preparing the DNP student must be not only on skills development but also on understanding how to select and evaluate systems and patient care technology and to consider legal, ethical, and regulatory issues that may impact its use.

The Health Resources and Services Administration (HRSA),[6] which funds many training grants in nursing, has recognized the importance of educating health care providers to deliver care through telehealth. In response to the need for education and more health care models to address population needs, the HRSA developed the Office for the Advancement of Telehealth (OAT). The purpose of the OAT is to promote education and the delivery of health care using telehealth technologies and health information services. They realize that telehealth is important for addressing the needs of those in rural and remote areas where care is limited and for increasing health care access for all populations.

ESTABLISHING AN EDUCATIONAL PROGRAM

Establishing a telehealth educational program can be very challenging. The development of telehealth education in many programs has been impacted by faculty who may feel unprepared to provide the education. This is often due to limited exposure to telehealth, limited knowledge regarding telehealth, and/or lack of comfort with the technology.[7,8] In order to provide telehealth education, a faculty champion must be identified. The champion must understand the importance of educating students and providers in telehealth and be committed to breaking down barriers to telehealth education. The champion would be responsible for spearheading the development and implementation of the telehealth education. Specific responsibilities for the champion include the following:

- Obtaining buy-in
- Developing faculty expertise in telehealth
- Establishing objectives for the program

- Developing and implementing the program using the multimodal approach
- Obtaining needed resources (equipment/technology/personnel)
- Evaluating outcomes

Faculty Buy-In/Support

Telehealth use has increased drastically in the past 5 years, with more emphasis being placed on the need to provide education to the providers of tomorrow. This is creating a problem for many programs where faculty have not encountered telehealth. As a result, faculty may be resistant to adding this new content to their programs—programs that are already overwhelmed with content. Many faculty members question where the content would fit, what it would replace, and whether it is even needed. However, changes in educational expectations are making it mandatory to begin integrating telehealth and technology with the curriculum.

It can be quite difficult to obtain support from faculty who are resistant to the integration of telehealth within the curriculum. Specific strategies may include the following:

- Providing faculty with articles on the impact of telehealth in health care
- Bringing in outside experts to provide presentations
- Encouraging conference attendance where telehealth content is provided
- Sharing the emphasis on technology and telehealth as identified in the American Association of Colleges of Nursing Essentials and practice competencies
- Discussing the importance of addressing the essentials and competencies for accreditation
- Seeking funding for education that supports the development of telehealth education (eg, from HRSA)

Developing Faculty Expertise

For successful telehealth programs to be implemented, the faculty providing the education must develop expertise in telehealth and telehealth education. Approaches to developing the needed expertise include attending telehealth educational programs (eg, conferences, workshops, webinars), working with a mentor, visiting existing telehealth educational programs, and/or reviewing professional journal articles and books (such as this book).

Organizations/Conferences

Professional conferences are often faculty members' first encounter with telehealth. Professional conferences provided by organizations such as NONPF, American Academy of Nurse Practitioners, and the Virginia Association of Doctors of Nursing Practice have provided plenary sessions, preconferences, and breakout sessions on telehealth and telehealth education. In order to get a more in-depth understanding of telehealth, there has been a great increase in telehealth organizations and their associated conferences. These conferences often bring together providers and faculty from many professions, telehealth experts, policy makers, and vendors. Some of the best known are the American Telemedicine Association (ATA), the Center for Telehealth and e-Health Law (CTel), the Society for Education and the Advancement of Research in Connected Health (SEARCH), and the regional conferences provided by the 12 Telehealth Resource Centers (TRCs) throughout our country. Each organization has a slightly different focus regarding telehealth, such as advancing and integrating telehealth into health care, addressing legal and regulatory issues, researching the impact of telehealth, or connecting regional leaders and providers in telehealth:

- ATA: This association brings together thought leaders and experts from the telehealth industry to address issues impacting telehealth. Their focus is on changing how people think about health care. The annual ATA conference provides opportunities for participants to network with experts in the field, learn about new technologies, and obtain information to improve telehealth delivery and policy/reimbursement issues that are impacting the field of telehealth. Their web address is www.americantelemed.org/.

- CTel: This organization was developed to address legal and regulatory issues impacting telehealth. It brings together venture capital firms, legal minds, health care providers, insurance companies, and universities with an interest in telehealth. Their web address is http://ctel.org/.
- SEARCH: This society brings together health care providers, researchers, and academics who are engaged in research and research collaborations in telehealth/connected health. Their web address is https://searchsociety.org/.
- National Consortium of Telehealth Resource Centers: Individual federally funded TRCs have been developed to cover the 12 regions of the United States. These centers provide free regional information, education, and collaboration to assist in the expansion of telehealth within their regions. Many of the TRCs have annual conferences that allow for networking and provide a mechanism for addressing regional telehealth issues. Their web address is https://www.telehealthresourcecenter.org/.

These are only a sampling of the many organizations that focus on enhancing the use of telehealth. They provide excellent sources of information and opportunities to increase involvement in telehealth.

Mentoring/Program Visitation

Mentoring can provide faculty with the expertise needed to develop and implement telehealth within advanced practice registered nurse (APRN) programs. Mentors can be identified through conference networking, literature reviews, and referral sources. Important criteria to consider when selecting a mentor include whether the mentor has done the following:

- Developed telehealth educational programs
- Published in telehealth education
- Demonstrated experience in the area that you are interested in pursuing
- Provided a variety of approaches to use
- Provided assistance in overcoming barriers to telehealth education
- Connected you to additional resources

Mentors can be vital in assisting faculty to develop the curriculum needed for their academic program. Mentors can assist faculty in developing goals and objectives for telehealth education programs and can provide learning opportunities (eg, didactics, workshops, hands-on experiences, simulations, and clinical rotations). The ability to provide faculty with didactic content and methods for delivering the content (eg, learning modules, videos, lectures, webinars) is most beneficial in a mentor. Many mentors are willing to share the content they have developed, provide the education, or assist in implementing the didactic programs. Mentors can also assist faculty in implementing competency-based evaluations. They can assist the faculty in overcoming barriers to the implementation of telehealth education by providing background information, literature, and research on telehealth in order to create buy-in; connect faculty with funding sources (eg, grants, vendors); provide educational opportunities for faculty and students; and expose the faculty to successful programs.

One example of a successful mentoring program was between a faculty member at Old Dominion University (ODU) and the Medical University of South Carolina (MUSC). MUSC provides faculty with opportunities to apply for a scholars program. The purpose of the program is to have the MUSC faculty member receive mentorship from faculty from another university. A faculty member involved in the development of the telehealth curriculum for the DNP program at MUSC received the funding to have a faculty member with expertise in telehealth at ODU serve as her mentor. The mentorship included the following:

- A review of the DNP curriculum and discussion of opportunities to integrate telehealth within the curriculum
- A visit by the MUSC faculty member to 2 different telehealth workshops at ODU (one for DNP students only and one for interprofessional teams)
- Discussion of content to be implemented within the MUSC DNP curriculum
- Brainstorming in relation to barriers encountered
- The development of a regional conference at MUSC for nursing programs interested in starting telehealth programs
- Opportunities for publications

A second collaboration occurred between ODU and the University of Cincinnati (UC) College of Nursing. Two psych-mental health nurse practitioner (PMHNP) faculty at UC worked with the faculty member from ODU to develop an educational program for PMHNP students with a focus on providing mental health counseling through videoconferencing. This mentoring involved the following:

- A review of the curriculum and plan for telehealth integration within the curriculum
- Development and evaluation of an assessment tool for evaluating confidence in using video-conferencing to provide mental health counseling
- Participation by the UC faculty in an ODU workshop using standardized patients and videoconferencing
- A review of their program outcomes
- Statistical analysis
- Assistance with presentations and publications

For the past several years, HRSA has requested that all recipients of their funding collaborate with other recipients to facilitate the program outcomes and benefits from one another's knowledge and experiences. This has resulted in many nursing programs establishing collaborative arrangements with one another. Some grant recipients have even subcontracted to other programs to fill voids within their programs. This has resulted in arrangements similar to the ones described here, as well as opportunities where faculty provides educational programs, workshops, and didactic lectures at the other schools.

Professional Journal Articles/Books

As programs are being developed and implemented, professional journals are seeking opportunities to publish on telehealth. In fact, some journals, such as the *Journal for Nurse Practitioners,* have run special issues on telehealth. Such journal articles provide an excellent source for learning about telehealth, as well as identifying mentors and collaborators. A current push is to develop textbooks that can further assist in the development of telehealth educational programs.

For Reflection 1:

Preparing Faculty to Implement Telehealth Education

 Think about an educational program you have been involved in. Consider how you could encourage the faculty to integrate telehealth education within the program. What barriers would need to be overcome? What would be the benefits of the telehealth education?

Telehealth Course Objectives/Competencies

Nursing programs are required to respond to the requirements of the accrediting bodies responsible for oversight of nursing curriculum. As such, they must provide the educational programs needed for the students to be prepared for practice in the ever-changing health care environment. The Master's and Doctoral Nursing Essentials[4,5] provide such guidance for educational programs in nursing. At present, they have recommendations regarding telehealth but do not provide detailed guidance.

Currently, very few professions have attempted to address the competencies that would be needed by providers of telehealth. The NONPF Telehealth Position Statement[1] has addressed the needed competencies. Their perspective is that telehealth competencies should be consistent with competencies required for in-person care. They list the following competencies as suggestions for nurse practitioner students regarding providing care via telehealth:

- Telehealth etiquette and professionalism while videoconferencing
- Skills in using peripherals, such as otoscope, stethoscope, and ophthalmoscope
- An understanding of when telehealth should and should not be used
- An understanding of privacy/protected health information regulations
- Proficiency in the use of synchronous and asynchronous telehealth technology
- Knowledge of appropriate documentation and billing of telehealth technology
- An ability to collaborate interprofessionally using telehealth technologies
- Proficiency in taking a history, performing an appropriate physical exam, and generating differential diagnoses using telehealth[1]

Based on the specific role, there may be additional competencies that would be pertinent. Programs should explore the use of telehealth in their field and establish needed experiences and expected learning outcomes as needed.

The Multimodal Approach to Telehealth Nursing Education

In order to educate nurses of the future, an idea of what that future may look like is essential. Heath care of the future will involve reconceptualizing our concepts of health, nursing care, and the leadership role of the advanced practice registered nurse in a highly technological age.[9] The goal of telehealth education is to create programs that foster the ability of students to develop the knowledge, skills, and attitudes (KSAs) needed to use telehealth in practice. Yet, there is an identified shortage of health professional programs that actually provide telehealth education within their curriculum. Those programs that do provide telehealth education tend to offer primarily didactic programs.[10] Purely didactic programs expose students to content but do not provide for the development of the needed skills and comfort required to prepare the graduate to advocate for and use telehealth as described in the MSN and DNP Amercian Association of Colleges of Nursing Essentials.[4,5]

A multimodal approach to telehealth nursing education guides the contents of this book by focusing on educating APRNs to translate telehealth technologies into practice and building nursing KSAs using telehealth technologies. Educating students using a multimodal approach that addresses the varying learning styles has been most effective in educating students in telehealth. The 4 areas of essential nursing telehealth education identified and actualized in the multimodal telehealth nursing education approach include (1) didactic introductory and advanced telehealth education, (2) experiential telehealth simulation experiences, (3) clinical telehealth project immersion and experiences, and (4) formal preceptorship/practicum experiences.[7,10-12] Didactic education includes incorporating telehealth theory and practical knowledge elements into current curriculum, developing specific basic and/or advanced telehealth courses, and including interprofessional telehealth courses. Telehealth experiential learning includes telehealth simulation

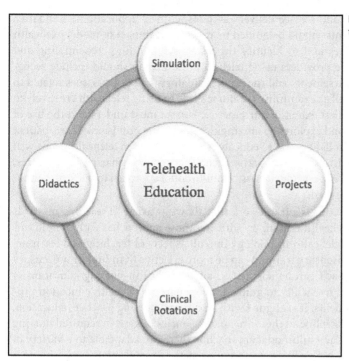

Figure 3-1. The multimodal approach to telehealth education.

experiences and/or hands-on skills labs and clinical telehealth experiences. Formal clinical telehealth experiences can be fostered through clinical preceptorship experiences and through telehealth mentors for doctoral projects. Figure 3-1 outlines the multimodal approach presented in this book.[9]

The multimodal approach is centered on identified APRN telehealth learning needs and is supported by the literature.[7,8,11-20] It is aligned with nurse practitioner competencies; interprofessional education competencies; and Master's, APRN, and Doctoral Essentials and is based upon recommendations from the IOM and the Affordable Care Act.[3-5,21-23] Specific content focuses on understanding the following[7,10-12,18,24,25]:

- How telehealth is defined
- The various telehealth modalities
- Regulations
- Security/Health Insurance Portability and Accountability Act (HIPAA)
- Reimbursement
- The role of the APRN
- Patient and provider satisfaction
- Telehealth etiquette
- Interprofessional collaboration

These content areas are addressed in detail in the various chapters of this book. Incorporating telehealth education into APRN education can provide advanced knowledge of telehealth and telehealth technologies through a variety of platforms, including dedicated telehealth courses, addition of telehealth education and skills to curriculum, provision of clinical experiences through preceptorship in telehealth and via DNP project mentors, and exploration of issues surrounding nursing telehealth practice. APRN telehealth education should include didactic and experiential learning, including hands-on telehealth experiences that students can use to integrate telehealth into nursing practice. Telehealth education includes education regarding basic telehealth technology and terminology, current technologies and service delivery systems, clinical applications, standards, and guidelines in telehealth. Students should be guided to analyze the impact of model telehealth programs on patient care outcomes and to identify the issues surrounding credentialing and licensure of nurses and health care providers using telehealth. Education should include recognizing the current status of reimbursements and the legal, regulatory, and policy issues related to implementation of telehealth, as well as examining the nurse's role in using telehealth creatively to address provision of care to the fullest extent of our practice. Nurses must understand the use of telehealth technologies in practice and explore the nursing role, including provision of care, patient education, and RPM. Interfacility collaboration to educate APRN students in telehealth lends well to telehealth itself because telehealth is a collaborative arena that requires sharing of resources, technologies, and interprofessional experts for success. A multimodal approach to telehealth nursing education is therefore recommended.

At its core, the multimodal approach is a framework that allows a variety of teaching methods and models to be used to teach telehealth nursing by infusing those approaches with a multisensory experience by incorporating telehealth technology into all aspects of teaching and learning. Shams and Seitz suggest that "multisensory training can be more effective than similar unisensory training paradigms."[26] This approach can be adapted to allow telehealth nursing education of practicing APRNs and can be used by faculty to guide development of telehealth education programs and education of APRN students. It is aligned with traditional nursing practice, education, and requirements of the nursing discipline so there are no deficiencies or gaps in required nursing knowledge taught to the student. The multimodal approach is therefore adaptable to a variety of teaching and learning models and is flexible as to teaching methods, making it applicable to a variety of teaching and learning platforms. Traditional lecturing and demonstration, case studies and presentations, high- and low-fidelity simulation experiences, standardized and virtual patient scenarios, collaboration via interprofessional work groups, interactive patient situations, theory alignment and development, and experiential and traditional pedagogy methods are able to be incorporated and used in this approach through the lens of a multisensory environment using the technology as a tool in learning. Importantly, the multimodal approach is aligned to traditional approaches with the addition of multifactorial heightened sensory stimulation to stimulate learning. Using all senses in learning has been shown to increase development of critical thinking, fostering the desire to learn and acquire knowledge.[26-28] Telehealth technology is, in large part, a visual and auditory tool that can be used in nursing practice but can also be used in nursing education to facilitate learning about telehealth nursing practice. It brings uniqueness to nursing education by melding multiple sensory experiences for learning purposes. The multimodal approach is therefore based on a multisensory experience for the learner, using the technology to increase knowledge through sensory stimulation in all avenues of learning.

Areas for further collaboration and growth can be actualized through using the hub-and-spoke model borrowed from telestroke (stroke telemedicine) to connect larger schools of nursing with telehealth programs/networks to smaller schools of nursing with no such telehealth resources. This networking would enable larger university schools of nursing to collaborate with smaller schools of nursing to provide telehealth expertise and educational opportunities to students. Maximizing resources and potential education and experience benefits students; therefore, using telehealth technology can expedite the infusion of telehealth education and experience to APRNs. All nursing programs need to be immersed with education and practice skills to translate in-person nursing to the virtual environment.[7] This can be accomplished by the alignment of traditional nursing education with the educational needs of practicing in the virtual environment with incorporation of telehealth knowledge, skills, and experiential and simulation experiences using the technology. The multimodal approach affords nurses this opportunity for fully immersed telehealth education.

Didactic Programs

Didactic programs, an essential component of telehealth education, are the most commonly used method for educating students on telehealth in the university environment.[9] In fact, in many educational programs, it is the only method of telehealth education. Didactic programs can be delivered in forums such as in-person lectures, narrated presentations, webinars, videos, and modules/online courses.[10,29] These didactic courses are best used to provide the learner with the knowledge needed to use telehealth. The biggest limitation to telehealth education that is solely didactic is that the learner is not able to develop the skill level or comfort needed to provide telehealth.

Didactic programs provide the easiest, quickest, and cheapest methods for providing the learner with information regarding telehealth. They can provide the learner with information on the history of telehealth (Chapter 1); the definition of telehealth and common telehealth terminology (Chapter 2); the technology needs for telehealth (Chapter 4); regulatory issues and reimbursement (Chapter 5); the role of the APRN in telehealth (Chapter 6); examples on the uses of telehealth (Chapter 7); ethical issues, including telehealth etiquette/human factors (Chapter 8); and the use of telehealth in providing interprofessional care (Chapter 9).[7,8,10-12,17,24,25]

Many universities provide a face-to-face didactic session where the learner is provided information on telehealth as part of an existing lecture or as a standalone lecture. This tends to expose the learner to telehealth but is often limited in the depth that it provides. Didactic learning is an essential part of telehealth education; however, in order to truly prepare a learner for telehealth, it is recommended that didactic content be enhanced with experiential learning opportunities. Specific approaches include simulations, hands-on experiences, clinical rotations, and telehealth projects.

In order to provide the learner with education on telehealth etiquette/human factors, ODU has developed video modules that show poor, fair, and excellent examples of telehealth etiquette. These videos can be used to educate the student on appropriate telehealth etiquette, prepare the learner for a hands-on telehealth experience where videoconferencing is the target telehealth methodology, provide for discussion board activities, and enhance the ability of the learner to evaluate and troubleshoot less-than-optimal telehealth encounters. These modules have even been used to prepare students for in-person group exercises where they are responsible for preparing for and then providing a telehealth encounter using appropriate etiquette. Chapter 8 will go into more detail on this experience.

The Karen Rheuban Center for Telehealth at the University of Virginia (UVA) has developed modules for providers in various specialty areas. These modules, known as the Telehealth Village, provide the learner with an overview of telehealth related to specific content areas. For instance, there is a module on telemental health that provides the learner with information he or she would need to know to establish and deliver a telemental health program. These modules are developed using a narrated PowerPoint approach.

Simulation

Simulation activities allow the learner to practice using telehealth equipment in a safe environment where mistakes do not compromise a patient's safety. It allows the student to experiment and make mistakes in a nonstressful environment. All too often, simulation activities with telehealth do not occur within an academic setting. Instead, they occur once the provider is in practice. Much of this education is provided by the vendors that install the equipment and teach the providers/support staff to use it. This approach often focuses on turning on and using the equipment from the technical perspective. Too often, it does not address the patient-provider or provider-provider interaction. As academic programs begin to implement hands-on experiences in telehealth, new educational approaches are being generated. These include hands-on practice sessions, simulation activities, standardized patient encounters, and interactive challenges.

Hands-On Practice Sessions

Programs are beginning to realize the importance of providing students with opportunities to practice with telehealth equipment. One of the most readily available approaches is with video-conferencing equipment. Most academic settings already have access to WebEx (Cisco) or Zoom. These 2 videoconferencing platforms can be purchased with HIPAA-compliant security that allows for 2-way live patient encounters. It is imperative that students understand the importance of using a videoconferencing platform that is HIPAA compliant. Students can practice conduct-ing videoconferencing sessions with each other. Prior to these sessions, it is important that the students are exposed to telehealth etiquette.[30] It can be provided prior to the videoconferenc-ing encounter through in-person education or videos and then reinforced during the encounter. Students' performance can be evaluated based on their telehealth etiquette. Tools for this type evaluation will be presented later in this chapter.

In order to prepare students to use specific telehealth devices, the easiest approach is to pur-chase several telehealth devices and provide the students with practice opportunities. The devices should be purchased based on the needs of the specific profession. For instance, if the students are hospital based, devices such as the telehealth cart might be appropriate. If the students are military, they might want to provide experiences with the telehealth travel kits. It is often easy and inexpensive to provide students with peripherals that can be used on smartphones. These may include electrocardiogram (ECG) monitors, pulse oximeters, blood pressure cuffs, otoscopes, ophthalmoscopes, and even ultrasounds. Students who care for patients with chronic illness such as congestive heart failure or diabetes may want to practice with RPM devices.

Faculty can provide students with written patient scenarios and then have them consider the use of the equipment for the case.[10-12,30] Students can practice using the equipment on each other to develop comfort with the technology and can brainstorm on how the equipment can be used to enhance the assessment and care for a specific patient population. In these situations, it is impor-tant for students to consider the benefits and barriers to the use of the technology and how to overcome the barriers.

Erickson et al[13] had students connect through videoconferencing technology to a laboratory that provided information technology (IT) at a local hospital. The students were then instructed on the use of videoconferencing cameras, stethoscopes, digital otoscopes, and examination cameras. This opportunity allowed them to practice with the technology.

Case-Based Telehealth Simulations

Some programs have students participate in telehealth exercises where they use the equipment based on a patient case that has been provided.[10,30] This allows the students to consider the uses for telehealth as they practice developing hands-on skills. The goals of these programs are to aid the learner in developing a deeper understanding of the uses for technology in health care and exploring the numerous ways telehealth can be used for provider, patient, and caregiver education and support.

One telehealth program provided hands-on experiences to students in which they were given a case of a stroke patient and then rotated through stations that provided various types of tele-health equipment. The purpose of the program was to assist students in understanding the use of telehealth in reaching out to rural and underserved populations. At one station, the students were provided smart tablets to explore services provided for stroke patients and families using websites. Another station provided the students with opportunities to focus on store-and-forward data transmissions such as diagnostic scans that could then be incorporated into the medical records. The final stations focused on the use of decision-making technologies and mobile applications that could be used by providers and patients addressing stroke management.[31]

Standardized Patients

Standardized patient encounters allow learners to have hands-on experiences with equipment at the same time they are applying the use of technology to a clinical situation. Standardized patient encounters can provide learning opportunities through simulated cases and allow for formative evaluations. Standardized patient encounters can also be used to evaluate the students' knowledge, skills, and abilities through Objective Structured Clinical Exams. The simulations often occur using trained standardized patients or even fellow classmates. The case scenarios are built so that the students must consider the function of the equipment, the abilities of the patients, and the desired outcome. It also allows for the student to address benefits and barriers encountered by the patient. Of utmost importance is that these simulations allow the learner to become acquainted and comfortable with using telehealth equipment prior to encountering a patient in need and to receive feedback about their ability to provide care using technology.

One of the most easily instituted telehealth simulation experiences focuses on videoconferencing skills. Videoconferencing can be provided by platforms such as Zoom or WebEx, platforms that are often readily available for use in university and clinical settings. During education on videoconferencing, it is important to address telehealth etiquette/human factor skills. Telehealth etiquette is addressed in detail in Chapter 8. A student can be placed in a room with a computer that is equipped with Zoom or WebEx. A standardized patient who has been trained to portray a specific scenario can be placed in a separate room with a computer. The student is then able to conduct a history and physical on the patient by observing him or her through the computer screen.

Rutledge et al[31] conducted a telehealth simulation workshop for 60 APRN students who were broken into groups of 5 to 6 students. The students were instructed to interview the standardized patient and their caregiver through the videoconferencing platform. The students interviewed the patient and their caregiver regarding the patient's health status following a stroke. They conducted a physical exam by having the patient lift a book with each hand, ambulate in front of the screen, and write on a piece of paper and hold it up. The students were surprised at how easily they could establish a rapport with the standardized patient and conduct a meaningful physical assessment. This was a perfect setting for practicing telehealth etiquette in order to improve the encounter.[31]

FOR REFLECTION 2:

Implementing Telehealth Simulation

 Suppose you are responsible for providing an educational program for a group of health care professionals. What didactic content would you provide? How would you provide that content? What experiential learning activities would you provide? What would be your goal of the education?

Practice Experiences

Clinical experiences with telehealth are needed in order to assist the learner in truly understanding the role of telehealth in health care. Opportunities can be provided enabling the learner to participate in telehealth from either the delivering or receiving side. Practicum experiences can occur as the result of a defined telehealth rotation or participation in practicum sites that provide telehealth to their patient population.

Telehealth-Focused Rotation

Clinical rotations are being integrated into educational programs to give students real-life exposure to telehealth. However, these rotations can be greatly enhanced by having students complete an assignment on the rotation. The objectives of the experience for the students include the following:

- Understanding the purpose of the telehealth program at the site
- Outlining the steps needed to set up a successful telehealth program
- Identifying the technology/telehealth devices needed
- Describing the population served
- Discovering the benefits and barriers to the program and how they were overcome
- Considering how a similar program could be instituted in their clinical site

In order to have students participate in a telehealth rotation, they can be expected to identify a program in their region that either provides or receives telehealth services. The students can be given a list of potential sites, as well as access to their state's telehealth resource center.[32] Students can be expected to set up their individual rotations and have them approved by their faculty. Rotations are 4 to 8 hours in duration. During rotations, students participate in telehealth encounters and interviews the staff in order to gain insight into the program. A 2-page paper is completed that addresses the objectives outlined previously.[31] In some programs, students are able to use telehealth to obtain patients' histories and reviews of systems, as well as to conduct physical exams using medical peripherals.[18] Examples of sites that have been used include primary care, mental health programs, state corrections systems, and specialty care such as cardiology, stroke (telestroke), and HIV.[31]

Incorporation Within the Clinical Practicum

Some students participate in clinical/practicum rotations in sites that offer telehealth. Many APRN programs find care provided via telehealth as acceptable for clinical hours; however, the provision of telehealth must meet the same requirements as in-person clinical experiences. As such, students should be involved in conducting patient encounters, not just observing. Patient visits may include obtaining a medical history, reviewing the systems, assessing the patient (using videoconferencing and/or telehealth medical peripherals such as blood pressure cuffs, pulse oximetry, otoscopes, or ophthalmoscopes), obtaining a diagnosis, and documenting the visit. Mental health and/or health and wellness counseling may be done using videoconferencing platforms as well.

Projects

Projects allow students to obtain better insight into the use of telehealth technologies and peripherals within a setting. Some projects encourage students to evaluate telehealth programs; others have students develop telehealth approaches. Examples of telehealth projects that can occur in clinical settings include evaluation of telehealth sites and plans for future development of a telehealth program. Projects that address the development of telehealth approaches include website development and mobile application development.

Website Development

Websites can be an important telehealth tool for providing patients/caregivers with content regarding health care issues, access to others dealing with similar health care issues, and information on support programs. In order to develop expertise with websites, some programs have had students either review/critique websites or develop and implement new websites. The goal is to have students understand how to implement websites as an asynchronous method of providing patients/caregivers with knowledge and support.

One approach to enhancing knowledge related to websites has been to have students review and critique websites that address a specific health care issue. For example, there are websites that have been developed to assist patients with chronic diseases such as diabetes. Students are expected to do a search of websites that address a chosen chronic illness. They then identify a reputable site that they would recommend to a patient. They are expected to identify the purpose of the site, determine who the site targets, describe the content found on the site, list the advantages to the site, and describe ways the site can be improved. This assignment helps students understand that providers should stay abreast of websites that address the patient population they serve and be able to recommend specific sites.

Another project that involves the use of websites as an asynchronous educational tool involves having students develop a website for a patient population.[33] There are many free website development programs available to students. One academic program asked interprofessional teams of students to develop a website for a patient population of their choice.[33] The following were the requirements of the website:

- The information being provided was at a third-grade level
- An interactive component was offered
- Links were provided to 3 additional types of media (eg, YouTube videos, Prezi presentations)
- It contained blogs
- The roles for the various professions were included

Students were required to develop the website at a distance without any in-person contact. This aided them in developing comfort in using synchronous videoconferencing to connect with various professions. After a week, the student groups were required to present their websites to faculty and other teams using WebEx. This further supported the role of videoconferencing as a useful tool in telehealth.[33]

Mobile Applications

Mobile applications, or apps, are playing a significant role in health care as a means for providing information, collecting clinical data, and tracking performance. There are also programs available that allow students to develop apps at no charge. One project that has been completed by students has been the creation of a health care app. Teams of students chose health care topics and then developed apps that would work well for their patient populations. The response to the app assignment has been very powerful as a means to improve interprofessional collaboration and provide a resource to patient populations.

Accessing Resources

One of the greatest barriers to setting up a telehealth education program is accessing the resources needed to provide the experience. The cost of starting a telehealth program has been identified as one barrier to programmatic implementation. Ali et al[7] found that the programs that used equipment as a tool for teaching telehealth were only able to do so with funding from grants, such as through the HRSA. Many schools have been fortunate in obtaining grant funding in order to buy equipment that may be needed. This funding has also been beneficial in assisting with faculty education. Some of these opportunities are still available and can be pursued. A second approach is to obtain donations in order to purchase needed equipment and/or receive appropriate faculty education. Donors can include alumni, community partners, and foundations. A third method is to work closely with vendors in order to obtain equipment or best use the equipment you have for lower costs. One of the more costly issues related to telehealth equipment is paying the platform fee needed to run the equipment. Many vendors are accustomed to selling equipment to health care providers where revenue is generated. The vendors should be educated on the difference between using telehealth equipment in education vs its used for providing care.

A second issue it that of space. Often there is limited space for adding a new educational activity. This can be addressed through discussions with the university administration, as well as by seeking donors for buildings on or external to the campus. Finding space and setting it up for multiple users may work well. For instance, many programs begin by incorporating telehealth into the space used for simulation programs.

Beginning a program can be as simple as using WebEx or Zoom, which is offered free of charge to faculty and students. This approach can be used to foster videoconferencing as a mechanism for delivering telehealth. Then apps can be added to a smartphone to introduce the learner to other technologies. For programs that have limitations in faculty and staff exposure to telehealth knowledge, contracting the education out to other experts or programs that are well equipped for such education may be the answer. As mentioned previously, it is not uncommon to have one program contract this learning from existing telehealth educational programs.

FOR REFLECTION 3:

Obtaining Telehealth Resources

You are interested in starting a telehealth educational program. Funds are limited. What resources will you seek to obtain? How will you go about obtaining the resources needed to start the telehealth program?

Evaluating Telehealth Education

In order to determine whether students are meeting the expectations/competencies related to the telehealth education, a number of tools have been developed, with some being published. Tools have been developed to assess knowledge, confidence, satisfaction, and usen. Other tools are used for observing the student's performance and may be completed by faculty and/or standardized or even real patients. The use of several tools may be required in order to assess the KSAs of the students.

Telehealth Etiquette Knowledge

The Telehealth Etiquette Knowledge (TEC) scale can measure telehealth etiquette. This scale is an 11-item knowledge test that is anchored using a 5-point Likert scale with scores of 1 (Strongly Disagree), 2 (Disagree), 3 (Undecided), 4 (Agree), and 5 (Strongly Agree). The TEC scale measures etiquette in its entirety using all items as well as 2 separate constructs: (1) telehealth knowledge (questions 1 through 5) and (2) human factors (questions 6 through 11). Internal consistency with Cronbach's alpha scores above 0.70 for the entire tool as well as the 2 constructs has been achieved.[34] The tool was assessed for validity by a panel of experts during its development. The TEC scale has been used to conduct pretest and posttest assessments of telehealth educational programs as well as baseline assessments to understand learning needs. Items on the tool include proper dress, HIPAA security, use of equipment, and proper preparation for a visit.

Telehealth Etiquette Observation Checklist

Uniformed Services University developed an observational tool that faculty used to observed telehealth etiquette during a mock patient videoconferencing encounter.[17] The tool was scored as yes/no based on whether the students performed each activity appropriately. Questions were established to evaluate the role of each participant in the telehealth encounter: patient, provider, and telepresenter. It consisted of 17 items that measured the setup of the room (2 questions), patient engagement (patient's ability to interact; 5 questions), provider telehealth behavior (8 questions), and telepresenter behavior (2 questions).

Telehealth Confidence Scale (Videoconferencing)

Faculty at the UC College of Nursing developed a tool to measure confidence in using videoconferencing as a means of providing care to patients through a videoconferencing platform via the Practice/Telehealth Confidence Scale. The tool has 2 components: confidence in providing care via videoconferencing and confidence providing care in person. The items for each component parallel each other. This allows the evaluator to determine if students are developing comfort in videoconferencing that equates to that of an in-person visit. The tool consists of 12 items with 5 choices, from Strongly Disagree to Strongly Agree, measuring the in-person confidence. Twelve additional items scored the same measure of confidence with videoconferencing. The tool was assessed by an expert panel when it was developed and has achieved Cronbach's alpha score of >0.80 for the 2 scales. This tool has been used to assess confidence in PMHNP students following an online telehealth educational program using standardized patients for mental health assessment. It has also been used during an interprofessional telehealth workshop.

Future Tools

Nursing programs are developing more tools to assess student performance in telehealth. These tools vary on the specific aspect of telehealth that is being evaluated. Tools can assess technique or KSA. Tools vary on how the data are obtained. For instance, some tools provide assessment of students by trained standardized patients or, at times, actual patients. Others provide for observations by faculty or student peers, or even self-evaluation.

CLINICAL OVERSIGHT

One of the greatest issues impacting APRN education is the oversight of clinical experiences. With the increase in online education, there is concern regarding the assessment of clinical proficiency of the APRN students. Are the graduates that are entering the workforce ready for practice? Organizations such as NONPF believe that there should be oversight of all students in the clinical sites.[35] However, many educational programs struggle with providing the faculty oversight, often done by conducting site visits. Issues include distance (eg, cost of travel, time from work), availability of faculty to conduct the visits, observing students when they are scheduled with patients that demonstrate their expertise, and consistency with the site visit. With the goal of ensuring that APRN graduates are ready for practice, new approaches that use telehealth for oversight are increasing. In fact, NONPF supports the use of telehealth as a means of completing clinical site visits at a distance.[1] Through the use of telehealth, programs are able to provide less costly site visits, standardize the evaluation of the students at a distance, and evaluate students when they are with appropriate patients. With the use of appropriate telehealth platform and medical peripherals (eg, stethoscope, otoscope, ophthalmoscopes), faculty should be able to assess students using the same expectations as with an in-person visit. In fact, by being able to listen to heart sounds or observe the fundoscopic exam with peripherals, the assessments and student description can be even better evaluated. Contact with the preceptors can also be conducted at a distance using videoconferencing platforms such as Zoom or Webex. Considerations for conducting a telehealth site visit include obtaining consent from the patient prior to the encounter because some states require written consents for use of telehealth and being sure the system is HIPAA compliant.

This same process can be used when assessing a student's physical assessment skills. For example, a few schools now require students to complete a physical on a patient (friend or family member) and submit it to the faculty using store-and-forward asynchronous methodology. To do this, the student can set up a videoconferencing platform and record their history gathering and physical assessment. The recorded assessment is then forwarded to faculty. Some programs have even had students review the videos of each other in small groups and provide feedback. Results have shown that students perform as well or better on physical assessment when assessed with standardized patients at a later point.[36]

The Advanced Practice Nurse Preceptor Link and Clinical Education Telehealth Network

Advanced telehealth technology used in clinical nursing education enables faculty to conduct virtual site visits, provides preceptor support and education, and enables a unique way of providing faculty oversight at the clinical practice site, albeit remotely. An innovative model of APRN clinical education is via a telehealth education network, which can facilitate improved preceptorships and clinical oversight of the student as well as increased engagement with the preceptor. The Advanced Practice Nurse Preceptor Link and Clinical Education (APN-PLACE) telehealth network is an HRSA-funded preceptor education program connecting students and preceptors at rural and underserved practices with faculty at schools of nursing via advanced communications technologies. APN-PLACE can be used by APRN faculty to address rates of practice-ready new APRN graduates and clinical preceptor shortages. APN-PLACE is designed to provide advanced communications between faculty, students, and preceptors using videoconferencing and peripherals. Student performance in the clinical setting can be evaluated remotely using the technology. Support and education for preceptors is also enabled via the telehealth network, as students are introduced to nursing care in the virtual environment. The network provides opportunity for students and faculty to meet as frequently as needed without encumbrance of faculty traveling to the remote clinical practice site:

> These changes shift the model from one in which faculty communicate, teach, and mentor students and preceptors only through in-person contact, to one where faculty can connect, observe, and educate students and preceptors frequently, easily, and spontaneously using live videoconferencing.[37]

The network creates virtual classrooms in which faculty can engage with and teach students and preceptors by way of the virtual site visit in clinical practice settings, remotely. The technology used in the network can vary, from a dedicated telehealth clinical room, to a videoconference enabled conference room, to a simple handheld mobile device. Digital diagnostic equipment or peripherals (such as a digital stethoscope) used at the practice site by the student and observed remotely by the faculty can increase real-time learning. The goals of APN-PLACE are to use these advanced communications and technologies to provide student oversight and preceptor education and support, such as education on how to better prepare students, providing opportunity for real-time discussions. Peer support networking enables preceptors to come together to engage in discourse on successful precepting strategies and techniques.

Remote student assessment by faculty supports the requirement of overseeing the student in the practice site, providing expert supervision in the clinical practice setting.[38] Use of medical peripherals enable the faculty to not only become familiar with the student's assessment skills, but also to provide real-time feedback on the student's knowledge and techniques. Timely remediation is therefore possible and expedited. The increased access and connection between the faculty, student, and preceptor using these advanced technologies creates more frequent communications, improving learning of the student and preceptor.

The network also provides opportunities for the student to engage in clinical telehealth experiences by participating in direct care delivery using telehealth technologies. Learning to practice in the virtual environment with standards-based practice guidelines expands the care opportunity for the student and the patient. Students can therefore participate in care delivery in virtual environment and gain important skills and knowledge. This knowledge and skill set can improve the nurse's ability to assimilate telehealth nursing practice to their own practice. An innovative approach to transforming and actualizing the role of telehealth nurse is therefore possible by use of the telehealth education network.

GROUP EXERCISE

Clinical Oversight

You are developing a program using telehealth to provide oversight for students at remote clinical sites. Describe what assessments you would like to observe. What equipment will be needed at both the student site and faculty site? How would you go about planning for the session? What expectations would you have of the students?

EXAMPLES OF EDUCATIONAL PROGRAMS

Specific education programs educate nursing students as well as faculty and practicing APRNs regarding telehealth technologies, and the application to nursing practice are presented. Telehealth education can be applied to and integrated in a variety of ways using the multimodal approach as demonstrated here.

Telehealth Immersion for Interprofessional Teams at Old Dominion University

ODU has been offering a 2-week telehealth immersion experience to an interprofessional team of learners since 2014.[33] This program was developed as a result of funding from HRSA with the goal of preparing teams of providers/students from varying disciplines to work together effectively using telehealth. This experience educated the students to use the expertise from varying professions regardless of the barriers related to distance. The immersion experience included the first 3 of the 4 components of the multimodal approach educational framework. It includes didactics, hands-on experiences, and projects. The program has grown since 2014 and now serves students from 11 professions (family nurse practitioner, clinical nurse specialist, physical therapy, speech and language pathology, clinical counseling, 4th year medicine, athletic training, dental hygiene, social work, pediatric nurse practitioner, and pharmacy) and 4 universities. Approximately 1,500 students have participated in the experience so far.

The same experience is provided 5 times each year in order to allow the students to schedule the experiences at a convenient time. No more than 80 students sign up for each session, with a set number of spots allotted to each profession. The experience meets differing requirements for the varying programs. For instance, programs such as nursing, medicine, and pharmacy make it a required experience in order to graduate. Other programs such as physical therapy make it a 1-credit course.

During the first week of the 2-week immersion experience, the students complete modules on interprofessional collaboration and telehealth. The students are placed in groups of 5 to 6 students from the different professions. As teams, they respond to the modules through discussion boards. The modules include videos, assigned readings, web links, narrated PowerPoints, and interactive activities. Content includes an overview of telehealth and use cases, an introduction to telehealth etiquette, legal and regulatory issues, and telehealth resources available. Readings are included to help students apply telehealth to their profession.

The students are expected to come to campus for one 8-hour telehealth experience. During the session, the students meet in groups to interview standardized patients with a substance abuse disorder, first in person and then via videoconferencing. This allows the students to better understand how effective videoconferencing can be as a tool for caring for patients. After each session, the students process the encounter and also consider telehealth etiquette issues. The discussions include lighting, positioning, HIPAA, distractions, background noises, and colors.[12,34] Nonverbal and deliberate empathy statements are emphasized to replace touch.

The students are then given patient cases and explore using various pieces of equipment to address the patients' needs. The equipment includes the following:

- Smartphones with medical peripherals
- Visions screener that assesses visual acuity
- Medication dispenser for regulating medications at a distance
- Telehealth cart
- RPM equipment
- Robot (VGo)
- Travel kit

This gives the students an idea of the breadth of telehealth equipment and its many uses. Students practice sending patient information using both synchronous and store-and-forward techniques.

The students complete the rotation by completing a telehealth project. The project consists of developing a website that could be used to address a need they encounter in health care. They have 5 days to complete the website, which is done using distance technology such as WebEx and Weebly for the development of the website. After 5 days, the teams meet with other teams and a faculty member in order to present their websites using WebEx. Selected websites are then used for community outreach.

Uniformed Services University

Uniformed Services University provided a 9-hour telehealth course for 149 third-year medical students.[30] The course included a pretest, asynchronous didactic lectures, in-person telehealth instruction, a mock telehealth patient encounter, hands-on use of equipment, and a posttest. Content included patient selection, risk management, telehealth etiquette, ethics, and safety. The course was divided into 4 hours of asynchronous lectures with activities; 3 hours of interactive in-person instruction; 2 30-minute mock patient encounters using videoconferencing; and then the hands-on equipment practice tied to common maladies. Students alternated in performing the roles of patient, telepresenter, physician, or observer during the mock encounters. The program was instrumental in increasing the students' interest in providing telehealth services. Knowledge scores related to telehealth increased significantly after the program.[30]

Hack-a-thon

Thirty-five students, including nurse anesthesia, nurse practitioner, clinical nurse specialist, and nurse executive students, participated in a one-day workshop that included a telehealth "hack-a-thon." The students were assigned to teams of 5 to 6 students from varying nursing tracks. In order to focus the presentations on a patient population that was addressed by all professions, substance abuse disorder was targeted. The students were given 2 hours to develop a 15-minute presentation that they would provide to their classmates and a team of "end users." The objectives of the activity were to introduce the students to various telehealth technologies, have the students demonstrate how to evaluate telehealth equipment for use with a specific populations, stimulate the students to research telehealth equipment in order to understand its benefits and barriers, and understand cost and regulatory issues. The groups were assigned to one of the following devices:

- iPhone with peripherals
- Telehealth cart
- VGo robot
- TytoCare
- RPM equipment
- Travel kit

At the beginning of the session, the students were given a demonstration on how the device they were assigned was used. They then had an opportunity to practice using the devices. The remaining time was spent brainstorming, researching, assigning roles, and developing their sales pitch. At the end of the 2 hours, all students met together and then, as a group, proceeded to each room for the presentation. Each device was presented to the "end users" and the other students. The "end users" then asked questions and evaluated the presentation. The programs enabled the students to develop a greater appreciation for telehealth in practice and in working as a team to address the task.

Etiquette/Messy Room

It is vital for students to understand telehealth etiquette/human factors when conducting a telehealth visit. In order to assist students in understanding telehealth etiquette, a workshop was provided where teams of students were required to prepare a telehealth room for a session with a patient. The student had been provided with videos and modules to review on telehealth etiquette prior to the workshop. Each team of 6 students was sent to a telehealth delivery room that was set up with a computer for a videoconferencing session. The rooms were in turmoil, with chairs out of place and food, drinks, and trash spread throughout. A sticky note was covering the camera and the lighting in the room was poor. The students were given 10 minutes to get the room set up for the telehealth visit while focusing on telehealth etiquette. At the end of the 10 minutes, the students started the videoconferencing session with a faculty member in another room. This videoconferencing session lasted 2 minutes. The student performance in the rooms was videotaped along with the videoconferencing session. The tapes were then reviewed and the findings presented to the students. The students were amazed at how many mistakes they made in addressing telehealth etiquette and, more importantly, the impact the poor etiquette had on the visit.

Mental Health

Two faculty members from the UC College of Nursing received a grant to design, implement, and evaluate a telemental health simulation experience for graduate-level PMHNP students. The faculty members were both from the post-Master's PMHNP certificate program. One was also in clinical practice and used telemental health with patients. The goal of the project was to prepare students to use telemental health for patients with mental health and/or substance use disorders upon completion of the program.

The PMHNP program is offered via distance learning, and students are located throughout the United States. The majority are family nurse practitioners, but others are from areas such as nursing education, hospital administration, and women's health. Forty-nine students, 24 in the fall semester and 25 in the spring semester, who were enrolled in the final clinical course in the program took part in the educational project. Their requirements for the course included performing comprehensive diagnostic assessments and planning, implementing, and evaluating evidence-based treatments for patients receiving care from either PMHNPs or psychiatrists.

Students in the course were offered an extra-credit assignment at the end of the semester. The assignment involved watching a prerecorded videotaped session of one of the students in the class doing a telemental health diagnostic assessment and treatment planning session with a standardized patient. The 2 students who conducted the sessions, one each semester, were recruited by faculty based upon the high quality of their work throughout the program. They played the role of a PMHNP interviewing a standardized patient who played the role of a person seeking treatment for heroin addiction. The scenario had been written by a faculty member on the grant who was the lead instructor for the course. Students in the course also viewed a recording of the student, faculty, and standardized patient debriefing after the session.

To evaluate the project, faculty created a 25-question survey tool based upon Bandura's model of self-efficacy.[39] Students completed the survey before and after watching the videos. They rated their confidence in conducting a telemental health visit and provided evaluative comments on the students who played the role of nurse practitioner. There was a significant increase in confidence on several measures, such as the ability to convey empathy and prescribe appropriate medications following the review of the PMHNP/patient telemental health encounter. The overall increase in confidence in assessing, diagnosing, and providing treatment for a patient via telehealth also reached significance. Students offered thoughtful feedback to their peers in the nurse practitioner role, as well as consideration of what they would have done differently. One of the students in the role play had this to say about what she learned: "This experience, via the telehealth simulation project, allowed me to troubleshoot technology needs, practice interviewing skills, and evaluate my own learning."

Medical University of South Carolina College of Nursing

The main telehealth focus in the MUSC College of Nursing has been on the integration of telemedicine into the DNP curriculum. Initially, a 1-day immersion event was provided where students were given lectures in the morning on such content as telehealth definitions, roles, practices, laws, regulations, licensing, credentialing, and equipment. The afternoon session included hands-on experiences with various types of telehealth and RPM equipment. The day ended with a mock telehealth visit. The immersion day was well received, but student feedback indicated that it was a lot of information to assimilate in 1 day. As a result of the feedback, the telehealth components were broken up and scaffolded throughout the DNP curriculum.

In planning the integration of telehealth content throughout the DNP curriculum, course content was examined, and, when applicable, telehealth concepts that were related to the core information was placed within the class (Figure 3-2). For example, the nursing informatics class gives an introduction to computers and how they and other information management and analytical sciences can be used within the health care setting. Telehealth is introduced within the textbook used for the course, so this appeared to be the most appropriate place to introduce telehealth, its definitions, and its equipment and IT needs. The majority of the telehealth information was made into modules, which consisted of a pretest and posttest and a prerecorded lecture (45 to 60 minutes long). The lecture was locked until the students completed the pretest. Students were encouraged to view the lectures as many times as they liked and, once comfortable, complete the posttest. The modules were required for each course, and students were required to score at least a 75% on the posttests to keep from having a point deducted from their final class grade.

In other courses, students were given telehealth-related articles to read and then participated in a discussion with their group. A scenario was given and students chose 1 of 5 or 6 questions to answer (students were in groups of 5 to 6; each student had to choose a different question). Each member of the group had to respond to at least 2 students' answers with a substantive response. These modules were graded using the same process used with the other discussions within the course. The telehealth modules were either pretest/posttest and lecture to be done within a certain time frame within the semester or built within the course as discussion questions, with a duration of 2 weeks during the semester.

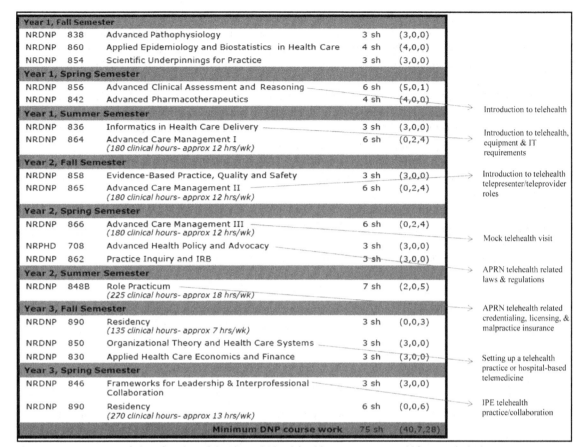

Figure 3-2. Assessment of plan of study and deciding which telehealth components would fit into which classes.

Hands-on telehealth activities were also built into the DNP curriculum. During the students' Advanced Clinical Assessment and Reasoning course, the telehealth cart was introduced to the students during their on-campus learning intensives where they are given a short introduction to the cart and its use. They were then provided with opportunities to use the medical peripherals, including the Horus scope and its otoscope lens attachment, to assist the student in performing a proper otologic exam (eg, being able to successfully find the tympanic membrane). The Welch Allyn panoptic ophthalmoscope with the iExaminer bracket was also used to help students find the red eye reflex, blood vessels, and optic disc/cone. During the third learning intensive, students viewed a video of the telepresenter and teleconsultant/provider roles and then visited MUSC's Center for Telehealth Learning Commons to have hands-on activities with the Avizia 310 cart and its medical peripherals, as well as practice the telepresenter and teleconsultant/provider roles. During their last learning intensive, the students participated in a mock telehealth visit using standardized patients. MUSC College of Nursing is currently developing telehealth-related clinical opportunities for the students during their last 3 semesters, involving school-based telemedicine clinics.

University of Virginia School of Nursing

A graduate nursing–level 3-credit course titled An Introduction to Telehealth has been offered at UVA School of Nursing for the past 6 years. The course is offered to APRN students as well as PhD nursing students, and bachelor of science in nursing (BSN) and registered nurse (RN)-BSN students with permission. This hybrid class uses a technology-enhanced course format to provide a rich learning environment for students, using a variety of senses known to improve learning as aligned with the multimodal approach, including didactic, experiential telehealth simulation experiences, and clinical telehealth project immersions and experiences. Ninety-nine students will have completed the introduction course by the end of 2019 and gained telehealth certification. The course is evaluated at the end of the class by a 20-question Likert scale tool (5=Strongly Agree, 1=Strongly Disagree) that evaluates contribution of telehealth education toward gaining/improving telehealth KSA and future interest using telehealth in practice. Results are consistently scored between 4.8 and 5.0 for improved KSA toward telehealth and 5.0 for interest using telehealth in practice. Students report that the hands-on skill-building lab bring things into perspective for them as the process, technical quality, and engagement using nursing presence in the virtual environment now allows them to actualize telehealth in their practice to improve outcomes, making this a valuable learning experience.

For the Introduction to Telehealth course, students meet at the start of class and work in small groups to explore a patient's journey through an inpatient hospitalization and how telehealth can be used postdischarge via remote monitoring programs. Throughout the course, students engage in the asynchronous online learning environment through a flipped classroom format for 4 modules (12 weeks) of discussions related to the following:

- The history of telehealth, related concepts, services, and technologies
- Telehealth clinical applications, model programs, standards and guidelines for successful clinical services, modalities, specific technology, and the evidence supporting telehealth practice
- The nurse's role in telehealth nursing and integrating nursing practice in the virtual environment
- Legal and regulatory issues surrounding telehealth practice

Telehealth experts join in the discussion to impart real-world experiences to students. Students engage in projects, including four 2-page papers, where they apply telehealth concepts and technologies to a selected health care arena to develop telehealth programs. Additionally, during the course, students are provided opportunity to engage in telehealth projects by participating in UVA's Project Extension for Community Healthcare Outcomes, which gives students experiential involvement and insight on how telehealth programs work to improve patient care outcomes.

The course culminates with module 5, which certifies students as telehealth telepresenters by completing UVA's Telehealth Village Certified Telehealth Telepresenter Program. For this module, students complete online modules, then attend an in-person class for a hands-on skills lab where they engage with telehealth simulation experiences and role-play using telehealth. The hands-on lab enables practicing with the actual technologies, such as computer-based HIPAA-compliant videoconferencing platforms, telehealth carts, mobile telehealth boxes, mHealth/mobile applications, and medical peripherals, including TytoCare exam kits, Horus HD digital scope systems, and Thinklabs digital stethoscopes, thus improving confidence and enhancing retention. The effectiveness of the program is derived from the use of the multimodal approach, simulation experiences, and hands-on skills and confidence-building experiences using the technologies in gaining telehealth nursing KSA. Finally, in conjunction with this course, students can take a 3-credit independent study course in telehealth, which provides an advanced didactic, experiential, and clinical project immersion and engage them in formal precepted practicum experiences, fulfilling all elements of the multimodal approach.

CONTINUING EDUCATION IN TELEHEALTH

Many providers have been through preprofessional programs that did not prepare them in telehealth. Yet, they find themselves in positions that require them to participate in telehealth. All too often, the needed education occurs in the clinical setting and is provided by vendors and their IT staff.[10] Fortunately, there are many opportunities being developed for providers to obtain the needed education or to keep up with current trends in telehealth. One of the most accessible venues is through 14 regional TRCs.[9] These centers have been designed to provide telehealth knowledge and collaborations throughout the various regions in the country. Many of the TRCs provide an annual conference where regional leaders in telehealth provide insight into their programs and mentorship to those new to telehealth.

Professional organizations are beginning to add content to their conferences and are bringing in telehealth vendors to help their participants keep abreast of changes in telehealth. In addition, there has been discussion regarding the need to develop more certification programs in telehealth. With the growth of telehealth as a mainstream approach to health care, a clear approach to telehealth education has not been mandated. However, more discussion is being directed toward the competencies needed to provide telehealth. Many of the approaches discussed in this chapter can be used by providers to learn about telehealth and to keep abreast of new trends and changes in health care.

CONCLUSION

With the nation's focus on improving access to care, telehealth is becoming an acceptable alternative or enhancement to the traditional in-person care model. However, academic centers have been slow to integrate the needed education within their curriculum. As the literature and accrediting agencies embrace and support telehealth, academia will be required to integrate telehealth within their programs. Most health care professions, such as medicine, physical therapy, and mental health, are beginning to feel the push. Yet, as integral players in national health care reform, it is vital for APRNs to embrace and even lead the movement to create telehealth supported models of care. Likewise, academic APRN programs must develop and implement educational programs needed to empower graduate students with the KSAs required for telehealth delivery.

In order for successful educational programs to be implemented, there should be a champion that is able to break down barriers or obstacles to their implementation. Specific focus should initially be on increasing faculty support for the integration of telehealth content within the program, and then developing their expertise. The champion would then be responsible for developing the plan for telehealth integration and then implementing it. This will require obtaining needed resources in the areas of equipment and personnel.

Telehealth education is best provided using the multimodal approach, which includes didactic education, experiential activities, project implementation, and practicum/clinical experiences. Numerous educational models using this approach have been developed and can serve as excellent resources for new programs. Many programs can serve as mentors and collaborators with the champion and faculty.

Academia is faced with graduating students from health care professions that are prepared to overcome the barriers inherent in health care. Telehealth is advancing as one of the most successful models for increasing access to care and allowing APRNs, including those in remote areas, to connect with other providers to deliver optimum care. Academia is now developing and implementing the needed educational programs, often with the support of existing successful programs. Now that many programs have been implemented, there is no need to pursue the journey alone.

THOUGHTFUL QUESTIONS

1. What are the components of a successful telehealth educational program? How can a successful program be developed and implemented in your academic/practice site? What specific content should be included?
2. Telehealth is new to health care educational programs. What are some of the barriers that can interfere with the integration of telehealth content within academic programs? How can these barriers be overcome?
3. A number of programs have successfully implemented telehealth educational programs. What type program would work well in your academic/practice site?
4. How would you go about obtaining mentors to assist you in implementing a telehealth program?

CASE STUDY

Barbara is a faculty member responsible for overseeing the family nurse practitioner (FNP) program at her university. The program is an online/hybrid program, with students coming to campus once a semester. Barbara recently attended a conference where telehealth was discussed. She realized that she needed to make sure the FNP students were prepared to use telehealth in practice when they graduated. When the FNP students come to her program, they participate in standardized patient encounters to develop clinical skills. These encounters occur one-on-one between the FNP and the standardized patient. Barbara would need to restructure the experience in order to include telehealth. The graduate program director is resistant to making any change to the curriculum, further complicating the process.

Questions

1. How should Barbara overcome the graduate program director's resistance?
2. Describe the program that Barbara could implement. Include content and methodology.

REFERENCES

1. Rutledge C, Pitts C, Poston R, Schweickert P. NONPF supports telehealth in nurse practitioner education: 2018. National Organization of Nurse Practitioner Faculties. https://cdn.ymaws.com/www.nonpf.org/resource/resmgr/2018_Slate/Telehealth_Paper_2018.pdf. Published 2018. Accessed February 8, 2020.
2. Thomas A, Crabtree MK, Delaney K, et al. Nurse practitioner core competencies content: 2017. National Organization of Nurse Practitioner Faculties. https://cdn.ymaws.com/www.nonpf.org/resource/resmgr/competencies/2017_NPCoreComps_with_Curric.pdf. Published 2017. Accessed February 15, 2020.
3. Institute of Medicine. *The Future of Nursing: Leading Change, Advancing Health.* Washington, DC: The National Academies Press; 2011. https://www.nap.edu/read/12956/chapter/1. Accessed February 15, 2020.
4. American Association of Colleges of Nursing. *The Essentials of Master's Education in Nursing.* http://www.aacnnursing.org/portals/42/publications/mastersessentials11.pdf. Published March 21, 2011. Accessed February 15, 2020.
5. American Association of Colleges of Nursing. *The Essentials of Doctoral Education for Advanced Nursing Practice.* https://www.aacnnursing.org/Portals/42/Publications/DNPEssentials.pdf. Published October 2006. Accessed February 15, 2020.

6. Health Resources & Services Administration. Telehealth programs. https://www.hrsa.gov/rural-health/telehealth/index.html. Updated August 2019. Accessed February 15, 2020.

7. Ali NS, Carlton KH, Ali OS. Telehealth education in nursing curriculum. *Nurse Educ.* 2015;40(5):266-269.

8. Zayapragassarazan Z, Kumar S. Awareness, knowledge, attitude and skills of telemedicine among health professional faculty working in teaching hospitals. *J Clin Diagn Res.* 2016;10(3):JC01-JC04.

9. Douthit N, Kiv S, Dwolatzky T, Biswas S. Exposing some important barriers to health care access in the rural USA. *Public Health.* 2015;129(6):611-620.

10. Rutledge CM, Kott K, Schweickert P, et al. Telehealth and eHealth in nurse practitioner training: current perspectives. *Adv Med Educ Pract.* 2017;8:399-409.

11. Edirippulige S, Armfield NR. Education and training to support the use of clinical telehealth: a review of the literature. *J Telemed Telecare.* 2017;23(2):273-282.

12. Haney T, Kott K, Fowler C. Telehealth etiquette in home healthcare: the key to a successful visit. *Home Healthc Now.* 2015;33(5):254-259.

13. Erickson CE, Fauchald S, Ideker M. Integrating telehealth into the graduate nursing curriculum. *J Nurs Pract.* 2015;11(1):e1-e5.

14. Gallagher-Lepak S, Scheibel P, Gibson CC. Integrating telehealth in nursing curricula: can you hear me now? *Online Journal of Nursing Informatics.* 2009;13(2):1-16.

15. Rutledge CM, Haney T, Bordelon M, Renaud M, Fowler C. Telehealth: preparing advanced practice nurses to address healthcare needs in rural and underserved populations. *Int J Nurs Educ Scholarsh.* 2014;11(1):1-9.

16. Rutledge CM, Renaud M, Shepherd L, et al. Educating advanced practice nurses in using social media in rural healthcare. *Int J Nurs Educ Scholarsh.* 2011;8(1):1-14.

17. Silva AS, Rizzante FA, Picolini MM, et al. Bauru School of Dentistry Tele-Health League: an educational strategy applied to research, training and extension among applications in telehealth. *J Appl Oral Sci.* 2011;19(6):599-603.

18. Sevean P, Dampier S, Spadoni M, Strickland S, Pilatzke S. Bridging the distance: educating nurses for telehealth practice. *J Cont Educ Nurs.* 2008;39(9):413-418.

19. Gray D, Rutledge CM. Using new communication technologies: fostering interprofessional collaboration and telehealth skills in nurse practitioners. *J Nurs Pract.* 2014;10(10):840-844.

20. Strehle E, Bateman B, Dickinson K. Medical students pediatric cardio vascular examination by telemedicine. *Telemed J E Health.* 2009;15(4):342-346.

21. National Organization of Nurse Practitioner Faculties. Advanced practice: curriculum guidelines and program standards for nurse practitioner education. 1995. https://www.nonpf.org/.

22. National CNS Competency Task Force. Clinical nurse specialist core competencies: executive summary 2006-2008. https://nacns.org/wp-content/uploads/2016/11/CNSCoreCompetenciesBroch.pdf. Published 2010. Accessed February 24, 2020.

23. Patient Protection and Affordable Care Act, 42 USC §18001 et seq (2010).

24. Bulik R. Human factors in primary care telemedicine encounters. *J Telemed Telecare.* 2008;14(4):169-172.

25. van Houwelingen CT, Moerman AH, Ettema RG, Kort HS, Ten Cate O. Competencies required for nursing telehealth activities: a Delphi-study. *Nurse Educ Today.* 2015;39:50-62.

26. Shams L, Seitz AR. Benefits of multisensory learning. *Trends Cogn Sci.* 2008;12(11):411-417.

27. Shams L, Wozny DR, Seitz AR. Influences of multisensory experience on subsequent unisensory processing. *Front Psychol.* 2001;2:264.

28. Proulx MJ, Brown DJ, Pasqualotto A, Meijer P. Multisensory perceptual learning and sensory substitution. *Neurosci Biobehav Rev.* 2014;41:16-25.

29. South Central Telehealth Resource Center. Telehealth etiquette [video]. http://learntelehealth.org/video-items/telehealth-etiquette/. Accessed February 15, 2020.

30. Jonas CE, Durning SJ, Zebrowski C, Cimino F. An interdisciplinary, multi-institution telehealth course for third-year medical students. *Acad Med.* 2019;94(6):833-837.

31. Rutledge CM, Haney T, Bordelon M, Renaud M, Fowler C. Telehealth: preparing advanced practice nurses to address healthcare needs in rural and underserved populations. *Int J Nurs Educ Scholarsh.* 2014;11.

32. National Consortium of Telehealth Resource Centers. Find your TRC. http://www.telehealthresourcecenter.org/who-your-trc. Accessed February 15, 2020.

33. Sweeney Haney T, Kott K, Rutledge CM, Britton B, Fowler CN, Poston RD. How to prepare interprofessional teams in two weeks: an innovative education program nested in telehealth. *Int J Nurs Educ Scholarsh.* 2018;15(1).

34. Gustin TS, Kott K, Rutledge C. Telehealth etiquette training: a guideline for preparing interprofessional teams for successful encounters [published online ahead of print April 23, 2019]. *Nurse Educ.* doi:10.1097/NNE.0000000000000680.

35. National Task Force on Quality Nurse Practitioner Education. Criteria for evaluation of nurse practitioner programs: 2012. 4th ed. Washington, DC: National Organization of Nurse Practitioner Faculties; 2012. https://cdn.ymaws.com/nonpf.site-ym.com/resource/resmgr/docs/ntfevalcriteria2012final.pdf. Accessed February 15, 2020.

36. Higgins K, Le-Jenkins U, Kirkland T, Rutledge C. Preparing students to be ready for practice: an innovative approach to teaching advanced physical assessment skills online. *J Am Assoc Nurs Pract*. In press.

37. Schweickert PA, Rheuban KS, Cattell-Gordon D, et al. The APN-PLACE telehealth education network: legal and regulatory considerations. *J Nurs Reg*. 2018;9(1):47-51.

38. Patton CW, Lewallen LP. Legal issues in clinical nursing education. *Nurse Educ*. 2015;40(3):124-128.

39. Bandura A. *Self-Efficacy Beliefs of Adolescents*. Charlotte, NC: Information Age Publishing; 2006.

4

Telehealth Technology

Richard L. Rose II, CTC, CWTS
Patty Alane Schweickert, DNP, FNP-C
David Cattell-Gordon, MDiv, MSW
Samuel Collins, MSc
Rebecca L. Steele, MSN, RN, CNL
Christianne Nesbit, DNP, AGNP, PMHNP
Michele L. Bordelon, MSEd
Brian Gunnell, BS, CTC

CHAPTER OBJECTIVES

Upon review of this chapter, the reader will be able to:

1. Identify the modes for integrating telehealth technologies into health care and advanced practice nursing.
2. Compare telehealth technologies and differentiate their use.
3. Examine telehealth service delivery systems and networks.
4. Describe future considerations for health care technologies and for incorporating the medical internet of things and artificial intelligence into health care.

Since the conception and development of the first simple tool, humans have steadily discovered and developed new inventions to improve life. Each new discovery has served as a foundation for further innovation. It is the partnering and assimilation of the various technological advances and achievements that has enabled this knowledge to be directed toward improving health. In today's modern society, technology is pervasive, from online banking to watching videos on our smartphones. Technology is advancing as well, from remotely monitoring patients to performing remote surgery using telepresence. The ability to project an image of oneself onto a screen to a patient far away in order to communicate with him or her, let alone perform a surgical procedure, seemed like fantasy only 50 years ago. Television series such as *The Jetsons* and *Star Trek* contain prime examples of these advanced technologies that were once fiction and are now part of our daily reality.

Schweickert PA, Rutledge CM, eds.
Telehealth Essentials for Advanced Practice Nursing (pp 71-95).
© 2020 Taylor & Francis Group.

Today, it may seem like fantasy to some to be able to use a variety of mobile, wearable, and/or implanted internet-connected devices to monitor health indicators, receive direct care and disease management, and track live health-related data to manage and prevent disease via the medical internet of things (mIoT). Telehealth technology is inherently changing health care and nursing practice because it provides an entirely new realm of patient interaction and collection and analysis of data in the virtual care environment. Creating this new practice arena is complex; the transition of in-person nursing knowledge, skills, and practices must be carefully integrated into telehealth advanced nursing practice. Also, new skills must be identified and learned. Questions must be addressed regarding how the nurse-patient relationship can be actualized in the virtual care environment to ensure that the essence of nursing practice is preserved and aligned with advanced practice nursing. However, before nurses can begin assimilation of telehealth in nursing practice, it is important they develop a strong understanding of the technologies, the application of the technologies to practice, the issues surrounding implementation, the network of connectedness of devices, and the implications for health care and nursing practice.

TELEHEALTH TECHNOLOGY IN HEALTH CARE

The discussion of broadband, smart devices, artificial intelligence (AI), robotics, and advanced digital technologies permeates planning and application to a multitude of human ventures. Digital technology is involved in commerce, education, sports, recreation, government, and many aspects of family life. The forces driving this adoption are inevitably impacting health care. Although the use of digital technology is still in relatively early development within health care, the application of telemedicine is spreading rapidly and is becoming integrated into the operations of health systems, hospitals, specialty practices, home health agencies, private provider sites, schools, and businesses, as well as consumer's homes and workplaces. Telehealth is applied to every patient group across the continuum of care, from high-risk pregnancies, to newborns, to children with complex care needs. Telehealth is used in every facet of health care, from an individual's chronic disease, such as diabetes mellitus, to wellness management of population health, through end-of-life care. Telehealth happens within single facilities, across networks of partner sites, and within consortia and global interactions.

FOR REFLECTION 1:

Technology in Nursing: Tools of Practice

Consider current technologies used in nursing and how familiarity and confidence is gained using these technologies in practice. When using telehealth in nursing practice, what are some of the similarities and differences of telehealth technologies as compared with other technologies in nursing practice that should be assessed and explored?

TELEHEALTH TECHNOLOGIES

Among the overall modes of telehealth technology, 2 primary types of technology serve as the foundation for use in health care. These include store-and-forward and real-time videoconferencing technologies. An integration of these technologies can be used in remote patient monitoring. Additionally, mobile devices, sensors, wearables, implantables, and health apps are being used in increasing frequency to improve personal health and personal health knowledge (Table 4-1).

Store-and-Forward Technology (Asynchronous)

Transfer of patient data (diagnostic and physiologic) from the patient site (source) to a remote site for evaluation and interpretation can be achieved via store-and-forward technologies.[1] Using store-and-forward technology, data are obtained and stored at the source site, then transmitted, or forwarded, to the remote intended site. Physiologic data (eg, blood glucose, blood pressure, oxygen saturation, patient weight), diagnostic radiologic and medical imaging (eg, wound, retinal, dermatology, and pathology images), electrocardiograms (ECGs), patient symptom survey data, and education are common uses of store-and-forward technology.[2] This type of technology is useful when the patient requires assessment with the collected data but does not require the patient to be present during the assessment of the data to receive care. The benefits of this type of delivery model include time savings, increased frequency of care, and secure information sharing. The clinician's ability to review a patient's diagnostic imaging or physiologic data asynchronously uses the patient's time wisely by decreasing travel time and repeated trips to the provider. Enabling more frequent assessments without unnecessary patient visits saves provider time. Additionally, diagnostic images and physiologic data can be transmitted and reviewed prior to a telehealth visit, allowing the clinician time to prepare for the visit. This can improve the quality of the visit by assimilation of all available patient information in preparation for the encounter. For example, a patient could transmit a month of home blood pressure measurements, daily weights, or glucose measurements so that the clinician could review this data prior to the telehealth visit. Furthermore, asynchronous services increase remote or rurally located patient access to a specialist that might not exist in their geographic region.

Real-Time Videoconferencing (Synchronous)

Videoconferencing technology enables real-time 2-way audiovisual interactions between patients and providers or 1 provider to another using television monitors or screens, cameras, microphones, software, computers, and computer networks.[3] Videoconferencing uses broadband internet over internet protocol (IP) networks and voice over internet protocol technology that allows for transfer of video and audio connections simultaneously over the same line.[4] There are many examples of this type of technology available, such as Apple FaceTime and Microsoft Skype, with which most consumers have some familiarity. Applications like this and how they are used may or may not be Health Insurance Portability and Accountability Act (HIIPAA) secure, causing a complex arena of technology security to navigate. These tools are invaluable in their application to health care because they enable people and patients to connect remotely in the virtual care environment for consultation, treatment, and timely health care management and education. This approach can be especially useful when seeing the patient is important for assessment, as in acute stroke, and for patients who have needs that are timely or have barriers to receiving care in person. For example, one of the most common uses of videoconferencing is in the area of mental health counseling. This allows the patient to receive needed counseling remotely, at the time that he or she needs it.

TABLE 4-1

TELEHEALTH SERVICES AND ASSOCIATED TECHNOLOGIES

SERVICE	PURPOSE	TECHNOLOGIES	EXAMPLES
Patient consultation	Provider and patient connect remotely for primary care or specialty consults, or for direct patient care Provider consult to patient and to intensive care unit care team	Live videoconferencing Store-and-forward	Telestroke Neurology, mental health, pediatrics eICU
Clinician consultation	Provider-to-provider consultation	Live videoconferencing Store-and-forward Email	eConsults Interprofessional video-collaboration
Remote patient monitoring	Provides frequent physiologic monitoring Enables health surveys and patient education	Live videoconferencing Store-and-forward Email Wireless monitors/devices Internet/web based	Post-hospital discharge monitoring Chronic disease monitoring Monitoring of high-risk patients Monitoring of older patients
Mobile health (mHealth)	Health monitoring and adherence Health education	Live videoconferencing Store-and-forward Wearable wireless monitors/devices Health apps	Health apps that produce EKG readings or measure blood glucose Medical peripherals for smartphones Wearables such as FitBit, Apple Watch
Web-based services	Remote conferencing Webinars Live videoconferencing Web conferencing for telehealth programs, education, and administration Online meetings Mobile collaboration	Cloud computing Live videoconferencing Internet Store-and-forward	Desktop and mobile platforms such as Zoom or Jabber

Currently, a statewide videoconferencing program is being established in Virginia in order to improve the care of children with mental health concerns. This videoconferencing platform will allow primary care providers (physicians and nurse practitioners) who care for children to receive consultation with a mental health provider in order to best plan the care, offer emergency counseling to the patient in the office with a mental health provider at a distance, and receive education from experts through programs such as Extension for Community Healthcare Outcome, which is a grand rounds style of case review between clinicians and university medical center experts for departing knowledge that can improve the clinician's ability to care for patients locally. Additionally, this delivery model is also ideal for remote or underserved areas where certain specialties might not be readily accessible or available.

Although synchronous care does have many positives, it also has some limitations, including meeting certain levels of criteria for reimbursement, being resource intensive if the clinician or patient does not have the appropriate technological setup to support such a visit, and being time consuming if not properly planned, tested, and prepared prior to clinical encounters. With this type of technology in place, clinicians can expand their reach, which in turn can mean taking on a greater patient load than what is typical of a traditional clinic. Despite the challenges of the synchronous care delivery model, it is necessary to continue to refine the technology and push the limits of what is possible so that those who need the care can have access and those who provide the care can meet the requirements for implementation and reimbursement.

Remote Patient Monitoring

Remote patient monitoring (RPM) allows for more frequent patient monitoring and trending of physiologic data. This approach can use both synchronous and asynchronous methods of connecting. RPM connects patients and providers by an RPM telemedicine system that is installed in the patient's home and transmits data to a provider site for assessment. A variety of monitors, tools, and technologies can be combined to form unique remote monitoring programs. This approach allows for the provider and the patient to engage in a live videoconferencing session after the patient data are collected and evaluated through the RPM.[5,6]

RPM is especially promising for improving chronic disease management,[7] diagnostic testing, and posthospitalization assessment for the patient from home. RPM is being used to assess for changes in patients' conditions who are in senior living facilities or in their homes. Specific emphasis is on monitoring individuals with chronic conditions and frail older adults in order to assess for complications and provide interventions before the conditions escalate. This type of care delivery system allows clinicians to continue to monitor patients beyond the clinic or hospital walls, enabling them to provide timely interventions, which in turn can reduce patients' risk to acutely decompensate. Many health systems, as they evolve to meet the demands of tighter reimbursement models, are focusing their efforts on helping patients transition safely home following hospitalizations or procedures by using RPM.

Additionally, RPM can be developed to meet the needs of specific patient populations, ensuring the data points are relevant and necessary for their continued care management. For example, a patient with congestive heart failure may be equipped with home monitoring devices that assess their oxygen saturation (pulse oximeter), weight (scale), and blood pressure (automatic blood pressure cuff). By transmitting these data daily to a provider or staff, changes in the patient's condition can be readily assessed and treatment implemented before the patient compensates further. This can be as simple as increasing the patient's diuretic remotely and further assessing for improvement of the condition. Other commonly managed conditions include the glucose monitoring of patients with diabetes, heart rate and ECG monitoring of patients with arrhythmias or other cardiac conditions, and fall assessments for older adults.

Even caregivers are embracing the use of RPM as they attempt to keep their family members in their homes. Some of these technologies include devices that assess for falls, door monitors to track whether a family member with dementia is leaving the house, or medication dispensers that regulate the medication dosage at a distance, dispense the appropriate dosages, and notify the patients when the medication is needed. A dissolving tracking pill that is dispensed with a medication and then notifies the caregiver when the medication is taken is also being developed.

Many technology companies are working in the health care space to leverage existing technology from wearables, such as the Apple Watch and the FitBit, to manual-entry methods using smart devices, such as tablets or smartphones. The opportunities with remote patient monitoring are endless but require thought on when to start and end a patient episode and how to ensure the patient can handle and engage with the technology providing the most accurate data-collection methods.

Some of the downfalls of this style of telehealth delivery include lack of interoperability and accessibility, and false alarms leading to increased resource use. Many of the companies vying in the arena of RPM are separate entities and not a part of the current electronic health record (EHR) software that clinicians often use. This will likely change in the future as EHR companies learn to accommodate these technologies and see them as integral to patient care. When looking at accessibility, the concern not only applies to the provider's ability to easily access the data the patient is submitting, but also to the patient's ability to leverage the technology. Currently, there are many pockets where internet service or cellular connectivity is absent. As dependency on these technologies increases, service providers will need to make those areas of isolation more accessible. Finally, if a patient is not properly trained on how to use the technology, the clinician may have an increased number of false alarms that in turn could potentially lead the patient to seek care for concerns that are unnecessary.

Mobile Health

Mobile health, or mHealth, enables individuals to access health education, personal health data, or health care from mobile devices such as smartphones, personal tablets, and wearable or implanted devices. Many of these devices are enhanced with mobile apps or sensors that measure, monitor, and calculate personal physiologic data and selected behaviors. They enable people to self-engage with measuring physiologic data and healthy behaviors and allow monitoring of essential physiologic parameters for those with chronic disease. With the growth in cellular network coverage areas and the steadily increasing number of people using mobile and wireless devices, advances in these technologies have great potential to aid in the transformation of traditional health care to that of fully connected mHealth platforms.[8]

Health education includes technologies that engage the patient in a deeper understanding of their health. The users benefit because these devices are accessible and largely available. The abundant accompanying mobile health care apps provide for general information sharing, data collection, provider information resources, and more. These apps, much like health education, can be extremely detailed or very vague, yet the benefit of these types of delivery systems is that the information is at the user's fingertips and can empower the user to feel more aware or engaged with his or her health. The additional benefit is that health systems or providers can create content and easily deliver the information in a manner that is more up to date than the traditional paper handout or brochure. Finally, it can be a cost savings for the clinician to use an app or education material that already exists and does not require developing or editing.

Individuals are using mHealth today by monitoring their activity levels and sleep quality, assessing their vital signs, accessing health care information, and tracking physiologic information such as blood glucose or weight. Providers are also becoming accustomed to using mHealth in their day-to-day practice. Providers are now able to purchase peripherals and apps that allow them to obtain and transmit data on their patients. Examples include ECG strips, blood pressure cuffs, ophthalmologic and otoscopic assessments, and ultrasounds. This has enhanced the ability of providers to perform more comprehensive assessments when they perform home visits or in the clinician's office when data need to be transmitted. For instance, the provider of a patient with diabetes can examine the retina using the ophthalmoscope and transmit the data to the ophthalmologist for interpretation; the patient with chest pains can have an ECG done in a home or office that is not equipped with an ECG machine; or the provider can obtain pictures of skin lesions and send them to the dermatologist for consultation. With so much information available, how can a patient be sure the information he or she is engaging with is accurate and up to date? This question is one that will always be a challenge as the world of mHealth and health education expands.

EMERGING TRENDS IN TELEHEALTH TECHNOLOGY

Telehealth is growing at an exponential rate, with new approaches being developed every day. However, the explosive growth of this industry is not without challenges. Cyber security is paramount among these challenges, as is reimbursement of services, parity laws, providing evidence to support telehealth practice, standardization of processes and technology interfaces, digitization of all medical records, ability for EHRs to be able to interface and communicate with other health-related technologies and devices, and coordination of data and care delivery. Of specific interest are the new medical peripheral devices that can enhance remote home monitoring, mHealth, and both synchronous and asynchronous care delivery systems. Electronic consults (eConsults) are also on the rise as a means of connecting providers asynchronously. In addition, the number of internet-connected devices, like wearables and implantables, passive and active sensors and monitoring devices, and mobile health applications in a connected network of the internet of things (IoT) and the mIoT are increasing. The maturing fields of predictive analytics, AI, and precision medicine, as well as the increasing gamification of apps and devices, are also changing the face of health care.

Medical Peripherals

Telehealth medical peripherals are some of the latest innovations to enter the medical device arena. Nurses have long used medical devices in the traditional nursing care environment, like the stethoscope to assess lung, heart, and vascular sounds. In telehealth, nurses also need a way to physiologically assess patients remotely. Medical peripherals are diagnostic tools used by providers in conjunction with telehealth equipment for physiologic assessment of patients. Common devices include digital stethoscopes, otoscopes, ophthalmoscopes, thermometers, ECGs, scales, and dermatology scopes. Other devices include ultrasound, spirometer, colposcope, and retinal cameras. Most of these devices use store-and-forward technologies, and some use a combination of both store-and-forward and synchronous technologies to obtain and transmit data.

Electronic Consults

eConsults are an asynchronous exchange that takes place between health care providers. Although not limited to primary care providers consulting specialists, eConsults are often used to facilitate specialist input on patient problems without requiring a referral and additional in-person visits for the patient. In many ways, an eConsult is the standardization and digitization of the curbside consult. By creating standard work in the midst of all of the myriad forms of contact means between providers emails, staff messages, phone calls, hallway conversations, and other means, eConsults can enable safer and more efficient consult methods that are conducted and remain referenceable in the EHR.[9]

There are several models of technology that can support eConsults, from live video to secure email or modules built into an EHR. This allows for a trackable and billable model for providers to exchange information online. Technology being used in these consults ranges from very basic store-and-forward patient information transfer via the internet to advanced imaging transfer, such as in diabetic retinopathy screening with new cameras synced to mobile devices for obtaining retinal images. The model of electronic consults is shown to improve referral appropriateness, clarity of consult question, and provider satisfaction. eConsults often use templates that are developed with input by specialist responders to guide and produce quality, thorough clinical questions. In a successful program, the consulted provider has the option to respond in a timely manner or deem the question too complex or inappropriate for an eConsult; he or she may elect to decline response or convert the eConsult to a standard referral visit.

The service benefits patients, primary care providers (PCPs), and specialists alike. For patients, there is clear reduced cost in medical expense in avoiding unnecessary additional visits, but also savings and satisfaction from reduced travel and a reduction of less apparent expenditures like time away from work, school, and coordinating child care. Generalists gain the benefits of increased access to specialty expertise and faster turnaround for subspecialty inquiries[10] while also benefiting from the inherent education benefits of care guidance and documentation that can be revisited.[11] The specialist, via the templates, is able to facilitate a focused clinical question containing what exactly is required to most effectively provide input and is now able to document and have his or her efforts recognized for the large amount of consults he or she frequently provides.

The eConsult service addresses many of the larger health system's aims of reducing no-show rates; specialists engaging in higher-yield, higher-complexity clinic visits; and PCPs gaining further access to ongoing education and opportunity to increase patient satisfaction and quality of care. eConsults also can be used to reduce specialty clinic wait times by reducing the low-acuity instances taking up much needed clinic slots.[12]

Use cases for eConsults are wide ranging, with typical consult questions including a PCP asking endocrinology about thyroid nodules or a clinician reaching out to cardiology after an abnormal ECG. But when paired with store-and-forward technology, dermatologic images or even fundus photos can be captured in the primary care setting and sent to dermatology, ophthalmology, neurology, or wherever most appropriate.

Part of the appeal of the service is that it is customizable to a specific need or institution. Essentially, it is about providing the best means for interprofessional exchange (Table 4-2). With time in the EHR adding up, much to the dismay of many providers, it is important to note that eConsults are augmenting and streamlining work that is often unaccounted for but being performed. Health systems are growing in scale both geographically and in scope of care. eConsults are a means of keeping providers engaged with one another to promote care coordination in an environment where not everyone sees each other in the cafeteria; it is a revitalization of close primary and subspecialty collaborative care.

Gamification

One of the greatest challenges in health care today is related to lifestyle diseases; noncommunicable diseases have surpassed preindustrial causes of disease, accounting for over 70% of all deaths globally.[8] It has been estimated that up to 75% of all US health care costs are due to chronic disease caused by individual lifestyle choices.[13] Lifestyle diseases are those directly associated with modifiable health behaviors. Our modern lifestyle of unhealthy diets, sedentary existence, and tobacco and drug abuse can lead to chronic diseases, including heart disease, stroke, diabetes, drug addictions, and pulmonary disease. The best treatment for lifestyle diseases is prevention; therefore, efforts to motivate people to take actions toward this end are important. In the digital age, individuals have become accustomed to, and expect, ease of access and use of all things, along with a stimulating experience.

Gamification involves applying principles of game design to increase engagement and increase the fun of commonplace activities. The concepts of gaming have been woven into the fabric of many standard activities in daily life, from collecting tokens at the local coffee shop to collecting points when grocery shopping. An example of the use of technology to change behavior using

TABLE 4-2	
ELECTRONIC CONSULT EXEMPLAR: SWINFEN CHARITABLE TRUST, UNITED KINGDOM	
WHAT IT IS	Swinfen is an eConsult system, a virtual hospital that never runs out of beds, has no political master, and welcomes every patient. It is a free service run mainly by nurses on a 24-hour system, 7 days a week, 52 weeks a year. It was established 1998 by Lord and Lady Swinfen. It set up the first telehealth eConsult link in 1999 to a hospital in Bangladesh.
PURPOSE	Swinfen connects doctors, nurses, and medical workers in the developing world to a growing panel of global medical consultants/specialists who offer free advice, diagnosis, and recommend treatment to give patients the best possible care.
HOW IT WORKS	A case is submitted by practitioner via secure internet-accessed server. A nurse reviews information and forwards it to the appropriate specialty provider. The specialist signs in to the server, reviews case, submits response. Referrer logs back into the server to obtain the response.
NURSING LEADERSHIP	At present, there are 4 nurses leading operations: • Mrs Robyn Carr, New Zealand, a leader in Nursing Health Informatics, New Zealand • Lieutenant Colonel Rtd Lynda Bardell, ex-Queen Alexandra's Royal Army Nursing Corps • Mrs Loveday Ellis, Semi Rtd, Former senior nurse in London, England • Lady Swinfen, ex-Lieutenant, Queen Alexandra's Royal Army Nursing Corps
REACH	Swinfen has involvement in 365 hospitals and clinics in 78 countries. Over 700 consultants and 618 referrers use the system.
TECHNOLOGY	Email for messages Digital cameras for clinical pictures Phone Fax
BENEFITS	Establishing a diagnosis Reassurance Changing patient care management Avoiding overseas travel Contributing to medical education using a small carbon footprint

gamification is the Volkswagen initiative, aptly named "The Fun Theory."[14] As part of this initiative, an interactive musical stairway called the Piano Stairs were installed in an underground station in Stockholm, Sweden, alongside the escalator. The main objective and mission of the initiative was to encourage behavioral changes through fun activities.[13] Results showed that when faced with the choice between climbing stairs and riding the escalator, subway commuters chose the Piano Stairs 66% more often. Other examples of health-related game design techniques and principles include apps that enable the user to track activities with bars, awards, badges, medals, or comparison to other individuals or groups. Many use social networks to stimulate friendly competitions among other users. Some well-known examples of devices and games that use this concept include Pokémon Go, the Nintendo Wii, and the FitBit.

The gamification of health is an emerging field that is increasingly being woven into the mobile health app arena, as wellness apps and wearable technologies are becoming more a prevalent attempt to make engagement in healthy lifestyle behaviors more fun. In 2016, evidence showed that 4% of health apps included gamification.[15] In 2018, it was shown that gamification was used by 64% of mobile applications.[16] Systematic reviews of the literature on gamification for health and well-being reveal positive impact in health and well-being, particularly for health behaviors.[17] e-Health applications have been shown to yield more short-term than long-term engagement using these extrinsic rewards. "Gamification can be effective in promoting and sustaining healthy behaviors, tapping into playful and goal-driven aspects of human nature."[15] However, clinical benefits have not been fully evaluated and more research is needed because the potential of gamification is yet to be achieved. Increased immersions into the essential physical and physiological experience are based on game theory.[15(p2)] Notably, there is a gap in apps that focus specifically on health behaviors that directly affect clinical outcomes.

Wearable Technology and Drones

Wearable technology has become more accessible and more useful in monitoring health status over the past few years. People are living longer, with 1 in 4 having multiple chronic conditions.[18] The popularity of this technology is growing, with the market for these devices expected to reach $150 billion by 2027. This technology has immense potential to help monitor various health conditions, provide feedback to encourage health promotion activities, and alert others if a sudden change in condition has occurred. Even the off-the-shelf products available today can provide useful health applications.

Smart watches, depending on the brand and cost, have the capability of easily monitoring heart rate, heart rhythm, location, and overall activity, including steps taken each day. These devices have been used to not only measure current activity level but also predict health outcomes such as readmission rates for individuals with specific health issues or overall mortality in post-surgical oncology patients.[19] Devices such as wearable watches or fitness bands can also easily identify a fall using the accelerometer function built into them. This allows quick detection that the wearer has had a fall, and help can be obtained quickly. Additionally, the ability to use location software can be helpful in instances of an older adult with dementia, or a child who has wandered away from home. This service alone can be life-saving; statistics show that the sooner a person wandering from home is found, the higher the survival rate, especially for those with dementia.

Other wearable technology is rapidly progressing in design and use. There are now conductive fabrics that can be assembled into clothing capable of measuring heart rate, respirations, body temperature, and skin conductance. These various measures can be helpful in many health care applications. For example, skin conductance has been used to measure changes in the autonomic nervous system that can occur during periods of emotional stress or anxiety.[20] Measurements of heart rate, temperature, and respirations can quickly indicate a change in health status and help promote rapid interventions.

The increase in technologies has gone far beyond individual use. Once only used for military reasons, drones are now being used for health care purposes. These pilotless devices can fly from one point to another to deliver medicine, blood products, and laboratory specimens and even provide rapid delivery of automated external defibrillators.[19] Much of the benefit of drones comes from their ability to reach areas that are hard to access or have limited resources. As an example, in rural areas, drones have been helpful in delivering medications and laboratory testing equipment that greatly impacts the speed of diagnosis and treatment. The future of drone technology is being tested now. It can be used to help older adults by attaching a manipulator arm or videoconference capabilities to the drone, which can help them with day-to-day activities.[19] The videoconference capability will also allow for telehealth visits, either in remote sites or in an urgent situation.

Internet of Things and Medical Internet of Things

For the health care data generated by connected devices to be useful, they must be analyzed together to produce results that can improve health care decision making. Big data analytics and IoT are interconnected because data generated from connected devices (big data) can be organized and analyzed together, producing big data of IoT. Kevin Ashton first described the IoT in the 1990s as he contemplated whether a radio frequency identification chip could be attached to a tube of lipstick for inventory purposes. [21] He subsequently worked on a project at the Massachusetts Institute of Technology to connect radiofrequency identification tags to the internet. The IoT is a cyber-physical network of internet-linked smart objects, devices, sensors, and apps that are able to obtain, store, exchange, analyze, and apply data.[22] The mIoT involves these activities in the health arena.

In their most basic forms, the mIoT and the IoT entail electronic devices connecting to other electronic devices to share information. Although electronic devices have been able to communicate with one another since the electric telegraph in the 1830s,[23] the current pace of technological innovation is explosive, and the rapidity of development is unprecedented. Additionally, today's smart devices, sensors, and apps collect and transmit a vast sum of data coupled with the components of the IoT, including advanced analytics, multilayer computing, AI, new and widespread applications, capabilities like automization and optimization, and connectivity to process and make sense of the individual, big data, and mIoT big data to improve health and health care of the future.[23] IoT advanced analytics involves analysis of huge amounts of data to identify insights, patterns, and behaviors not otherwise discoverable with smaller volumes of data. Descriptive (organize and describe), predictive (forecast), and prescriptive (determine actions) analytics of things (AoT), big data analytics, and now IoT data analytics will bring new ideas, answers, and solutions to health care. Computing in the mIoT can evolve from cloud to AI-enabled cognitive output, surpassing present ability and function.

AI, which will be explored further in the following section, is a data-driven science based upon intelligent algorithms, which can be used in many ways in health care. One way is by using augmented reality, which can assimilate all of a person's connected device data and present them in an individualized virtual reality format. AI is also being developed for improved automation of devices and systems, cognitive computing, and deep learning (a subset of predictive analytics).[23] Machine learning, machine-to-machine communications (perhaps the beginning of the IoT), the neural network, speech and facial recognition technology, voice assistance, and virtual reality all are under the umbrella of AI.[23]

Going forward, perhaps the internet of everything will become prominent, focusing technology more on people, process, data, and things, linking the person more closely to the IoT.[24] Additionally, all health care arenas could have their own IoT, such as the pharmacy (pharma) IoT focused on pharmacologic issues, including smart devices, clinical trials, and patient care.[25] For example, pharma IoT could use sensors and personalized technologies for insulin and asthma medication management and administration, directed at improving the pharmacological management of the patient.[25] Nursing could also have an IoT-specific arena. Advanced practice registered nurses (APRNs) could be leaders in the development of the nursing IoT or the nursing internet of everything, focused on nursing care of the patient in the cyber world. Nursing roles such as nursing prescriptive analytics expert, APRN mIoT data analyst, nursing IoT expert, and APRN cyber-health manager may be developed. It is even conceivable that nursing education programs will include tracks such as the Doctorate in Cyber Nursing in the future.

It is estimated that up to 40% of all IoT technologies will be health related by 2020, accounting for a $117 billion industry.[25] Challenges for IoT going forward include connectivity, device management, data storage and analytics, security of data, and reimbursement and policy issues.[25] Other issues important for success include device and network interoperability and interconnectivity and how to integrate existing silos and islands of data into big data IoT data.[25] Optimization of current and future platforms is necessary to enable advances in predictive analytics. Also, the importance of protocols and standards development and adoption across services and platforms can improve quality and safeguard data and data use. Finally, challenges related to perceived lack of nurse-patient privacy in the virtual care environment, general protected health information security concerns in the cyber world, questions about forming a trusting relationship with the patient in the virtual care environment, and the need to gain confidence and trust using the technology and results of data from the IoT need to be explored.[26]

Artificial Intelligence

Like a lot of technology innovation, opinions often precede or even preclude actually knowing what a technology is or is not, and AI is no exception. AI is, at its core, a science based on intelligent algorithms, with algorithms essentially being governing parameters that delineate operational sequence. *Machine learning* is a subfield within AI that functions on the idea that a computer system learns from data sets and makes inferences and decisions that it might not have been explicitly programmed to execute. These data sets can come predefined, as in images of a specific bone labeled fractured or not (also called *supervised learning*), or undefined, such as a large set of images where the system can highlight differences with no such up front classifications (*unsupervised learning*). *Deep learning* is another term used; biological neural networks inspire it, and these artificial neural networks can work from data sets both supervised or unsupervised. There is a wide array of use cases for AI in health care, from diagnostics to population health, imaging, and beyond. With data pooled in EHR, AI can be used to do massive chart reviews and flag problems like diabetes, osteoporosis, hypertension, and others.

AI has big potential in routine screenings. Let's take a specific problem and look at the application. Diabetic retinopathy is one of the leading causes of blindness in working-age adults in the United States,[27] and patients often have no symptoms until later stages. This means routine and regular screening is imperative. Some research institutions are piloting AI systems that have reviewed numerous positive and negative diabetic retinopathy screening images and have been taught to provide diagnosis and improve early detection. This has potential to scale the screening parameters to enable staff and facilities beyond ophthalmology departments to reach more patients and get patients with diabetic retinopathy seen for interventions sooner.

We hear "unintended consequences" often in technology and health care innovation conversations. The internet transformed connectivity and globalized the world, but a fundamental difference with AI is that with humans being left out of the decision-making loop and with systems teaching themselves in ways that may not be entirely understood, consequences may be not only unintended but also entirely unpredictable. Bill Gates expressed his caution about this:

> I am in the camp that is concerned about super intelligence. First the machines will do a lot of jobs for us and not be super intelligent. That should be positive if we manage it well. A few decades after that though the intelligence is strong enough to be a concern. . . . [I] don't understand why some people are not concerned.[28]

There is a common argument that supposes a highly intelligent system is set to do a task that is seemingly benign and it artificially "thinks" through the problem and enacts a malevolent means (by our human judgment) to the end goal; this is often termed *perverse instantiation*. Caution and optimism, per usual, are together both reasonable and necessary. Health care providers have to be vigilant and aware of AI developments. The core principles of care delivery and patient advocacy do not change just because care delivery methods do. The efficacy of care for human beings suffers when it is dehumanized. Providers have to remain central to and drive innovation conversations so that patients, too, remain central.

THE TELEHEALTH NETWORK

In the telehealth arena, a network refers to 2 or more devices that can communicate. The technology and devices chosen for telehealth programs enable formation of the telehealth network, which provides the communications pathway inherent in telehealth. Often, telehealth programs connect many devices within the same program. Telehealth programs use these devices to enable patients and providers to communicate and to transmit patient health information and physiologic data from patients to providers and monitoring centers. Transmission of data requires connectivity, either wired or wireless, and telehealth encounters have different bandwidth requirements for successful interactions. In addition to choosing the correct technology and connectivity for the program network, other telehealth network considerations include data storage (private or cloud based), building redundancy in the network, systems testing, knowledge of how to troubleshoot when problems arise, and technical standards.

Connectivity

In the world of telemedicine, network systems and connectivity require fast connections to ensure high-quality interactions. These interactions use a variety of types of broadband connectivity. Broadband refers to the degree of bandwidth, which is the range of frequencies in a wavelength.[29] Therefore, broadband connectivity refers to high-speed data transmission that can transmit a broad spectrum and quantity of data all at once. The most common types of internet broadband connections are cable modems, which use the same connection as cable television, and digital subscriber line (DSL) modems, which use existing telephone lines. Today, broadband is provided through many different formats both wired and wireless. Some examples of wired internet connections include DSL, cable, and fiber.[30] These types of networks bring connectivity to the facility or home via a physical connection. Cable and DSL have the greatest coverage; however, the fiber network has grown over the past few years. Alternatively, wireless internet enables connectivity through transmitted radio waves rather than through physical wires connected to a computer or other device.[30]

Wireless connectivity is reliable and becoming more widely available. Wireless connections typically involve cellular-enabled devices using today's 3rd generation (or 3G), 4G, long-term evolution (LTE), and 5G networks. Wireless methods allow for connectivity into many more locations, such as enabling neurologists to connect to patients in the ambulance for prehospital acute stroke assessments.[31] These mobile networks offer greater flexibility that allow users to connect from more locations; however, this mobility presents new challenges around security and HIPAA compliance because users are no longer in a fixed location. This also brings up new issues with ensuring quality because users may no longer be in a controlled environment. That being said, it is clear that the capacity of the upcoming 5G networks will offer new opportunities and ways to connect from more locations.[32]

With all the choices in connectivity available, the main consideration in choice is determined by what technology is needed to accomplish the intended outcome. To determine the bandwidth needed, the American Telemedicine Association (ATA) has developed standards for connectivity in each of their practice guidelines.[33] For example, telepsychiatry encounters require a minimum bandwidth of 384 kilobytes per second (kB/s). Services that require more detail, such as in telestroke assessment, have a higher need for bandwidth with clearer resolution of the video, and minimum upload and download speeds of 768 kB/S are needed to achieve the quality of visualization using high-definition video.[34] In general, connectivity requirements of telehealth encounters using internet video technologies are dependent upon the type of service delivered, the specifics of the encounter, and the assessment needs as to what bandwidth and resolution meet the minimum quality needed to conduct the encounter.[35] Today, there are many options for connections, with the fastest growth occurring in mobile and cellular-connected devices.

Aligning Use of Technology With Program Need

Although each telehealth service delivery system is unique and presents its own benefits and challenges, it is important to understand that the purpose of these technologies is to enable better, timelier care to those who need it most. Now more than ever, many of those in health care are trying to disrupt the current system to create models of care that are smarter, faster, more effective, and less costly. It is important to remember that although these systems might not be perfect, use by APRNs can result in better outcomes.

A major barrier to successful telehealth program development is the ability to align telehealth with program needs. This includes the appropriate use of equipment to produce desired outcomes. Too often, sites purchase technology they never use due to its inability to function as expected or its inability to support the required service. Technology choice and acquisition can be difficult due to the variety, complexity, functionality, cost, setup, activation, integration, and maintenance needed to operationalize equipment for a telehealth program. It is therefore important that the chosen technology has the ability to perform the activities needed to accomplish the specific goals of the program. Difficulty arises when translating this to actual practice. How does one know what each piece of equipment can and cannot do? How can you tell if the equipment is compatible with existing systems? How can you verify that the telehealth equipment will produce positive outcomes? How can you ascertain that the technology is a good match for the target population? Unfortunately, one telehealth solution is not the right solution for all, despite similar problems or goals.

Health care is the largest employer in the nation,[36] and each health system, rehabilitation hospital, Federally Qualified Health Center, state health department, and clinic is unique. Each serves a distinctive community of people with different health-related issues/needs. Providers developing and/or practicing using telehealth networks should therefore be cognizant of the nuances of the technology and devices as well as the population they will include in the program to be sure that the technology serves the intended purpose and is feasible for said population. Development of successful telehealth networks requires identification of gaps in care through rigorous needs assessment and stakeholder group development so that the chosen technology meets the identified needs of the program.

Success in choosing appropriate telehealth networks requires that program needs are identified, goals and objectives are established, personnel and resource barriers are understood, and financial commitment is established. The needs of the programs must be well aligned with the functionality and feasibility of the chosen technology. Depending upon the complexity of the program and network, a systems-level knowledge of network operations may be needed to design, develop, and start the telehealth network. Partnership with internet and communication technology experts and specialists are often needed. This may include telehealth systems engineers responsible for building the program's network, integrating the telehealth networks into the existing infrastructure, and providing ongoing network maintenance and upgrades. Telehealth systems experts can also provide instruction, education, and support for users; scalability so that programs can grow or downsize providing the right amount of services; and built-in system measures to ensure compliance with regulatory statues and laws, as well as established standards for telehealth care.

FOR REFLECTION 2:

Where Is Telehealth Needed?

Consider the ways in which telehealth technology can be applied to addressing gaps in practice that have been identified through needs assessment.

Technology Infrastructure and Data Storage

When thinking about the technology needed to support telehealth programs, there are a few different approaches. In the past, the health care industry focused on costly on-premises infrastructures that allowed for tight security controls; however, more recently, systems are shifting more and more to a hybrid or cloud system. Hybrid systems leverage both on-premises deployed systems along with cloud technology. These systems lead to complex discussions around security and data protection.[37] With more data being collected and new companies entering the field with new data sets, security is one of the biggest concerns in telehealth. New data housed in new locations managed by companies with no experience in handling PHI can be difficult to discern when choosing data storage systems. Additionally, although the majority of the encounters that revolve around telehealth are not recorded because they are conducted just as traditional in-person encounters are conducted, some encounters are recorded for specific health care purposes. If recording is planned, understanding how to secure and manage the data is important because there are different regulations for data in motion vs data at rest. Although data at rest is sometimes considered to be less vulnerable than data in transit, attackers often find data at rest a more valuable target than data in motion.[38]

Telehealth programs and organizations need a place to store the data collected and processed by the technology. Every telehealth program will have different technology needs based on the specifics of the program and what devices, technologies, and data are involved. There are 2 basic types of data storage: on-premises/private vs the cloud. On-premises data storage refers to data that are stored on a server that is maintained by an organization, private company, or group. For example, in the on-premises system, the telehealth data storage server is usually located on the premises of the program facility. In this system, the telehealth devices, equipment, and infrastructure could be as simple as a device connected to the internet or complex with multiple systems comprising the network. These systems could include multipoint video solutions that allow more than 1 participant at a time, voice over internet protocol networks, or a series of security devices. On-premises networks are usually more expensive and require information technology (IT) expert support to maintain them due to systems engineering needs and maintenance requirements. This type of solution works well in large medical centers with IT experts on staff that need a robust and scalable system for a multitude of specialties and remote sites. The on-premises solution also allows for more back-end control of the system and enterprise user management. When considering an on-premises data storage solution, it is best to engage the site's IT department at the start of the program because this can save a lot of time and resources when the server, infrastructure, technology, and devices are set up and integrated within the practice.

Alternatively, the cloud is a system of data storage that uses remote servers whereby users access the data via the internet. The servers are typically owned and maintained by large outside companies such as Microsoft, IBM, Amazon Web Services, Adobe, Google, Oracle, and Verizon. There are 3 main types of cloud storage systems: public, private, and hosted.[32,39] In the public cloud data storage model, the cloud provider is responsible for providing access to the data and running any agreed-upon applications, as well as backing up data and providing data security and server maintenance. The private cloud enables users to manage their own programs and applications, giving more direct control over which software and hardware is used and over regulatory compliance with data privacy and security. The private cloud gives users the ability to individualize the data system and gives better regulation of access and location of data. In the hosted cloud system, data are stored on a separate server, where no other data are stored. In this way, the provider manages the data, and access is given to the user although the user does not maintain the server. The servers are remote from the users, and access is achieved over the internet.

The cloud may still require engineering staff and support because the computers that support the network live off site in the cloud. They may still require expertise to manage and operate. The biggest benefit to the cloud is moving the hardware expense from a capital expense to an operational expense. This approach also helps mitigate the hardware replacement cycle and maintenance expense use because they require less IT expertise on site.[33,40] Cloud systems can be used for data storage or they can accommodate complex data access, processing, and storage needs from large, multifaceted telehealth systems of care with a variety of interconnected technologies. With cloud storage, users typically pay only for cloud services used, helping lower operating costs, run infrastructure more efficiently, and scale as data storage needs change. Cloud solutions are generally cheaper to set up because the user does not have to purchase and maintain hardware and software, but can become costly over time because many require monthly fees.

When looking at cloud solutions, be sure the service is HIPAA compliant and assess user costs, annual fees, and system requirements to be sure the service is a good match for the needs of the program. Other benefits to cloud services include easy accessibility via the internet, backup of data so there is low potential for data loss, and cost savings of not having to supply power to run the storage system.[32,39] Disadvantages include relying on an outside entity for data security and data privacy, as well as potential difficulty accessing data during peak user times. There are many different solutions to help telehealth programs address data storage needs. Talk with local practitioners already connecting through telehealth, attend a telehealth conference, or contact the regional Telehealth Resource Center (TRC) for more information.

Organizations of any size will often find they have to manage a mix of on-premises and cloud solutions. Some of these applications are standalone, and some use more of a hybrid approach that integrates cloud and on-premises solutions. This hybrid approach is used by Zoom and Cisco WebEx, where a video system in a conference room at a hospital can connect to a cloud-based videoconference, allowing for more flexibility and availability of services.

Building in Redundancy

Many telehealth networks rely on an interdependence of systems. For example, videoconferencing relies on the electrical grid for power and the communication system for the audio and visual components and functioning.[41] Designing robust telehealth networks that can withstand network or device malfunction or failure is necessary to ensure that telehealth provides consistent, equivalent care without interruptions. Network or device failure or malfunctions can cause interruption of care and erode patient and provider confidence in using telehealth. It is therefore necessary to provide redundancy in the network to be able to avoid care interruption or downtime due to equipment failure or network outages. This is especially important for on-premises systems because the users and their IT staff would be responsible for maintaining the functioning of the system in the setting of network, programs, or equipment malfunctions or failure. In cloud models, redundancy is routinely built in to prevent systems failure, so loss of data is rare.

Redundancy in computer networks represents an alternative pathway via duplicate process and components that can be used as a backup for the telehealth encounter to continue despite system or component failure.[42] These systems and processes are built into the network to provide consist network communications. "Redundant design is a primary approach to enhance the reliability and robustness of the system."[43(p1)] Redundancy is important for stability and consistency of telehealth networks. For example, including use of a backup cellular service could be a component of the redundancy of your system if your site loses internet connections frequently. Other examples of redundant systems include backup storage for personal computer hard drives in case of hard drive failure, or alternative power supplies, which are especially important when using telemedicine to prevent interruption of care and communications. Attention to redundancy in telehealth networks will enable robust systems to develop supporting consistent telehealth care without interruptions or loss of health care data.

Testing

Testing is a great way to not only assess technology systems to ensure operational readiness but also to become familiar with using the technology at the program and remote facility. Testing network systems and equipment involves IT systems testing and user testing. Systems network testing is usually performed by the IT staff to ensure the communication systems and devices are properly functioning and connected to one another, allowing planned communications and data collection. User testing confirms that users can turn equipment on and connect to remote or program sites, as well as perform basic troubleshooting as needed. Devices, peripherals, and other equipment should also be tested frequently and before each telehealth encounter. Testing not only helps ensure equipment is operational, but also ensures the remote partner site's equipment is working correctly. Testing is an opportunity to learn more about the system's strengths and weaknesses.

Having strong knowledge of systems networks and limitations can assist in development of network testing procedures and protocols to avoid problems with function or use of the technology. For example, during systems testing, you discover that only 5 participants can be connected at one time, when the system was planned to accommodate more. A videoconference is planned for 10 participants later that week. Upon troubleshooting, perhaps you discover the technology and network has a system limitation that will not allow more than 5 sites at a time to connect. Your knowledge can help direct the conversation to another solution, maybe 2 conferences with 5 participants each. Such system limitations are frequently discovered during testing of the equipment and network and can fortunately be addressed prior to the start of a telehealth program. It is recommended that systems are tested each day and/or before every videoconference.

Each remote site connection is unique, and successful testing at one site does not ensure success at another. It is thus advisable to test systems after any network changes, after equipment additions or relocations, and after additional remote sites are added to a network. Testing also ensures providers and staff become familiar and experienced using the technology, thus building confidence in telehealth delivery.

Troubleshooting

Troubleshooting problems with advanced telehealth technologies, computers, and other electronic equipment is a systematized means of assessing and remedying difficulties with or malfunctioning of the technology. It is preferred that issues with function and use of telehealth technologies be identified during testing, where they can be further assessed and corrected before they are needed for care or program activities. However, problems can also arise during use, and it is therefore important that all users have some basic knowledge of how to assess, identify, and potentially correct and resolve problems that arise. Experience in troubleshooting telehealth systems is an asset and is gained by increasing knowledge of networked systems and gaining experience using the technologies. Many issues can be resolved with basic troubleshooting skills, but others may require more extensive investigation by IT experts. Basic troubleshooting can generally be accomplished by problem identification, gathering more information and excluding variables that could be affecting the problem, forming a hypothesis as to what is causing the problem, and taking corrective actions.

Therefore, the first step in troubleshooting is to clearly identify what the specific problem is and to identify which components are not working correctly. For example, identify whether the video or audio is not working or whether there a device or network issue. Learning to identify which component is not working can help to focus on the problem area and help identify problems needing IT support. Next, assess the identified issue and gather more information. Rule out any variables that could be causing the problem. After identifying the issue, assess for things that could be affecting its proper functioning. For example, check to be sure the device or system is plugged into the power source and that it is turned on and connected properly. Form a hypothesis as to why it is not working. Then, take action on any fixes that you can perform that may be causing the issue. An example would be not receiving audio. A few basic troubleshooting items include checking that all connections are secure and plugged into the correct ports and outlets, looking to see if volume is turned up on your equipment, checking for external speaker volume, and/or checking to see if the other site has a muted microphone. If these basic troubleshooting activities do not resolve the issue, more advance troubleshooting may be needed. This troubleshooting could include connecting to another site to see if the problem can be replicated, following the audio cable to the jack to ensure a proper connection, and/or connecting an external speaker device to see if sound can be produced through a different speaker. After resolving your issue, the issue and resolution should be recorded in a logbook or electronic file so it may be reviewed should the issue present in the future. Keeping a log of issues and resolutions not only helps resolve the issue faster, it can also help identify patterns of failure and allow sites to address the problem so failures can be prevented going forward.

Technical Standards to Achieve Desired Outcomes

In order to determine the evidence for and suitability of technology in the provision of care, there are many questions that need to be reviewed. The following are some foundational elements for providers to know to ensure that standards are met:

- Establishing sufficient bandwidth. Although this varies with regard to the technology and use case, the minimum standard for a face-to-face is 768 kB/s; the goal is 2 megabytes per second (mbps).
- Ensuring HIPAA-complaint security standards by applying all needed firewalls and end-to-end encryption at 128-bit advanced encryption standard
- Using standards-based technologies defined as Session Initiation Protocol to ensure device-to-device connectivity. Systems using H.323 protocols are viable, although this is declining.
- Establishing organizational standards on telehealth etiquette and skills training to ensure privacy and quality
- Using Food and Drug Administration–approved devices when necessary to ensure quality video and audio equipment
- Ensuring all encryption and privacy standards apply when moving to mobile devices
- Ensuring a business associate agreement is in place when acquiring a telehealth platform; this is especially pertinent when using cloud-based computing and videoconferencing.
- Developing best-practice comparisons for technology acquisition and reliance upon resources such as the federally funded TRC

- Maintaining performance standards and measures for quality such as patient satisfaction, packet loss, and audio quality
- Providing redundant systems when practicing clinical telemedicine
- Ensuring regular testing, monitoring, on-call, and protocol provision

Although technology is getting easier to acquire and apply, these underlying standards are fundamental when the use is focused on clinical outcomes. There are widely available resources to support the development of these technical practice standards from the ATA and the Health Resources and Services Administration–funded TRCs. These components are essential to successful and safe practice.

In order to ensure desired outcomes, there are also a whole host of administrative requirements around telehealth, including proper consent, staff training, patients' rights around in-person care, and partnership agreements that should align with the technology standards, as well as with Centers for Medicare & Medicaid Services (CMS) conditions of participation and clinical practice guidelines. (See the core operational guidelines for provider-patient encounters offered free through the ATA.)

The end goal of the evidence (technical, administrative, and clinical) is for the experience of the users (provider and patient) to be safe, secure, seamless, and easy to use. A high-quality image, good audio, and ease of use properly administered are important to achieving equivalency in care. The summary focus for understanding the choice of telehealth technology is the primary question: does the technology ensure the opportunity for the desired outcomes?

CHOOSING TECHNOLOGY FOR A PRACTICE

In selecting the appropriate technology for a practice, it is imperative that the user determine whether the technology does the following:

- Provides services that are clinically equivalent to those delivered in person
- Is cost-effective
- Has research or evidence to support its use
- Has a high level of satisfaction by its users
- Provides for improved quality of care

Clinical Equivalency

The simple question everyone should ask in choosing telehealth equipment is whether the care provided using the telehealth technology is clinically equivalent with in-office care. As an example of research that answers that question, a study in the *Journal of the American Medical Association Network Open* looked at the following question: Does an online, collaborative connected-health delivery model result in equivalent improvements in disease severity compared with in-person care?[44] The researchers found that in a 12-month randomized clinical equivalency trial, adults with psoriasis randomized to the online model experienced improvement in disease severity equivalent to those randomized to in-person management. This online, collaborative, connected-health model was as effective as in-person management in improving clinical outcomes among patients with psoriasis. It is the kind of replicable study that demonstrates that telehealth delivery models emphasize collaboration, quality, and efficiency as essential for transforming chronic disease care in a patient-centered way.[44]

Cost-Effectiveness

Most of the peer-reviewed research about the cost-effectiveness of telemedicine that is based on large sample sizes and follows sound scientific rigor is relatively new, with many emerging in the past 2 years. These studies are consistent in finding that telemedicine saves the patients, providers, and payers money when compared with traditional approaches to providing care. Many of these studies assess the cost-effectiveness of specific telemedicine applications. The evidence suggests, however, that telehealth generates more use of health care, and so the outcomes are currently not clear.

In choosing specific technologies, the user may find it helpful to gather information from the vendor as well as other users related to any data on its cost-effectiveness. Cost-effectiveness should address the cost of equipment/network, reimbursement, saved travel time, health outcomes/decreased practice and hospital use, and efficiency/time saved by the provider. All factors should be considered because revenue generated will often not be the best means of measuring its cost-effectiveness.

GROUP EXERCISE

Design Your Own Telehealth Program

Choose an identified health care need in a rural or underserved population. Outline a simple telehealth program designed to address this problem in your population. Include components of a telehealth system of care to address the gap in practice that may include remote monitoring, synchronous and asynchronous technologies, mHealth, health education, apps, wearables, and/or eConsults, or in a way that uses gamification or AI to improve an identified outcome.

RESEARCH EVIDENCE

Telehealth should not be applied without a diligent process to ensure safe, secure, high-quality technology to support well-defined, clinical use cases. Therefore, it is critically important to ensure the evidence for telehealth and the adoption of digital solutions is reviewed and supported. This is especially true given the billions of dollars in investment in and rapid expansion of telehealth.

Within health care, there is a growing willingness to use telehealth capability to do the following:

- Increase access for specialty care
- Directly intervene in environments where the patients reside
- Innovate to provide care in remote locations
- Provide solutions for workforce shortages
- Offer care to prevent disease progression
- Ensure passive monitoring
- Help individuals, families, and populations manage their own care in partnership with providers, especially given the emergence of value-based care models

This desire for increased use is especially true because the evidence for the value of the technology aligns with clinical outcomes from virtual health practices.

In order to migrate quickly to this resource as an accepted, evidence-based methodology for care, it is essential to know if the technology that is applied has been assessed appropriately. Questions should include the following:

- Is the technology able to perform as advertised?
- Is it safe?
- Is it HIPAA compliant?
- Is it of sufficient quality?
- Is it standards based?
- Are the support mechanisms for troubleshooting present?
- Does it comply with the professional standards of care?
- Is it simple and easy to use?
- Most importantly, does it ensure quality outcomes?

Patient Satisfaction With Telemedicine

Patient and provider satisfaction studies with the use of telemedicine to access care and the use of telecommunications technologies to connect with specialists and other health care providers in order to meet unmet medical needs has been, while still nascent, consistently high. Results from patient satisfaction studies indicate exceptionally high levels of perceived satisfaction, often above the rates of expected satisfaction for traditional forms of health delivery.

Degrees of satisfaction may vary slightly with the specialty accessed through telemedicine, but overall, patients have responded well to its use. The source of satisfaction for most patients is the ability to see a specialist trained in the area most closely related to the patient's condition, the feeling of getting personalized care from a provider who has the patient's interest in mind, and the ability to communicate with the provider in a very personal and intimate manner over the telecommunications technologies. In selecting the technology and network for a practice, the user would benefit from obtaining information regarding data on patient and provider/staff satisfaction. This would minimize resistance and provide acceptance from patients. In addition, it would provide information on issues that may need to be considered in its implementation. See Chapter 7 for more on satisfaction in telehealth.

Telemedicine and Quality of Care

Scientific studies around quality of care indicate that the use of telemedicine for such applications as monitoring of chronic care patients or allowing specialists to provide care to patients over a large region have resulted in significantly improved care. For most telemedicine applications, studies have shown that there is no difference in the ability of the provider to obtain clinical information, make an accurate diagnosis, and develop a treatment plan that produces the same desired clinical outcomes as compared with in-person care when used appropriately.

The primary goal surrounding quality is found in achieving clinical equivalency. At the University of Virginia (UVA), for instance, outcomes from telestroke care can be measured in the speed with which patients receive care and the use of thrombolytics in the treatment of ischemic disease. What the program has found is that the telestroke network has moved from 0.05% use in rural partner facilities to 20% in 3 years in all eligible cases, which is equivalent to use within UVA's own emergency department.[45]

It is imperative that the user understands the effectiveness of the equipment as a health delivery tool and in improving the quality of care delivered. As such, the user should be well-informed about the successes in care that have been achieved with the equipment he or she is selecting.

Sufficient initial evidence exists on the application of appropriate technology to support the effectiveness of telehealth for specific uses, including RPM for patients with chronic conditions; communication, clinical care, and counseling for patients with chronic conditions; provision of acute, emergent care such as telestroke; inpatient transfer management; and the application of telemental health care. This list is impressive and growing. With new payment guidelines released in 2018 by the Centers for Medicare & Medicaid Services and with increasing use, new opportunities are emerging to study outcomes. For instance, the Agency for Healthcare Research and Quality has released an evidence map to show where outcomes research is pointing to potential areas for application.[46] This movement to systematic application is also being supported by the Centers for Disease Control and a multitude of government agencies. The evidence for telehealth is growing, and clinical providers need to evaluate that evidence and recognize that this is a health care market force that is here to stay. By 2017, 76% of hospitals in the United States used some form of telehealth.[47] Additionally, since the US COVID-19 outbreak in March 2020, telehealth usage has increased exponentially. Examples of this increase includes a North Carolina hospital system (serving North and South Carolina and Georgia) with a 500% increase in telehealth usage, and a 600% increase was reported by another hospital system serving Washington DC.[48] This is in the context of a market estimated in 2015 as being at 9.6 billion.[49] Providers seeking to have an engaged practice with optimal clinical outcomes now need to aggressively review the evidence, understand the standards required to build the capability, and look to providing the research on new use cases, especially within the context of advanced practice nursing.

CONCLUSION

Technology is changing the essence of virtually everything, including health care. Nursing is at a point at which it must make fundamental decisions about how to go forward in practice in a digital world. This moment requires a fundamental understanding of the nursing profession's relationship to technology and whether nursing will choose to own the technology and use it as a tool in nursing care or whether technology and AI mechanisms will own parts of the nursing care process and merge it into a nursing algorithm as part of massive technological advances in health care.

This moment is not about rejecting digital technology, but rather how to translate the caring nursing relationship with patients while using advanced technologies. It is about the need to convey the essence of nursing while using technology to deliver nursing care. Chapter 1 discussed the role of the telehealth nurse, and this chapter took that idea into the future as the IoT takes shape and transforms health care in ways that will make many of the past health care processes unrecognizable. Although the telehealth nursing role is important, it is more than just the actualization and visualization of a role. Telehealth nursing is a concept of imparting nursing presence and relationships using technologies to improve health. Nursing, therefore, is at the precipice as to whether technology gets incorporated into nursing or whether nursing gets incorporated into technology.

For nursing to retain its identity, nurses must gain knowledge and confidence developing and using these technologies and own the ability of technology to innovate and improve care. In this way, telehealth will not define or replace nursing care but will support and improve our ability to care for patients. For nursing to be well-positioned to remain significant in health care, we must conceptualize the partnership of technology to the art and science of nursing and gain proficiency and confidence using technology in nursing practice as a tool to connect with patients and provide nursing care.

THOUGHTFUL QUESTIONS

1. In what ways can nurses use store-and-forward (asynchronous) technology to improve outcomes in primary care?
2. How are the various telehealth technologies different but complementary?
3. How would you envision a telehealth program in primary care that uses gamification or AI? Describe how the technology is aimed at achieving an outcome.
4. What are the aspects of a telehealth network that are important to address for an effective telehealth program?

CASE STUDY

Ellie is a newly graduated primary care APRN who has joined a small, rural family practice group in a geographic part of the United States called the Stroke Belt, where the risk of stroke is over one-third higher than that of the general population. Many of the patients at this clinic experience transient ischemic attacks, and few seek timely help before it is too late for administration of life-saving thrombolytics and emergent advanced endovascular treatments and neurologic care. Ellie knows that stroke is often caused by risk factors that are modifiable and that her patients have lifestyles that have association with high vascular risks. Realizing the rurality of her patients, the generally low-moderate socioeconomic status of the community, and the average age of clinic patients of 65, Ellie considers how she could use telehealth technologies to decrease vascular risk factors in her patient population.

The clinic has strong past connections to the larger community through prior programs and functions, but the community has aged, and transportation and disability from the strokes is a barrier to attending the clinic programs, so few still attend. Ellie has performed a needs assessment and discovered that most people in the community do not know what a stroke is, do not know the symptoms of stroke, do not know what actions to take to decrease stroke risk, and do not know what actions to take when having a stroke. Most people in the community have broadband internet access with mobile devices or smartphones, or have access via a friend or family. The clinic does not have resources for large-scale, robust telehealth system development, but the clinic does have internet access and computers with cameras. They also have some technology funds that could be used to support a small-scale telehealth program focused on stroke and decreasing vascular risk factors in the local community, as well as providing education of stroke symptoms and what actions to take if they develop them.

Questions

1. What are the possible outcomes Ellie could focus on?
2. How can telehealth be used to attain the identified outcomes?
3. What are the benefits of using telehealth in such a patient population?

REFERENCES

1. Brinker TJ, Hekler A, von Kalle C, et al. Teledermatology: comparison of store-and-forward versus live interactive video conferencing. *J Med Internet Res.* 2018;20(10):e11871.
2. Rutledge CM, Kott K, Schweickert PA, Poston R, Fowler C, Haney TS. Telehealth and eHealth in nurse practitioner training. *Adv Med Educ Pract.* 2017;8:399-409.
3. Liu WL, Zhang K, Locatis C, Ackerman M. Cloud and traditional videoconferencing technology for telemedicine and distance learning. *Telemed J E Health.* 2015;21(5):422-426.
4. Sackett KM, Campbell-Heider N, Blyth JB. The evolution and evaluation of videoconferencing technology for graduate nursing education. *Comput Inform Nurs.* 2004;22(2):101-106.
5. Su D, Michaud TL, Estabrooks P, et al. Diabetes management through remote patient monitoring: the importance of patient activation and engagement with the technology. *Telemed J E Health.* 2018;23(1):3-17.
6. Vegesna A, Tran M, Angelaccio M, Arcona S. Remote patient monitoring via non-invasive digital technologies: a systematic review. *Telemed J E Health.* 2017;23(1):3-17.
7. Totten AM, Womack DM, Eden KB, et al. Telehealth: mapping the evidence for patient outcomes from systematic reviews. Rockville, MD: Agency for Healthcare Research and Quality; 2016. Technical Brief No. 26. Report No. 16-EHC034-EF.
8. World Health Organization. Telemedicine: opportunities and developments in member states. Report on the second global survey on eHealth. Global Observatory for eHealth Series – Volume 2. http://www.who.int/goe /publications/goe_telemedicine_2010.pdf. Published 2010. Accessed February 14, 2020.
9. Vimalananda VG, Gupte G, Seraj SM, et al. Electronic consultations (e-consults) to improve access to specialty care: a systematic review and narrative synthesis. *J Telemed Telecare.* 2015;21(6):323-330.
10. Keely E, Liddy C, Afkham A. Utilization, benefits, and impact of an e-consultation service across diverse specialties and primary care providers. *Telemed J E Health.* 2013;19(10):733-738.
11. Keely EJ, Archibald D, Tuot DS, Lochnan H, Liddy C. Unique educational opportunities for PCPs and specialists arising from electronic consultation services. *Acad Med.* 2017;92(1):45-51.
12. Liddy C, Moroz I, Keely E, et al. The use of electronic consultations is associated with lower specialist referral rates: a cross-sectional study using population-based health administrative data. *Fam Pract.* 2018;35(6):698-705.
13. Woolfe SH. The power of prevention and what it requires. *JAMA.* 2008;299(20):2437-2439.
14. Houpt S. The fun theory. *The Globe and Mail.* https://www.theglobeandmail.com/report-on-business/industry -news/marketing/volkswagen-goes-viral-with-the-fun-theory/article4292155/. Published November 13, 2009. Updated May 1, 2018. Accessed February 17, 2020.
15. Edwards EA, Lumsden J, Rivas C, et al. Gamification for health promotion: systematic review of behaviour change techniques in smartphone apps. *BMJ Open.* 2016;6(10):18.
16. Cotton V, Patel MS. Gamification use and design in popular health and fitness mobile applications. *Am J Health Promot.* 2019;33(3):448-451.
17. Johnson D, Deterding S, Kuhn KA, Staeva A, Stoyanov S, Hides L. Gamification for health and wellbeing: a systematic review of the literature. *Internet Interv.* 2016;6:89-106.
18. Balasingam M. Drones in medicine—the rise of the machines. *Int J Clin Pract.* 2017;71(9):e12989.
19. Barry SA, Emhoff SM, Rabkin AN, et al. Relation between aggression exposure during youth and later resting skin conductance levels. *J Aggres Maltreat Trauma.* 2017;26(4):354-371.
20. Guk K, Han G, Lim J, Jeong K, Tang T, Lim EK, Jung J. Evolution of wearable devices with real-time disease monitoring for personalized healthcare. *Nanomaterials (Basel).* 2019;9(6)LE813. doi: 10.3390/nano9060813
21. Maney K. Meet Kevin Ashton, father of the internet of things. *Newsweek.* https://www.newsweek.com/2015/03 /06/meet-kevin-ashton-father-internet-things-308763.html. Published February 23, 2015. Accessed February 17, 2020.
22. Meinhert E, Van Velthoven M, Brindley D, et al. The internet of things in health care in Oxford: protocol for proof-of-concept projects. *JMIR Res Protoc.* 2018;7(12);e12077.
23. SAS. *A non-geek's A-Z guide to the internet of things.* https://www.sas.com/content/dam/SAS/en_us/doc/ whitepaper1/non-geek-a-to-z-guide-to-internet-of-things-108846.pdf. Published 2019. Accessed February 17, 2020.
24. i-SCOOP. What the internet of everything really is—a deep dive. https://www.i-scoop.eu/internet-of-things- guide/internet-of-everything. Accessed February 17, 2020.
25. Dimitrov DV. Medical internet of things and big data in healthcare. *Healthc Inform Res.* 2016;22(3):156-163.
26. Laplante PA, Laplante N. The internet of things in healthcare: potential applications and challenges. *IT Professional.* 2016;18(3):2-4.
27. National Eye Institute. Diabetic retinopathy. https://nei.nih.gov/health/diabetic/retinopathy. Updated August 3, 2019. Accessed February 17, 2020.
28. Rawlinson K. Bill Gates insists AI is a threat. *BBC News.* https://www.bbc.com/news/31047780. Published January 29, 2015. Accessed February 17, 2020.
29. Tech Terms. Broadband. https://techterms.com/definition/broadband. Accessed February 17, 2020.

30. Federal Communications Commission. Types of broadband connections. https://www.fcc.gov/general/types-broadband-connections. Updated June 23, 2014. Accessed February 17, 2020.

31. Chapman Smith SN, Govindarajan P, Padrick MM, et al. A low-cost, tablet-based option for prehospital neurologic assessment: the iTREAT Study. *Neurology*. 2016;87(1):19-26.

32. Federal Communications Commission. The FCC's 5G fast plan. https://www.fcc.gov/5G. Accessed February 17, 2020.

33. American Telemedicine Association. Practice guidelines. https://www.americantelemed.org/resource/learning-development. Accessed February 17, 2020.

34. Lazar I. How to calculate videoconferencing bandwidth requirements. https://searchunifiedcommunications.techtarget.com/tip/Business-video-conferencing-setup-Calculating-bandwidth-requirements. Published November 11, 2016. Accessed February 17, 2020.

35. American Telemedicine Association. Core operational guidelines for telehealth services involving provider-patient interaction. https://www.americantelemed.org/resources/core-operational-guidelines-for-telehealth-services-involving-provider-patient-interactions/. Published October 3, 2018. Accessed February 17, 2020.

36. Thompson D. Health care just became the U.S.'s largest employer. *The Atlantic*. https://www.theatlantic.com/business/archive/2018/01/health-care-america-jobs/550079/. Published January 8, 2018. Accessed February 17, 2020.

37. O'Dowd E. Identifying health IT requirements for telehealth. HIT Infrastructure. https://hitinfrastructure.com/news/identifying-health-it-infrastructure-requirements-for-telehealth. Published May 29, 2018. Accessed February 17, 2020.

38. HIPAA encryption requirements. HIPAA Journal. https://www.hipaajournal.com/hipaa-encryption-requirements/. Accessed February 17, 2020.

39. O'Dowd E. Rural healthcare network connections require IT infrastructure support. HIT Infrastructure. https://hitinfrastructure.com/news/rural-healthcare-network-connections-require-it-infrastructure-support. Published August 15, 2018. Accessed February 17, 2020.

40. Level Cloud. Advantages and disadvantages of cloud computing. https://www.levelcloud.net/why-levelcloud/cloud-education-center/advantages-and-disadvantages-of-cloud-computing. Accessed June 6, 2019.

41. Buldyrey SV, Parshani R, Paul G, Stanley HE, Haylin S. Catastrophic cascade of failures in interdependent networks. *Nature*. 2010;464(7291):1025-1028.

42. TechTerms. Redundancy. https://techterms.com/definition/redundancy. Updated November 23, 2011. Accessed February 17, 2020.

43. Liu L, Yin Y, Zhang Z, Malaiya YK. Redundant design in interdependent networks. *PLoS One*. 2016;11(10):e0164777.

44. Armstrong AW, Chambers CJ, Maverakis E, et al. Effectiveness of online vs in-person care for adults with psoriasis: a randomized clinical trial. *JAMA Network Open*. 2018;1(6):e183062.

45. University of Virginia. Internal Records tPA utilization. Accessed June 6, 2019.

46. Agency for Healthcare Research and Quality. Telehealth evidence map. https://effectivehealthcare.ahrq.gov/topics/telehealth/research-protocol. Published August 11, 2015. Accessed February 17, 2020.

47. American Hospital Association. Fact sheet: telehealth. www.aha.org/factsheet/telehealth. Accessed April 28, 2020.

48. Roth M. 4 ways you haven't thought about using telehealth during the COVID-19 pandemic. HealthLeaders. www.healthleadersmedia.com/innovation/4-ways-you-havent-thought-about-using-telehealth-during-covid-19-pandemic. Published March 24, 2020. Accessed April 24, 2020

49. Drobac P, Morse M. Medical education and global health equity. *AMA J Ethics*. 2016;18(7):702-709.

Legal and Regulatory Issues in Telehealth

Karen S. Rheuban, MD
Kathy H. Wibberly, PhD

CHAPTER OBJECTIVES

Upon review of this chapter, the reader will be able to:

1. Discuss the legal and regulatory issues related to telehealth nursing education in the 3 areas of clinical education oversight, clinical practice, and use of technology.
2. Review the state and federal policies that guide telehealth practice and discern rural and urban similarities and differences.
3. Describe legal and regulatory considerations for telehealth program development and accreditation.
4. Summarize the evidence map of systematic reviews of research evidence for telehealth clinical practice related to improved outcomes.

In order for advanced practice registered nurses (APRNs) to develop, participate, and use telehealth in education and practice, attention to federal and state policies impacting telehealth nursing education and telehealth services is required. Telehealth is being used in advanced practice nursing education in a variety of ways, increasing the frequency of communications between faculty, students, and preceptors. Educators and students alike must be aware of the implications of using advanced telecommunications technology in clinical education. For example, faculty connecting from a school of nursing to a remote practice site to observe a student interacting with a patient must be sure to use a secure connection, providing privacy of patient information per the federal laws aligned with the Health Information Portability Accountability Act (HIPAA). Additionally, for the faculty to oversee the student in the practicum site, whether in person or in the virtual care environment, the faculty must be licensed and credentialed appropriately for the

Schweickert PA, Rutledge CM, eds.
Telehealth Essentials for Advanced Practice Nursing (pp 97-119).
© 2020 Taylor & Francis Group.

clinical site in the state in which the faculty and student are engaging. These are but 2 of the many issues that must be addressed when conducting clinical telehealth nursing education.

Regarding clinical practice, increased acceptance of the concept of telehealth is permeating society as telehealth augments and complements health care and health care delivery. Twenty-first–century telemedicine services can be provided live, via high-definition interactive video-conferencing supported by high-resolution peripheral devices; asynchronously, using store-and-forward technologies; or through the use of remote patient monitoring (RPM) tools. Telehealth has been demonstrated to effectively mitigate the significant challenges of workforce shortages and geographic disparities in access to care while improving patient triage and timely access to care by the right provider at the right time. Where local specialty care services are not available, particularly in rural and underserved regions and Health Professional Shortage Areas, telemedicine offers timely access to care and spares patients the burden of long-distance travel for access to that care. APRNs need to be cognizant of state and federal rules and regulations pertaining to telehealth, including intricacies of urban vs rural telehealth policies.

Both urban and rural practitioners and patients can benefit from incorporating telehealth services into practice. Rural APRNs frequently practice in geographically isolated areas where there is a shortage of specialty providers, making patient-to-provider or provider-to-provider specialty consults unavailable. Additionally, in many rural primary care settings, the APRN is often the first contact for the patient. Incorporating telehealth into these practices can provide needed access to specialty consults for these geographically isolated patients and practitioners. Knowledge of telehealth and appropriate application of laws and regulations to advanced nursing telehealth practice in rural regions is therefore necessary. Additionally, although the challenges of unfavorable geography and distance tend to be uniquely rural, socioeconomic issues, health disparities, and other serious barriers to access to quality health care are also compelling in urban areas. Poverty, unhealthy behaviors, and adverse health status indicators are also highly prevalent in our urban communities. Wait times for access to specialty care services adversely impact urban insured beneficiaries as much as they impact rural insured. Isolated, vulnerable urban patients suffer from high rates of chronic illness. A bus ride across town with a long wait in an emergency department can be as challenging for an isolated, vulnerable urban patient as a long drive is for a rural patient. Knowledge of telehealth and appropriate application of laws and regulations to advanced nursing telehealth practice in urban regions complements the full scope of legal issues to consider.

Telemedicine supports an integrated systems approach focused on disease prevention, enhanced wellness, chronic disease management, decision support, and improved efficiency, quality and patient safety.[1,2] It is therefore important that APRNs be informed and proficient in legal rules, regulations, and considerations of telehealth practice and telehealth education. Successful telehealth programs comply with the myriad of federal and state rules associated with the delivery of safe, secure, high-quality telehealth services. The scope of these variations affects nursing practice; thus, familiarity with the policies that govern advanced nursing telehealth practice is essential. These policies include reimbursement, licensure, credentialing and privileging, informed consent, documentation in the medical record, HIPAA privacy and security laws, Stark Law and Anti-Kickback Statute, malpractice coverage, telecommunications, Food and Drug Administration (FDA) guidance, practice standards and guidelines, and the remote prescribing of drugs and controlled substances.

Federal law generally supersedes state law unless state law is more restrictive, and unless specific laws regarding delivery of telehealth care are defined, practitioners should adhere to current applicable regulations when using telehealth. Additionally, there remains a lack of conformity across the states regarding these policy issues, and as such, telehealth providers must understand the state-by-state nuances that impact telehealth practice for compliance with requirements and standards of care using technologies in health care. Knowledge of the legal and regulatory requirements will enable provision of high-quality care, which protects the patient and minimizes legal and malpractice issues. Finally, a review of the research for improving practice in the telehealth arena provides a solid foundation for further understanding of evidence supporting telehealth practice.

LEGAL AND REGULATORY ISSUES GOVERNING USE OF TELEHEALTH IN EDUCATION

Life today presents ever-changing scientific discoveries and technological advancements that fundamentally change the nature of social interactions, communications, and conceptualizations about health, health care, and health care delivery. Substantive changes in health care practices through use of evidence-based medicine and development of terminal degrees in many disciplines, such as in nursing with the Doctor of Nursing Practice degree, enables health care providers to adjust to the fluctuations in the health care milieu. Another substantial change in health care is occurring with the development and assimilation of advanced communications technologies into practice. Telehealth profoundly changes our ability to communicate, interact, and provide care to patients. This change in paradigm requires health care providers to learn not only how to operate this new equipment, but also to understand the full scope of foundational and related knowledge for practicing in the care environment. Therefore, health care students and practitioners alike need telehealth education to gain skills and knowledge to use telehealth in clinical practice. Additionally, because development and use of technologies generally precedes specific legal and regulatory guidance on their use, it is important to align telehealth practice within the existing laws and regulations governing such practices and to understand specific laws and regulations for telehealth in clinical practice and in clinical education. We are at a precipice in health care as technology inherently changes our ability to practice by adding an entirely new realm of practice: remote practice in the care environment. It is therefore important to review the current status of legal and regulatory issues related to telehealth education.

Nursing Education Arena

Shortages of primary care health care providers in rural regions of the United States compound the burden of accessing care for these patients, who often have additional health care disparities.[3] Increasing the number of practice-ready APRNs is challenging due to school of nursing faculty shortages and shortages of available preceptors and clinical practice sites.[4] Innovative, nuanced approaches to APRN education are needed to position APRNs to fill the gap of primary care providers. Toward this end, a new look at existing nursing clinical education paradigms shows opportunity in reconceptualizing academic-practice partnerships, incorporating simulation, and developing innovative models of clinical preceptorships, including telehealth education networks. With the incorporation of technology into clinical education models and networks, it is important to align these changes with current legal and regulatory practices that would impact these programs in the clinical education arena. State nursing practice acts govern nursing telehealth practice, and rules and regulations vary by state. Educators and students alike must be knowledgeable in the legal and regulatory considerations of using telehealth in clinical education. In the clinical education arena, existing laws that abide over in-person clinical education also govern use of telehealth in clinical practice and can be applied to 3 arenas: nursing, federal, and technology.[5]

Nursing regulations relate to the following:

- Licensure of the faculty educator, because the faculty often must be licensed in the state the student receives the clinical education;

TABLE 5-1
CURRENT LAWS AND REGULATIONS APPLICABLE TO TELEHEALTH NURSING CLINICAL EDUCATION

ARENA 1	ARENA 2	ARENA 3
Nursing (Clinical Education Oversight)	*Federal (Clinical Practice)*	*Technology (Technology in Health Care)*
State boards of nursing Professional licensure Licensure portability Nursing Licensure Compact *The Essentials of Master's Education in Nursing* *The Essentials of Doctoral Education for Advanced Nursing Practice* Specialty competencies	Nursing scope of practice HIPAA The Joint Commission telehealth standards Medicare conditions of participation standards	The Federal Communications Commission Health Information Technology for Economic and Clinical Health Act (HITECH) FDA guidance on mobile medical apps Stark Law and Anti-Kickback Statute

- Nurse Practice Acts in each state, because they address standards and scope of practice; and
- State boards of nursing laws and regulations, because they approve nursing education programs and regulate practice, discipline of nurses, and licensure.

Federal regulations include the following:

- Compliance with HIPAA, which has set national standards of protected health information (PHI) and requires electronic safeguards and security monitoring of cyber communications, and in some states requires informed consent to perform telehealth clinical educational encounters with patients
- The Medicare Conditions of Participation Standards, which apply to the credentialing and privileging of the faculty as telehealth provider when students are participating in direct care via telehealth[6]

Technology regulations include the following:

- The 2009 Health Information Technology Act,[7] which establishes privacy and security regulations for PHI and all clinical data and communications, including electronic transfer of health information and images
- FCC regulations on new technology broadcast communication device safety and effectiveness,[8] such as medical peripheral devices used in telehealth and in telehealth nursing education

Additionally, the FDA regulates mobile medical applications (apps), and when using apps in the education environment, faculty and students should adhere to this guidance (Table 5-1).[9] Finally, it is recommended to use a HIPAA-compliant platform when using a telehealth education network so that faculty can observe students at the practice site as they engage with patients.

FOR REFLECTION 1:

Privacy in the Virtual Care Environment

 Think about patient privacy considerations when caring for patients in person, and compare that with caring for patients in the virtual care environment. What are the privacy similarities in both practice settings? What are the differences?

Telehealth in nursing education presents additional concerns in licensure, such as licensure portability, or the ability to practice across state lines with a license from a different state. The Tenth Amendment of the US Constitution grants states the power to outline standards and licensure for health care practice in each state, but it does not give states authority to grant this licensure to other states.[10] The ease of providing care in a virtual care environment that transcends geographic boundaries must be reconciled with state laws and regulations. As such, it becomes essential that professional licensure portability and multistate privileges be clarified when using telehealth for clinical care and for education.[11] Nursing Licensure Compacts (NLCs) in telehealth, in which there is an agreement between states to recognize and accept a nursing license from another state, is also a topic for further clarification. Cross-state licensure remains a debated topic in telehealth practice, and the question of whether faculty would need to be licensed to conduct virtual site visits with students in states they were not licensed to practice in remains unanswered. Currently, faculty can conduct virtual site visits with students within their state of licensure. Clarification is needed to determine whether faculty in one state can provide clinical oversight via virtual site visits across state lines or within an NLC.

Additionally, despite fairly widespread adoption of telehealth into many clinical settings, telehealth educational programs of all health care disciplines, including nursing, continue to lag behind. Although a growing number of nursing education programs have started to include some course content and provide opportunities for exposure to telehealth technologies, few have required such content or mandated such clinical experiences. Lack of adequate telehealth nursing education and statements of specific laws and regulations are barriers to understanding the depth of legal and regulatory issues involved in the telehealth education arena. Challenges to incorporating telehealth into nursing programs include lack of defined telehealth education requirements by state boards of nursing and national professional nursing associations and credentialing agencies, as well as a dearth of concise sources specific to telehealth nursing education and telehealth nursing education approaches and models. "Educational programs have found it challenging to not only teach telehealth theory but also provide hands-on experiences with technology; this has proven especially difficult within a rapidly changing environment."[12(p404)] Therefore, it is necessary that nursing telehealth education be fully embraced and clearly defined by federal, state, and professional nursing entities so that professional competencies, required education and experiences, and legal and regulatory issues can be determined and implemented throughout advanced practice nursing education programs.

General Health Care Provider Arena

Most health care professional programs lack inclusion of formal telehealth education and experiences; therefore, many providers using telehealth gain experience in the clinical practice setting or via online telehealth certification programs. A well-defined, organized approach to educating

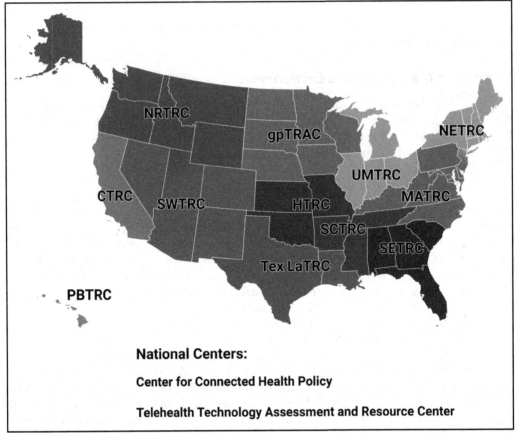

Figure 5-1. Telehealth resource centers. CTRC, California Telehealth Resource Center; GpTRAC, Great Plains Telehealth Resource Center; HTRC, Heartland Telehealth Resource Center; MATRC, Mid-Atlantic Telehealth Resource Center; NETRC, Northeast Telehealth Resource Center; NRTRC, Northwest Regional Telehealth Resource Center; SCTRC, South Central Telehealth Resource Center; SETRC, South Central Telehealth Resource Center; SWTRC, Southwest Telehealth Resource Center; TexLaTRC, Texas Louisiana Telehealth Resource Center; UMTRC, Upper Midwest Telehealth Resource Center. (Reprinted with permission from The National Consortium of Telehealth Resource Centers.)

the health care workforce has yet to be established, as have standard provider competencies when delivering care via telehealth during the virtual care visit. There now exists an ever-growing number of telehealth certification and training programs for interested providers. Many of these training programs are available online. The majority focuses their didactic content around tele-health technologies, HIPAA regulations, and other legal and regulatory issues. For example, the American Telemedicine Association (ATA) is an informative resource for information related to program startup, selection of technology for telehealth program development, and policy and regulations related to telehealth, as well as telehealth practice guidelines.[13] Telehealth Resource Centers (TRCs), a national clearinghouse for telehealth information related to use, policy, and program development, is also an excellent resource for telehealth provider information.[14] The 14 TRCs across the United States share training modules and certification programs related to use of telehealth technology (Figure 5-1). However, there is lack of programs to educate nurses on using telehealth in patient care or to educate providers to practice in the virtual care environment.

A subset of other online training programs focus on presentation skills and videoconference etiquette. The practice of telehealth requires health care professionals to learn a set of skills that are not always transferable from the in-person encounter. Bulik[15] explored 4 categories of behavior in a mixed-methods study and suggested that they be taught to telehealth providers to improve the overall patient-provider relationship with telehealth. They include behaviors in verbal, nonverbal, relational, and actions/transactions categories. Even smaller subsets of the existing training programs focus on clinical practice, helping clinicians understand how to integrate telehealth into clinical workflows and different emerging models of care (eg, interprofessional care teams, behavioral health integration). Therefore, the lack of standards, specifics, and conformity results in individual schools of nursing and facilities determining what training, education, and experiences are needed or required for student learning.

Legal and Regulatory Issues Governing Use of Telehealth in Clinical Practice

As health care provider educators embrace telehealth educational needs and legal and regulatory compliance issues for students, practitioner guidance related to telehealth clinical practice is also necessary. Because telehealth has been used in clinical practice longer than in professional health care provider educational programs, there are more specific and identified regulations that pertain to and address telehealth clinical practice. More rules and regulations also exist that cover telecommunications and many apply directly to telehealth communications. Additionally, HIPAA of 1996 and the HITECH Act of 2009 have established regulations for patient data privacy and security. Federal and state agencies continue to assess telehealth and provide legal and regulatory oversight for use of these advanced technologies in clinical practice. The telehealth regulatory environment is complex due to the myriad policies, rules, and regulations via state, federal, and private entities that must be understood in order to fully comply with privacy, security, and regulatory issues. A summary of relevant state and federal laws, regulations, and guidelines is presented as an overview to the legal and regulatory issues governing the use of telehealth in clinical practice.

Licensure

The determination of criteria and the issuance and enforcement of health professional licensure is a right delegated to the states. Other than for Veterans Health Administration (VHA) providers, there is currently no true physician or licensed independent practitioner licensure portability. The paradigm for telehealth is such that providers must hold a valid license in the state in which the patient is physically located.[16] Affirming that policy, the American Medical Association and the Federation of State Medical Boards (FSMB), along with other specialty societies, have developed model policies for telehealth.[17,18] The FSMB has developed an interstate licensure compact designed to expedite licensure in multiple states.[19] As of 2020, 29 states, the District of Columbia, 1 territory, and 43 medical and osteopathic boards in those states have signed on to the compact. Some states offer a special telehealth license or registration process to enable out-of-state providers to offer telehealth-only services in their states. Other states have created policies that allow for reciprocal agreements for providers working in adjoining states.

The nursing profession uses the enhanced Nursing Licensure Compact (eNLC), a model based on mutual recognition to enable licensure portability. Under the eNLC, overseen by the National Council of State Boards of Nursing (NCSBN), registered nurses (RNs) and licensed practical/vocational nurses (LPN/VNs) in member states can provide care to patients in other states without having to obtain additional licenses. The eNLC creates an expedited licensing process that gives nurses these privileges as long as they meet 11 uniform licensing requirements.[20] In addition, licensed nurses in 34 states can now use telehealth to treat patients in other states under the terms of the eNLC.[20] Regarding advanced practice nursing, the NCSBN approved the creation of a new interstate compact for APRNs in May 2015. The legislation states:

> The expanded mobility of [APRNs] and the use of advanced communication technologies as part of our nation's health care delivery system require greater coordination and cooperation

among states in the areas of APRN licensure and regulation. New practice modalities and technology make compliance with individual state APRN licensure laws difficult and complex.[21]

The APRN Compact will only be implemented after 10 states have enacted such legislation. As of 2020, only 3 states have passed such legislation to join the compact: Idaho, North Dakota, and Wyoming. Two states have pending legislation. Additionally, in an effort to uniformly regulate advanced practice nursing across all states, the NCSBN APRN Consensus Model has been developed to align APRN education, certification, accreditation, and licensure to uphold safe care while increasing population access to APRNs.[21] Included in the Consensus Model is a provision to allow for advanced practice nursing via the APRN Compact. States are given scores for achieving compliance with required items, such as independence of practice and joining the APRN Compact. Currently, 15 states have scored 100% for implementation status, 11 states have scored 75% to 96%, and the remainder scored 71% or less.[22]

FOR REFLECTION 2:

The APRN Compact

What are the advantages of the APRN Compact as related to nursing telehealth practice? What additional responsibility does licensure in the APRN Compact present? How would the APRN Consensus Model affect the compact?

In addition to licensure compacts for physicians and nurses, other professional areas are also in the process of developing interstate compacts. The Association of State and Provincial Psychology Boards finalized language for their compact (PSYPACT) in 2015. PSYPACT was created to facilitate telehealth and temporary in-person, face-to-face practice of psychology across jurisdictional boundaries and began its introduction into state legislatures in 2016.[23] PSYPACT became operational once it was enacted by 7 states. As of 2020, it has been enacted by 13 states and there is pending legislation in 17 states. The Federation of State Boards of Physical Therapy has developed a Physical Therapy Licensure Compact that covers physical therapists and physical therapist assistants. In 2017, the Physical Therapy Compact reached the threshold requirement of 10 states and finalized its rules and bylaws.[24] As of 2020, it has been enacted by 28 states.

Credentialing and Privileging for Telehealth

Currently, APRNs must be licensed in the state in which they practice and credentialed at the facility in which they practice. To ensure patient safety and high-quality care, credentialing and privileging remain important elements of telehealth nursing practice, much as they are with traditional nursing practice. *Credentialing* is the process by which hospitals verify the qualification of practitioners. *Privileging* is the authority given to practice at a health care facility within the scope of their qualifications at the commencement of their employment and at regular intervals. The process of credentialing and privileging a practitioner is time consuming and can be costly and impractical when large numbers of providers seek to provide telehealth-facilitated services in multiple hospitals. Telehealth was incorporated into the Joint Commission Standards for Credentialing and Privileging beginning in 2000 and in its 2012 subsequent revised standards.[25] In 2011, the Centers for Medicare & Medicaid Services (CMS) published new regulations in its hospital and critical access hospital Conditions of Participation standards that include proxy credentialing and privileging arrangements as a viable option to further facilitate the delivery of telemedicine services across the nation.[26] These standards allow, through a written agreement between hospitals, for the originating site to accept the distant practitioner's credentials and privileges and require clear articulation of the types of privileges granted, the sharing of quality data, and adherence to state licensure requirements. Streamlining these processes will enable more consistent practice requirements and increase portability of licensure for nursing telehealth practice, especially in the setting of upcoming APRN Compacts.

Malpractice and Liability

As with most new technologies and technological advancements, use precedes the laws and regulations governing said technologies. This is also true for telehealth practice, especially due to the surge in development and incorporation of telehealth technologies into health care practice and health care delivery in recent years. Substantial, agreed-upon standards and regulations do not yet exist for nursing telehealth practice, although work in these arenas continues to gain momentum. Generally speaking, there have been few malpractice claims brought against telehealth practitioners, although data are not available regarding confidential settlements. However, APRNs should be aware of whether their professional liability policy covers telehealth practice.

Of importance to the telehealth practitioner is that claims may be brought against him or her in the state in which the patient is resident. Thus, it is imperative that telehealth practitioners are assured coverage through their malpractice carriers, and in that process identify the types of services offered and locations of patients being treated. Some carriers and policies exclude telehealth from coverage. Therefore, additional coverage for telehealth practice, in particular when services are provided in states without medical malpractice caps, may be required. If practice will be taking place across state lines, it is also important to ensure that malpractice liability extends coverage to multiple states. Additional recommendations to limit liability include disclaimers and use agreements signed by the patient, notification of adverse events, conformance to practice guidelines, and the securing of informed consent. Thus, telehealth technology in advanced practice can be used responsibly and with confidence in relation to the professional liability inherent in all health care practices.

Standards and Practice Guidelines

Standards and practice guidelines have been developed for telehealth, conforming to existing laws, regulations, and guidelines used for in-person practice, without changing the practitioner scope of practice. For example, as stated in the Virginia Board of Medicine and Nursing document "Telemedicine for Nurse Practitioner Guidance": "These guidelines support a consistent standard of care and scope of practice notwithstanding the delivery tool or business method used to enable practitioner-to-patient communications."[27]

Telemedicine does not create a new field of health care, but rather allows duly credentialed clinicians to provide care at a distance using technology. That being said, the American Telemedicine Association and its more than 9000 member-supported special interest groups, committees, and discussion groups have developed standards and practice guidelines to address technical applications and clinical practice guidelines endorsed by specialty societies. Many of these standards and practice guidelines extend beyond the practice guidelines that currently exist for traditional health care and give guidance to the use of technology in a specific practice arena.[13]

Investment in Broadband Connectivity and Universal Service

High-bandwidth and high-quality connections remain the underpinnings of successful tele-health encounters. Even today, there remain gaps in broadband connectivity in certain rural regions of the country.[28] Following passage of the Telecommunications Act of 1996, the establishment of the Rural Health Care (RHC) Program of the Universal Service Fund has promoted expansion of broadband services for eligible health care facilities in rural areas by providing discounts for ongoing connectivity. However, other entities, such as emergency medical services providers, skilled nursing facilities, for-profit clinics, and solo practices, remain ineligible for support altogether.[29] In 2010, the FCC's National Broadband Plan recommended substantive changes to the RHC program and commented on a number of challenges and opportunities to integrate broadband communications services into sustainable models of health care delivery.[30] Beginning in funding year 2017, the program reached its funding cap of $400 million as authorized by the FCC following passage of the Telecommunications Act. The $400 million funding cap was an amount that was set in 1997 and never indexed for inflation. On June 25, 2018, the FCC issued an order that adopted rules to increase the annual RHC program funding cap to $571 million and to annually adjust the RHC program funding cap for inflation, beginning with fiscal year 2018.

Privacy and Security

A number of privacy and security concerns are raised when obtaining, accessing, storing, and transmitting patient PHI, and legal and regulatory compliance must be observed for protection of patient rights to privacy and safety. Telehealth practice adds advanced telecommunications technologies and devices as tools for practice; therefore, adherence to privacy and security of data in the virtual care environment is a high priority. In telehealth, risks to loss of privacy of PHI could potentially occur during transfer of data or in unauthorized access, just as it can during standard in-person care. However, with increased use of telecommunications and devices, it is essential that privacy and security be built into telehealth systems of care to prevent privacy and security violations. For example, home-monitoring sensors could potentially unintentionally transmit private data, such as whether a patient is home or not. Alternatively, collected data could be mistakenly shared with outside agencies. Rigorous attention to security and privacy issues in telehealth is an inherent part of integrating the technology into practice in order for patients and providers to have trust in the security of the patient health information in telehealth systems of care.

Although existing federal and state privacy and security rules are applied to telehealth technologies and practice, more comprehensive and specifically focused regulations must be developed to align with the growing telehealth practice going forward. More guidance is needed, such as rules that safeguard data at the patient endpoint, because HIPAA only pertains to care in the clinical setting. "Given HIPAA's limited applicability to patient facing telehealth systems, its protections will not apply to information collected by most digital tools provided to patients."[31(p218)] At present, all telemedicine programs and services must conform to federal and, in some cases, state privacy and security standards per HIPAA. This requires encryption of data stored and transported, access control of patient data, audit controls, a data breach response plan, and business associate arrangements with any entity that is tied to the covered entity carrying out its health care functions. The HITECH Act adds additional guidance and further defines the patient as a data source.[7] Also, oversight is provided by way of FDA authority to regulate mobile medical apps of those defined as medical devices.[31]

Remote Prescribing

Prescribing is an important element of telehealth practice, and APRNs should seek their specific state laws and statutes for guidance. Some state boards of medicine, nursing, and pharmacy allow health professionals with prescriptive authority to use interactive audio-video encounters as a means to establish a provider-patient relationship necessary to prescribe certain medications. Some states require that the remote practitioner comport with the standards of in-person care prior to prescribing. Other more restrictive states require an actual in-person visit prior to the prescribing of medications and/or controlled substances by the telehealth practitioner. Written guidelines are needed for understanding of appropriate telehealth practice for prescribing controlled substances.

The federal Ryan Haight Act,[32] enacted in 2008, added additional Drug Enforcement Agency (DEA) regulatory requirements and criminal provisions so as to combat unlawful internet prescribing. This act was the result of the death of a California teen who secured controlled substances though form-only online prescribing by a practitioner in another state. The impact on telehealth practice and remote prescribing is as follows[33]:

- No controlled substance may be delivered, distributed, or dispensed by means of the internet without a valid prescription acting in the usual course of his professional practice;
- The prescriber must have a license to practice medicine in the state where the patient is located at the time of the consultation.
- A prescription must be issued by (a) a practitioner who has conducted at least 1 in-person examination of the patient, or (b) a covering practitioner for (a).

Telemedicine exceptions to the in-person examination requirement include the following[33]:

- The patient is being treated at a DEA-registered hospital or clinic.
- The patient is being treated in the physical presence of a DEA-registered practitioner.
- The telemedicine consultation is conducted by a DEA-registered practitioner for the Indian Health Services.
- The telemedicine consultation is conducted during a public health emergency declared by the Secretary of Health and Human Services.
- The telemedicine consultation is conducted by a practitioner who has obtained a DEA special registration
- The telemedicine consultation is conducted by a VHA practitioner during a VHA-declared emergency.
- The telemedicine consultation is conducted under other circumstances specified by future DEA regulations.

In an effort to expand the use of telemedicine as a tool to mitigate the public health emergency of opioid use disorder, bills to amend the Ryan Haight Act have been introduced.[32] Recent communications (May 2018) from the Diversion Control Division of the DEA outline exceptions to the requirement that the practitioner must have conducted 1 in-person visit prior to prescribing medication assisted treatment using Schedule III to V controlled substances.[34] Practitioners including qualifying practitioners and qualifying other practitioners (medication-assisted treatment providers) must hold a valid DEA registration, must hold a license in the state where the patient is located, and must maintain adequate record keeping, and the patient must be physically located at a DEA-registered hospital or clinic or in the physical presence of a DEA-registered practitioner. APRNs should stay abreast of changes in telehealth practice laws and regulations in order to be in compliance with telehealth practice standards.

Stark Law and Anti-Kickback Statute

When providing telehealth services associated with any federal programs (eg, Medicare, Medicaid), providers must comply with applicable fraud and abuse laws.[35] The Stark Law prohibits a physician or family member from referring federal program beneficiaries to any entity in which the physician has a financial relationship. The Anti-Kickback Statute expressly prohibits any remuneration that induces referrals of items or services reimbursable by federal health care programs. *Remuneration* is anything of value. Attention should be given to the Stark Law and Anti-Kickback Statute when developing telehealth programs, purchasing equipment, and developing telehealth education networks. Safe harbor regulations define practices that are not specifically subject to the Anti-Kickback Statute. The Office of the Inspector General has favorably reviewed requests related to certain telemedicine services.[36] More than half of the states also have all-payer anti-kickback statutes with similar prohibitions.

Food and Drug Administration

The FDA has issued guidance on regulated medical devices, which are defined as "healthcare products intended for diagnosis, cure, mitigation, treatment or prevention of a medical condition intended to affect the structure or any function of the body."[37] Class I devices are of low risk and subject to less regulatory control, Class II devices require greater control and are subject to requirements that ensure safety and effectiveness, and Class III devices are the highest risk and require the highest level of regulatory control. Mobile apps are subject to regulatory oversight if they serve as extensions of a medical device; store, analyze, or transmit patient medical data; are used to diagnose and treat; or transform a mobile platform into a regulated medical device. As examples, apps that are subject to regulatory control include those that are used for patient self-management, track medication usage, perform calculations for clinical practice, or support remote examination tools.

GROUP EXERCISE

Tele-Mental Health

Suppose you are working as an APRN in a rural mental health care practice. Your clinic is considering providing telepsychiatry services to address mental health disease and the opioid crisis. Discuss the legal and regulatory concerns and considerations related to licensing for telepsychiatry and the remote prescribing of controlled substances.

STATE REGULATIONS

Although there are many similar telehealth programs in a variety of states, no 2 states have the same telehealth laws and regulations. This adds to the complexity of navigating compliance with clinical telehealth practice. For example, although Medicare is a federal program, Medicaid is both a state and a federal program; therefore, each state interprets and implements laws differently for telehealth practice. Issues of informed consent for telehealth encounters, documentation requirements in medical records, and reimbursement vary state to state. The following sections identify state-specific considerations for telehealth clinical practice.

Informed Consent

Principles of nonmaleficence, confidentiality, and patient consent are important to telehealth practice, just as they are to standard, in-person practice. Providing informed consent ensures patients have a clear understanding of the risks, benefits, and alternatives of intended assessments, treatments, and procedures. Requirements for informed consent in telehealth practice vary by state. Many states require telehealth providers to obtain patient informed consent either by statute, regulation, or guidance. Such consent may be written or verbal and should be documented in the patient's medical record. Consent for telehealth services can be incorporated into existing facility consents or be individualized and should do the following[38]:

- Inform the patient who the providers are, along with their credentials and their location
- Inform patients of what technology the encounter will use
- Include a description of the care to be given
- Describe potential benefits and risks of using telehealth, with emphasis on privacy and security
- Discern strategies for providing care if problems with the technology occur
- Discuss patient rights to stop or refuse any treatments at any time
- Indicate the process to raise a concern or complaint regarding telehealth care
- Include specific policies regarding care at the individual facility, such as scheduling and billing policy

Readers are advised to conform to their state requirements, a summary of which may be found on the TRC website.[39]

Medical Records Documentation

Medical records for telehealth encounters should mirror all the elements of the in-person medical record, including all data and communications associated with each patient, and may be in the form of an electronic health record. Records of the telemedicine encounter should be available just as for in-person care records and in alignment with existing laws and regulations related to patient health care records and data. Some states offer specific guidance on the management of all medical information transmitted during a telehealth encounter, and, as such, it is recommended that providers develop storage, retention, and medical record documentation protocols and policies that are congruent with laws in the state of practice.

Reimbursement

Payment coverage restrictions remain a major impediment to the broader adoption of telehealth by providers. Through the Balanced Budget Amendment of 1997 and the Benefits Improvement and Protection Act of 2000, Congress authorized CMS to reimburse for telemedicine services provided to rural Medicare beneficiaries across a broad range of Current Procedural Terminology (CPT) codes and services.[40] This enables providers, including APRNs, to function as referrer and consultant. However, those Medicare telehealth provisions, as established in the Section 1834(m) of the Social Security Act, limit eligible patient originating sites to rural and have not evolved to take advantage of subsequent analyses of best practices, outcomes data, and new paradigms of health care delivery, even following enactment of the Affordable Care Act.[41] The Medicare definition of rural for purposes of telehealth coverage requires that the patient must be in one of the following:

- Non-Metropolitan Statistical Area (MSA)
- Health Professional Shortage Area outside an MSA
- Rural census tract or county outside an MSA
- Entities participating in a federal telehealth demonstration project as of December 31, 2000

Recent changes in law allow for the provision of telestroke services to patients located in both urban and rural sites.[42]

In addition, Medicare restrictions on eligible originating sites are limited to the following types of facilities:

- Hospital
- Critical access hospital
- Office of a practitioner or a physician
- Community mental health center

- Skilled nursing facility
- Federally qualified health center (FQHC)
- Hospital-based or critical access hospital–based renal dialysis center

The home is not an eligible originating site for purposes of telemedicine services, with the recent exception of qualifying visits for dialysis patients. However, provider review of data obtained through RPM services in the home are now covered and not restricted by rurality.

CMS is constantly reviewing and updating rules related to telehealth care reimbursement. It is important for the APRN to be aware of changes to CMS regulations. For example, 2019 guidance from CMS Medicare Telehealth Services information indicates that CMS has amended telehealth geographic location and originating sites for acute stroke care.[43] CMS has also developed a new set of CPT codes for 2019 related to Virtual Check In, Remote Evaluation of Pre-Recorded Patient Information, Interprofessional Internet Consultation, and Chronic Care Remote Physiologic Monitoring.[44,45] These have been removed from the definition of telehealth so that they are not bound by the geographic restrictions. Additionally, CMS is working on guidance effective July 1, 2019, that would lift any originating site geographic site restrictions (including home as originating site) for telehealth for substance use disorders and for those with substance use disorders and co-occurring disorders. Another change beginning January 2020 is that Medicare Advantage plans will no longer be bound by geographic restrictions on telehealth but have the flexibility to offer the full array of telehealth benefits.[46] Finally, CMS is establishing what is called the Emergency Triage, Treat, and Transport Model.[47] The anticipated start date is January 2020, and it is planned to last for 5 years. This is a voluntary 5-year payment model that will allow ambulance teams to address emergency health care needs of Medicare beneficiaries following a 911 call. It will allow those who volunteer to use this payment model to either transport to a hospital emergency department or other destination, transport to an alternative destination (eg, primary care office or urgent care clinic), or provide treatment in place with a qualified health care practitioner, either on the scene or connected using telehealth.

In addition, Medicare, by statute, restricts eligible distant site practitioners to the following:

- Physicians
- Nurse practitioners
- Physician assistants
- Nurse midwives
- Clinical nurse specialists
- Certified nurse anesthetists
- Clinical psychologists, clinical social workers
- Registered dieticians and nutrition professionals

Other restrictions placed by Medicare include the mode of communication, requiring real-time interactive audio and video communications and not audio only. Store-and-forward (asynchronous) services are only covered in Hawaii and Alaska. Medicare lists and updates annually in the physician fee schedule eligible CPT and Health Care Common Procedure Coding System codes. Any service provided that is not covered by those codes will not be reimbursed.

Medicare reimbursement of telehealth services remains woefully limited. The Center for Telehealth and e-Health Law (CTEL) reported that in 2015, Medicare allowed $15,664,543 in distant site reimbursement and $1,937,453 in originating site charges nationwide.[43] Medicare payment data in the fee-for-service program are available from CTEL.[48]

There have been recent efforts to address some of these limitations. The Center for Medicare and Medicaid Innovation has funded pilot programs that incorporate broader telehealth reimbursement, although some accountable care organizations remain limited to the rural originating site restrictions. The American Medical Association Digital Medicine Payment Advisory Group is currently working to align telehealth taxonomies with use cases and make recommendations to the CPT Advisory Panel and the relative value units Update Committee.

The 2018 budget bill[49] includes improvements in telemedicine coverage as follows:

- Eliminates geographic restriction on telestroke services beginning in 2019
- Affords accountable care organizations greater flexibility to use telehealth services
- Expands telehealth services in Medicare Advantage Plans beginning in 2020
- Adds the patient's home and freestanding dialysis facilities without geographic restriction as eligible originating sites for monthly assessments by the nephrologist
- Extends the CMS Independence at Home demonstration for Medicare beneficiaries with multiple chronic conditions

Additionally, CMS finalized its 2019 physician fee schedule on November 1, 2018,[50] and incorporated significant telehealth-related changes. These changes expand Medicare telehealth services to include the following:

- New codes for chronic care management
- New codes for remote patient monitoring
- Expanded reimbursement for end-stage renal disease and acute stroke based on the Bipartisan Budget Act of 2018
- Proposed exemptions from some of CMS's telehealth requirements for the treatment of substance use disorder

Even more significantly, in its final rule, CMS stated its belief that the restrictions imposed by the Social Security Act apply only to the types of services explicitly delineated in the act: professional consultations, office visits, and office psychiatry services. In other words, it provided clarification that services using remote communications technologies outside of these specific categories are not subject to the same restrictions. These include things like virtual check-ins, remote evaluation of prerecorded information, and interprofessional internet consultation.

Medicaid

Currently, nearly every state Medicaid program provides some form of reimbursement for the delivery of telehealth-facilitated care to Medicaid beneficiaries. Medicaid innovations adopted by many states include coverage for video-based telemedicine consults and follow-up visits, coverage for remote monitoring, home telehealth, store-and-forward services, school-based services, and, in some states, eConsults (structured exchanges between primary care and specialty care providers within the electronic health record). Transformation from fee-for-service Medicaid to Medicaid managed care organizations requires consideration of the nuances of contracting with the managed care organizations but also affords additional opportunities for collaborative models of care coordination and outcomes analyses.[51-53]

Other Federal Payer

The Office of Personnel Management offers some telemedicine benefits for individuals covered under the Federal Employee Health Benefit Plans. The VHA has long integrated telehealth solutions, as has the Department of Defense.

Commercial Payer

Thirty-three states and the District of Columbia require that private insurance cover telehealth services. There is great variability among the state private pay statutes; some require coverage and others mandate coverage with payment parity. Many of the Employee Retirement Income Security Act plans have chosen to cover telehealth services. The reader is referred to the National Telehealth Policy Resource Center for specific language regarding individual state reimbursement policies.[54]

Temporary Changes in Telehealth Laws and Regulations During the COVID-19 National Public Health Emergency

Telehealth providers must stay abreast of changes to federal telehealth laws and regulations, as well as changes to state and professional regulations. This is vitally important especially in times of national emergencies. Changes during the COVID pandemic have been made regarding use of telehealth by the federal and state government, as well by as most states and many private insurers. On March 6, 2020, The Coronavirus Preparedness and Response Supplemental Appropriations Act 2020 (H.R. 6074) was signed into law. This act provided changes in laws for use of telehealth services during this national public health emergency so that people have easier access to care via telehealth services.[55] This was done to enable patients to see their providers without travel to brick-and-mortar health care facilities to mitigate spread or risk of contracting infection during the COVID-19 crisis. H.R. 6074 allows the Department of Health and Human Services to temporarily waive some Medicare limitations and requirements, and releases some financial restrictions.[56] CMS also expanded its telehealth services under the 1135 Waiver authority and Coronavirus Preparedness and Response Supplemental Act.[55] Goals of the relaxed regulations includes providing access to care while mitigating patient exposure to the coronavirus, especially for those in high-risk or vulnerable populations.

A summary of items changed for the duration of this waiver is presented below. The reader is advised to check for updates and changes as the situation changes rapidly. As of April 2020 these changes include[57]:

- Location of patient
  - The site restriction to rural locations is suspended. This means that authorized providers can connect with patients at any site as an originating site, including in the patient's home.
- Eligible services
  - The list of eligible services has been expanded.
- Eligible providers
  - H.R. 748 expands the list of eligible providers to FQHCs and rural health clinics (RHCs)
- Modality
  - CMS defines that telehealth services can be delivered from telecommunication systems including "audio and visual equipment permitting 2-way real-time interactive communication between the patient and distant site physician or practitioner" (p1)
- Out-of-pocket costs
  - The Office of the Inspector General has authorized providers to reduce or waive fees.
- Prior existing relationships
  - Relaxes the rules regarding telehealth services, remote monitoring, and virtual check-ins for new and established patients
- End-stage renal disease and home dialysis patients
  - The monthly face-to face requirements are waived, and patients with end-stage renal disease do not have to have monthly in-person evaluations of the vascular access site. Additionally, providers are relieved of the face-to-face National/Local Coverage Determinations.
- Nursing homes
  - In-person visit can be conducted via telehealth instead of previously required face-to-face visits.

- Hospice
  - The requirement for a face-to-face visit to determine continued eligibility is waived.
- Frequency limitations
  - The every 3 day frequency limitations for in-patient visits and the 30 day frequency limits for skilled nursing facilities and for critical care consults are lifted.
- Supervision
  - Allows for physician supervision via live video as well as other supervision changes.
- Stark laws
  - Allows hospital and providers to pay above or below fair market value for needed equipment, supplies, and services, and allows providers to support one another financially for continuance of health care operations.
- Modifiers
  - Allows providers to use point of service codes enabling reimbursement at the in-person rate using the "95" modifier, which indicates the encounter was a telehealth encounter.

Other Medicare and Medicaid changes include:

- Medicare Advantage
  - Medicare Advantage Organizations are allowed to expand telehealth coverage further than previously approved by CMS.
- Other technology-enabled services
  - Allows physical therapists, occupational therapists, and speech-language pathologists to bill for virtual check-ins. Telephone evaluation and management service are also allowed by phone.
- Medicaid
  - Gives permission to utilize telehealth in Medicaid programs, including telehealth and telephone consultations to replace in-person requirements if certain conditions are met.

Other federal changes include changes to the Ryan Haight Act:

- Drug Enforcement Agency changes
  - For the duration of this emergency the Drug Enforcement Agency–registered providers can prescribe controlled substances to patients who they have not met in-person requirements, provided they meet certain restrictions.
- HIPAA
  - The HHS Office for Civil Rights will show enforcement discretion and waive penalizations for HIPAA violations against providers who use certain described non-HIPAA complaint technologies during the covid public health emergency.

Private insurance changes include:

- Health plan changes
  - A number of private health care companies will enable providers and patients to use telehealth to access care. Examples include Aetna, Cigna, and BlueCross BlueShield.

FQHCs and RHCs changes include:

- Medicare
  - The Coronavirus Aid, Relief and Economic Security Act enables FQHCs and RHCs to be both the originating and remote site when delivering telehealth services

- Medicaid
  - Ability of FQHCs and RHCs to be a designated distant site will be different from state to state.
- Private payer
  - Differences between individual states and payer for telehealth services exists.

State COVID regulation changes include:

- Waiver of licensure requirements/renewals
  - Varies state to state
- Waiver of in state licensure requirements
  - Varies state to state

LEGAL AND REGULATORY CONSIDERATIONS FOR TELEHEALTH PROGRAM DEVELOPMENT AND ACCREDITATION

Many APRNs have independence of practice enabling them to open nurse practitioner–owned clinics and facilities that offer telehealth services, and others are in practices that currently use or will develop telehealth services. Starting a telehealth program includes several fundamental steps, and compliance with legal and regulatory issues must be observed. The first step is to assess the service needs and overall readiness of the organization. Clinical and community needs should be the driver of any telehealth program, and that need should be documented using data whenever possible. An environmental scan or market analysis may also be useful for understanding the market forces that might impact program implementation and highlight aspects of organizational readiness. The next set of steps includes developing and planning the telehealth program. Identifying the key program components, understanding and getting buy-in regarding workflows, establishing technology requirements, developing the business case/model, pilot testing the program and coming up with a plan for monitoring program performance, and evaluating its success should all come before full implementation. It is important to be aware of the laws and regulations governing telehealth practice so that appropriate incorporate technology, processes, and privacy and security features can be used in the program, enabling the program to comply with legal rules and guidelines for practice. Once a telehealth program is ready to implement, putting processes and procedures in writing will help to ensure a smoother roll-out and establish consistency and quality and aid in training. Consistent monitoring of the performance of the program and having regular checkpoints to determine quality improvement needs are also important.

There is a lack of consensus on whether accreditation of programs or credentialing of telehealth providers is necessary to ensure program and provider quality. Some would argue that telehealth is simply a tool and not a separate service. Therefore, things like accreditation and credentialing of telehealth providers creates a barrier to the delivery of health care. Nonetheless, several such programs have begun to emerge. For example, the Utilization Review Accreditation Commission Telehealth Accreditation[58] is the first independent third-party national program to define standards for both programs and providers. Additionally, the National Board for Certified Counselors, through its Center for Credentialing & Education, has developed a Board Certified-TeleMental Health Provider Credential as a way to establish credibility.[59]

Telehealth practice is growing at an ever-increasing rate, and the legal and regulatory arena will continue to evolve. It is important to stay current with the changes while encompassing existing standards in telehealth practice. Recommendations to provide high-quality, safe care that limits risk and malpractice exposure or violations to nursing practice include the following:

- Be sure to obtain correct licensure and credentialing specific to your state, the remote patient site, and the practice in alignment with the Nurse Practice Act.
- Obtain consent as required to conduct the virtual care visit.
- Always introduce yourself at the beginning of the visit with the patient and be sure to inform the patient if anyone else is in the consult room.
- Be compliant with HIPAA privacy and security of all forms of health care data and cyber communications.
- Be sure to use HIPAA-compliant technology and partner with telehealth and cyber security experts to be knowledgeable of your state's telehealth prescribing rules and regulations.
- When possible, conduct telehealth care in a dedicated telehealth work environment to ensure consistency in video and audio quality between the provider site and the patient site.
- Provide patient education to ensure patient comfort and proficiency using telehealth technology.
- Be aware of telehealth reimbursement policies for private insurers in your state, as well as Medicare and Medicaid policy.
- Obtain training and education to ensure confidence and proficiency when using telehealth technology in patient care.
- Use telehealth equipment frequently and conduct preconsult testing to ensure equipment works properly.

For more details on establishing clinical telehealth services and programs, see Chapter 6.

RESEARCH EVIDENCE FOR IMPROVED OUTCOMES

The evidence base for improved outcomes using telehealth is already quite substantive, and it continues to grow. The Agency for Healthcare Research and Quality (AHRQ) created a technical brief in August 2016 to provide an overview of the large and disparate body of evidence about telehealth for use by decision makers.[60] The approach used was to create an evidence map of systematic reviews published to date that assess the impact of telehealth on clinical outcomes. The technical brief concluded that there was sufficient evidence to support the effectiveness of telehealth for RPM for patients with chronic conditions; communication and counseling for patients with chronic conditions; and psychotherapy as part of behavioral health. The AHRQ has developed research protocols to look more in-depth at telehealth for acute and chronic care consultations and mobile health technology for diabetes.

Research catalogues have been developed by the Center for Connected Health Policy that reference the body of research on the efficacy of telehealth in specialty and subspecialty areas, such as telestroke, teledermatology, palliative care, telehealth and schools, and telehealth and prisons.[54]

Finally, the Northeast Telehealth Resource Center has also compiled webliographies of research publications across over 35 specialty and subspecialty areas, including cardiology, dentistry, diabetes management, emergency medicine, endocrinology, genetics, intensive care unit, and obstetrics.[61]

CONCLUSION

There are 2 areas related to telehealth legal and regulatory issues where tremendous opportunity exists for APRNs. First, in relationship to the widespread adoption of telehealth in practice, the education and training of APRNs in telehealth practice continues to lag behind. This is particularly true when it comes to clinical practice and helping nursing professionals understand how to translate in-person nursing knowledge, skills, and care to the virtual environment; employ proper videoconference etiquette in nursing telehealth practice; and integrate telehealth into both existing clinical workflows and within the context of emerging models of care (eg, interprofessional care teams, behavioral health integration). However, there has been quite a bit of recent activity around telehealth training for nurses. Should this growing interest continue, the nursing profession could be among the first of all health professions to adequately prepare its workforce to both integrate and innovate their clinical practice with telehealth technologies.

Second, when it comes to licensure, the nursing profession is one of few health professions who have an eNLC that truly enables licensure portability; however, the model is only applicable to RNs and LPN/VNs who practice within its 31 member states. Although the NCSBN approved the creation of the APRN Compact, it has not yet been implemented because presently only 3 out of the required 10 states have enacted the necessary legislation. Should the implementation of the APRN Compact come to fruition and reach or surpass the level of adoption of the eNLC, APRNs would have a significant opportunity to leapfrog over the other health professions when it comes to interstate telehealth practice.

In summary, there are complex federal and state laws and regulations that impact telehealth practice. These rules are still evolving, and in general, they have a difficult time keeping up with the rapid changes in technological developments and their emerging clinical applications. It is imperative that the telehealth APRN and all related health care entities remain informed and seek appropriate legal counsel in the development and scaling of any models of telehealth practice.

THOUGHTFUL QUESTIONS

1. Why is it important for APRNs to be familiar with the legal and regulatory telehealth arena?
2. What are the similarities and differences in using telehealth in practice and in nursing education?
3. As technology progresses, what factors need to be considered when addressing legal and regulatory policy development to cover changing telehealth services?
4. Regarding evidence that telehealth improves outcomes, review the AHRQ Technical Brief.[62] In what areas is there evidence to support the use of telehealth to improve outcomes?

CASE STUDY

Ten-year-old Abby is at the school nurse's office for the sixth time in the past month. She was up coughing much of the night. She was diagnosed with allergy-induced asthma several years ago. Abby is a terrific basketball player and a real asset to her middle school team, but during the early spring pollen season, Abby struggles to breathe and misses most practices and games.

Abby lives in a small, rural community where there is a part-time nurse practitioner at a rural health clinic and a part-time school nurse. Abby's family struggles to make ends meet. Her father works at the local orchard, and her mother works as a seamstress. They are both paid by the hour and do not receive health insurance benefits from their employer. They have difficulty affording the inhalers and nasal sprays recommended by the allergist.

(continued)

CASE STUDY (CONTINUED)

The school nurse is very concerned about Abby and feels she needs to be seen by someone. However, the school nurse also knows that Abby's family could not possibly afford an emergency room visit, nor could they afford to take the time off from work to bring Abby to the nearest primary care provider who, on this day, is about 30 miles away. The school nurse decides to called the local nurse practitioner. Unfortunately, as a part-time practitioner, this was a day when she was not in her office.

When her phone rang, the nurse practitioner was having lunch with her sister, who lived in the next town, 45 minutes away. The school nurse describes Abby's conditions over the phone, but the nurse practitioner does not feel she has enough information to make a recommendation without actually talking to and physically laying eyes on Abby. The nurse and nurse practitioner struggle with what to do, and eventually the nurse suggested that perhaps they could use Skype on their personal phones to conduct a telehealth visit. The nurse practitioner excuses herself and goes out to her car to ensure some privacy. She connects to the school nurse using Skype. Through Skype, the school nurse allows the nurse practitioner to see and speak with Abby. After a 10-minute conversation and observation of Abby, the nurse practitioner feels comfortable making the assessment that Abby does not need to go to the emergency room. She advises that the school nurse work with the parents to get a refill for her rescue inhaler.

Question

1. Did the school nurse and nurse practitioner do the right thing? Why or why not?

REFERENCES

1. Institute of Medicine of the National Academies. *Quality Through Collaboration: The Future of Rural Health.* Washington DC: National Academies Press; 2005.
2. Institute of Medicine. *The Role of Telehealth in an Evolving Health Care Environment.* Washington, DC: National Academies Press; 2012.
3. Douthit N, Kiv S, Dwolatzky T, Biswas S. Exposing some important barriers to health care access in the rural USA. *Public Health.* 2015;129(6):611-620.
4. Clabo LL, Giddens J, Jeffries P, McQuade-Jones B, Morton P, Ryan S. A perfect storm: a window of opportunity for revolution in nurse practitioner education. *J Nurs Educ.* 2010;51(10):539-541.
5. Schweickert P, Rheuban KS, Cattell-Gordon D, et al. The APN-PLACE telehealth education network: legal and regulatory considerations. *J Nurs Regul.* 2018;8(4):1-6.
6. Centers for Medicare & Medicaid Services. Telemedicine services in hospitals and critical access hospitals (CAHs) [memorandum]. https://www.cms.gov/Medicare/Provider-Enrollment-and-Certification/SurveyCertificationGenInfo/downloads/SCLetter11_32.pdf. Published July 15, 2011. Accessed February 19, 2020.
7. US Department of Health and Human Services. HITECH Act Enforcement Interim Final Rule. https://www.hhs.gov/hipaa/for-professionals/special-topics/hitech-act-enforcement-interim-final-rule/index.html. Updated June 16, 2017. Accessed February 19, 2020.
8. Federal Communications Commission. Wireless devices and health concerns. www.fcc.gov/consumers/guides/wireless-devices-and-health-concerns. Updated October 15, 2019. Accessed February 19, 2020.
9. US Food and Drug Administration. Device software functions including mobile medical applications. https://www.fda.gov/medical-devices/digital-health/device-software-functions-including-mobile-medical-applications. Updated November 11, 2019. Accessed February 19, 2020.
10. Hutcherson CM. Legal considerations for nurses practicing in a telehealth setting. *Online J Issues Nurs.* 200;6(3). www.nursingworld.org/MainMenuCategories/ANAMarketplace/ANAPeriodicals/OJIN/TableofContents/Volume62001/No3Sept01/LegalConsiderations.aspx. Accessed April 6, 2020.
11. Brous E. Legal considerations in telehealth and telemedicine. *Am J Nurs.* 2016;116(9):64-67

12. Rutledge CM, Kott K, Schweickert PA, Poston R, Fowler C, Haney TS. Telehealth and eHealth in nurse practitioner training: current perspectives. *Adv Med Educ Pract.* 2017;8:399-409.

13. American Telemedicine Association. Practice guidelines & resources. http://hub.americantelemed.org/resources/telemedicine-practice-guidelines. Accessed February 19, 2020.

14. National Consortium of Telehealth Resource Centers. Find your TRC. http://www.telehealthresourcecenter.org/who-your-trc. Accessed February 19, 2020.

15. Bulik RJ. Human factors in primary care telemedicine encounters. *J Telemed Telecare.* 2008;14:169-172.

16. Blackman K. Telehealth and licensing interstate providers. *LegisBrief.* 2016;24(25):1-2.

17. American Medical Association. AMA adopts new guidance for ethical practice in telemedicine [press release]. https://www.ama-assn.org/press-center/press-releases/ama-adopts-new-guidance-ethical-practice-telemedicine. Published June 13, 2016. Accessed February 19, 2020.

18. Federation of State Medical Boards. Model policy for the appropriate use of telemedicine technologies in the practice of medicine. http://www.fsmb.org/Media/Default/PDF/FSMB/Advocacy/FSMB_Telemedicine_Policy.pdf. Published April 2014. Accessed February 19, 2020.

19. Federation of State Medical Boards. Interstate Medical Licensure Compact Commission issues 3,000th license. www.fsmb.org/advocacy/news-releases/interstate-medical-licensure-compact-commission-issues-3000th-license/. Published November 8, 2018. Accessed April 28, 2020.

20. National Council of State Boards of Nursing. Enhanced Nursing License Compact (eNLC) [news release]. https://www.ncsbn.org/11945.htm. Published January 19, 2018. Accessed February 19, 2020.

21. National Council of State Boards of Nursing. Advanced Practice Registered Nurse Compact. https://www.ncsbn.org/APRN_Compact_Final_050415.pdf. Published May 4, 2015. Accessed February 19, 2020.

22. National Council of State Boards of Nursing. APRN Consensus implementation status. https://www.ncsbn.org/5397.htm. Updated April 23, 2018. Accessed February 19, 2020.

23. Association of State and Provincial Psychology Boards. Psychology Interjurisdictional Compact (PSYPACT). https://www.asppb.net/page/PSYPACT. Accessed February 19, 2020.

24. Federation of State Boards of Physical Therapy. Physical Therapy Liscensure Compact. www.fsbpt.org/Free-Resources/Physical-Therapy-Licensure-Compact. Accessed April 28, 2020.

25. The Joint Commission. Accepted: final revisions to telemedicine standards. https://www.jointcommission.org/assets/1/6/Revisions_telemedicine_standards.pdf. Published January 2012. Accessed February 19, 2020.

26. Centers for Medicare & Medicaid Services. Telemedicine services in hospitals and critical access hospitals (CAHs) [memorandum]. https://www.cms.gov/Medicare/Provider-Enrollment-and-Certification/SurveyCertificationGenInfo/downloads/SCLetter11_32.pdf. Published July 15, 2011. Accessed February 19, 2020.

27. Virginia Board of Medicine and Virginia Board of Nursing. Telemedicine for nurse practitioners. Guidance document 90-64. https://www.dhp.virginia.gov/nursing/guidelines/90-64.docx. Published July 18, 2017. Accessed February 19, 2020.

28. Federal Communications Commission. 2016 broadband progress report. https://www.fcc.gov/reports-research/reports/broadband-progress-reports/2016-broadband-progress-report. Published January 29, 2016. Accessed February 19, 2020.

29. Federal Communications Commission. Report and order: order on reconsideration and further notice of proposed rule making. *Fed Regist.* 2004;69(14). https://www.govinfo.gov/content/pkg/FR-2004-11-22/pdf/04-25629.pdf. Accessed May 11, 2019.

30. Federal Communications Commission. The national broadband plan: connecting America. https://transition.fcc.gov/national-broadband-plan/national-broadband-plan.pdf. Published March 17, 2010. Accessed February 19, 2020.

31. Hall JL, McGraw D. For telehealth to succeed, privacy and security risks must be identified and addressed. *Health Aff (Millwood).* 2014;33(2):216-221.

32. Lacktman NM, Ferrante TB. Congress proposes change to Ryan Haight Act to allow telemedicine prescribing of controlled substances. Foley. https://www.foley.com/en/insights/publications/2018/03/congress-proposes-change-to-ryan-haight-act-to-all. Published March 5, 2018. Accessed February 19, 2020.

33. Ryan Haight Online Pharmacy Consumer Protection Act of 2008. Pub L No. 110-425, 122 Stat 4820.

34. Drug Enforcement Administration. Use of telemedicine while providing medication assisted treatment (MAT). https://www.hhs.gov/opioids/sites/default/files/2018-09/hhs-telemedicine-dea-final-508compliant.pdf. Accessed February 19, 2020.

35. US Department of Health and Human Services. Comparison of the Anti-Kickback Statute and Stark Law. https://oig.hhs.gov/compliance/provider-compliance-training/files/starkandakscharthandout508.pdf. Accessed February 19, 2020.

36. US Department of Health and Human Services. OIG Advisory Opinion No. 18-03. https://oig.hhs.gov/fraud/docs/advisoryopinions/2018/AdvOpn18-03.pdf. Published May 31, 2018. Accessed February 19, 2020.

37. US Food and Drug Administration. Medical devices. https://www.fda.gov/Medical-Devices. Published May 31, 2018. Accessed February 19, 2020.

38. Krupinski EA. Telemedicine & informed consent: how informed are you? Southwest Telehealth Resource Center. https://southwesttrc.org/blog/2017/telemedicine-informed-consent-how-informed-are-you. Published February 1, 2017. Accessed February 19, 2020.

39. National Consortium of Telehealth Resource Centers. Informed consent laws. https://www.telehealthresourcecenter.org/toolbox-module/informed-consent-laws. Accessed February 19, 2020.

40. Centers for Medicare & Medicaid Services. List of telehealth services. https://www.cms.gov/Medicare/Medicare-General-Information/Telehealth/Telehealth-Codes.html. Updated November 1, 2019. Accessed February 19, 2020.

41. Special payment rules for particular items and services. 42 USC §1395m (2011).

42. Bipartisan Budget Act of 2018. Pub L 115-123, 132 Stat 64.

43. Centers for Medicare & Medicaid Services. New modifier for expanding the use of telehealth for individuals with stroke. MLN Matters Number: MM10883. https://www.cms.gov/Outreach-and-Education/Medicare-Learning-Network-MLN/MLNMattersArticles/Downloads/MM10883.pdf. Published September 28, 2018. Accessed February 19, 2020.

44. Centers for Medicare & Medicaid Services. Telehealth services. https://www.cms.gov/Outreach-and-Education/Medicare-Learning-Network-MLN/MLNProducts/downloads/TelehealthSrvcsfctsht.pdf?utm_campaign=2a178f351b-EMAIL_CAMPAIGN_2019_04_19_08_59&utm_term=0_ae00b0e89a-2a178f351b-353229765&utm_content=90024811&utm_medium=social&utm_source=linkedin&hss_channel=lcp-3619444. Published January 2019. Accessed February 19, 2020.

45. Center for Connected Health Policy. Finalized CY 2019 physician fee schedule. https://www.cchpca.org/sites/default/files/2018-11/FINAL%20PFS%20CY%202019%20COMBINED_0.pdf. Published November 2018. Accessed February 19, 2020.

46. Centers for Medicare & Medicaid Services. Contract Year 2020 Medicare Advantage and Part D Flexibility Final Rule (CMS-4185-F). https://www.cms.gov/newsroom/fact-sheets/contract-year-2020-medicare-advantage-and-part-d-flexibility-final-rule-cms-4185-f. Published April 5, 2019. Accessed February 19, 2020.

47. Centers for Medicare & Medicaid Services. Emergency Triage, Treat, and Transport (ET3) model. https://innovation.cms.gov/initiatives/et3/. Updated January 28, 2020. Accessed February 19, 2020.

48. Center for Telehealth and e-Health Law. http://ctel.org/. Accessed February 19, 2020.

49. Vitek T, Flood J, Willis S. Government affairs – the progress of telehealth bills in Congress. https://www.cmhealthlaw.com/2018/11/government-affairs-the-progress-of-telehealth-bills-in-congress/. Published November 16, 2018. Accessed February 19, 2020.

50. Centers for Medicare & Medicaid Services. CMS releases the CY 2018 physician fee schedule (PFS) proposed rule. https://ecqi.healthit.gov/ecqi/ecqi-news/cms-releases-cy-2018-physician-feeschedule-pfs-proposed-rule. Published June 19, 2019. Accessed February 19, 2020.

51. Thomas L, Capistrant G. State telemedicine gaps analysis: coverage & reimbursement. American Telemedicine Association. https://higherlogicdownload.s3.amazonaws.com/AMERICANTELEMED/3c09839a-fffd-46f7-916c-692c11d78933/UploadedImages/Policy/State%20Policy%20Resource%20Center/2017%20NEW_50%20State%20Telehealth%20Gaps%20%20Analysis-%20Coverage%20and%20Reimbursement_FINAL.pdf. Published February 2017. Accessed February 19, 2020.

52. Centers for Medicare & Medicaid Services. State waivers list. https://www.medicaid.gov/medicaid/section-1115-demo/demonstration-and-waiver-list/waivers_faceted.html. Accessed February 19, 2020.

53. Centers for Medicare & Medicaid Services. Telemedicine. https://www.medicaid.gov/medicaid/benefits/telemedicine/index.html. Accessed February 19, 2020.

54. Center for Connected Health Policy. https://www.cchpca.org/. Accessed February 19, 2020.

55. Centers for Medicare & Medicaid Services. Medicare telemedicine health care provider fact sheet. www.cms.gov/newsroom/fact-sheets/medicare-telemedicine-health-care-provider-fact-sheet. Published March 17, 2020. Accessed April 28, 2020.

56. H.R.6074 - Coronavirus Preparedness and Response Supplemental Appropriations Act, 2020. https://congress.gov/bill/116th-congress/house-bill/6074. Published March 6, 2020. Accessed April 28, 2020.

57. Center for Connected Health Policy. Telehealth coverage policies in the time of COVID-19 to date. www.cchpca.org/sites/default/files/2020-04/CORONAVIRUS%20TELEHEALTH%20POLICY%20FACT%20SHEET%20APRIL%206%202020.pdf. Published April 6, 2020. Accessed April 28, 2020.

58. Utilization Review Accreditation Commission. https://www.urac.org/. Accessed February 19, 2020.

59. National Board for Certified Counselors. https://www.nbcc.org/. Accessed February 19, 2020.

60. Totten AM, Womack DM, Eden KB, et al. Telehealth: mapping the evidence for patient outcomes from systematic reviews. Rockville, MD: Agency for Healthcare Research and Quality (AHRQ). 2016: Technical Brief No. 26. Report No. 16-EHC034-EF.

61. Northwest Telehealth Resource Center. Northwest Telehealth resource library. http://www.netrc.org/resources.php. Accessed February 19, 2020.

62. Agency for Healthcare Research and Quality. Telehealth evidence map. US Department of Health and Human Services. https://effectivehealthcare.ahrq.gov/products/telehealth/research-protocol. Published August 11, 2015. Accessed April 28, 2020.

6

The Role of the Advanced Practice Registered Nurse in Implementing Telehealth Practice

Katherine E. Chike-Harris, DNP, APRN, CPNP-PC, NE

CHAPTER OBJECTIVES

Upon review of this chapter, the reader will be able to:

1. Describe the various roles that the advanced practice registered nurse (APRN) can perform related to telehealth.
2. Describe the essential steps to developing and implementing a telehealth program and identify telehealth services and how they are applicable to patient outcomes.
3. Identify key stakeholders and discuss achieving and maintaining their support.
4. Identify barriers to implementing and sustaining of a telehealth program.

Telehealth has been used by APRNs since the 1970s to provide care.[1] Since this time, use of APRNs within telehealth health care delivery has expanded. In early 2000, it was suggested that telehealth could assist in the expansion of nursing practice by increasing the care that APRNs provide to patients through expansion of services, as well as enhancing the APRN's professional roles.[2-4] This has been demonstrated in current literature via the usage of nurse-led clinics to increase patient outcomes. For example, one study evaluated the effectiveness of a nurse practitioner–led clinic for the management of patients with congestive heart failure (CHF) through use of remote patient monitoring (RPM) and early nurse practitioner evaluation and intervention; this resulted in a reduction of CHF readmission rates well below the national average.[5] Another article reports on the success of a telehealth collaborative relationship between APRNs and perinatologists within a rural community to increase maternal-child health outcomes. Synchronous visits were conducted between the rural clinic APRNs and perinatologists and resulted in fewer missed prenatal visits and higher mean birth weight, indicating that this relationship was beneficial to high-risk pregnant patients.[6]

Schweickert PA, Rutledge CM, eds.
Telehealth Essentials for Advanced Practice Nursing (pp 121-140).
© 2020 Taylor & Francis Group.

Although there are numerous articles that demonstrate the effectiveness of a nurse-led tele-health clinic, literature describing telehealth clinics developed and implemented by APRNs are difficult to find. Is this due to the nonexistence of such programs or simply a lack in publishing? The latter may be more applicable. One telehealth graduate nursing educational intervention article described postgraduates of their Doctor of Nursing Practice (DNP) program who used telehealth within their careers. Two of the graduates developed and implemented a nurse-run clinic in a remote mountain region and incorporated a collaborative agreement with physicians and specialist consultations via telehealth.[7] One neonatal nurse practitioner developed and imple-mented an online telehealth program with mobile hotspots that provided communication between transport team and neonatologists during transport of neonates.[7] A DNP-prepared gerontological APRN graduate received grant funding to develop a website intervention consisting of an inter-professional team that provided online education to the caregivers of older adults with dementia.[7]

Another article described the successful use of teleconsulting between an APRN in a rural emergency department and emergency physicians of an academic medical center Level I trauma center. This collaboration was eventually expanded statewide and received the designation as a Center for Telehealth, and it is currently led by a DNP-prepared nurse as its chief telehealth and innovation officer.[8] This article also states that many of their telehealth specialty sites across the state, such as telestroke, teledermatology, telepediatrics, telepsychiatry, teleneonatology, and telcardiology, are staffed by nurse practitioners.[8] Thus, although the literature is not robust in describing or reporting telehealth clinics or programs developed by APRNs, these clinics do exist (see Chapter 7). APRNs are well positioned to impact patient outcomes because they are embed-ded within communities and should incorporate all aspects of telehealth within their practice.[9] It is, therefore, essential that APRNs be knowledgeable regarding the development and initiation of telehealth programs and services.

PLANNING FOR A TELEHEALTH PROGRAM

In order to successfully develop and implement a telehealth program, it is imperative that the APRN follow specific steps. Research indicates that if proper planning is not done prior to imple-mentation, the telehealth program will be less likely to succeed or be sustainable.[10] The minimum steps include identifying the purpose of the program and the populations to be served, the type of program that will be used, the stakeholders, the skills needed, the technology and resources required, and the barriers to overcome.

Purpose/Populations

When deciding to develop or welcome telehealth into a practice, decision makers must first ask themselves: Why should telehealth be implemented? What is the vision and the specific goals that is being sought? These goals will dictate the business model that will be used and assist with the development of a strategic plan.[11,12] Examples of telehealth care models are access to care, cost savings, and access to market.[11]

The access to care model serves to increase access to health care in areas that have barriers to health care, such as those populations in rural or remote geographical locations. When using this model, providers and/or decision makers must consider what type of care this population needs, such as primary care (limited or through the lifespan), high-risk pregnancy, or chronic disease management. Due to the geographical nature of some populations, plans must include strategies for reaching the populations. Should a satellite office be established in the area being accessed? Should a relationship be developed with a local clinic or hospital?

Is the main goal for telehealth reducing the overall cost of health care? With the cost savings model, the overall goal is to provide health care to populations that typically incur expenses for travel or who have limited resources. An example of the cost savings model is providing care to inmates,[13] thus removing the need for the prisoners to be transported to a clinic or hospital. Other populations that could benefit from this model include patients of skilled nursing facilities[14] or children with special needs.[15] Bringing health care to these populations via telehealth would eliminate the time and expense for travel, which can be complex related to the need to have vehicles with wheelchair access. School-based clinics can also benefit from telehealth,[16] both economically and medically, because a provider can be located within one school or office and offer care for children located in multiple schools within the same day.

A positive correlation exists between telehealth and increased type of care that can be offered. Developing and implementing a telehealth clinic that brings specialist consultation to a population is an example of the access to market model. Does a community have a high incidence of diabetes? Providing diabetes management and education, as well as RPM, via telehealth has been shown to be cost-effective while increasing patient self-management and compliance.[17,18] This is well received overall by patients[19] but requires patient engagement to be successful.[20] Specialists can also be brought into the school setting either asynchronously[21] or synchronously.[22]

Once the population that will be served is identified and the type of telehealth model is selected, it will be important to perform a health needs assessment to determine accessibility, perception, and affordability.[10] Examining data and trends of health care availability, accessibility, and use are important and should be guided by the community or patient needs rather than the provider or the technology.[10] The key processes in performing a health needs assessment are to discuss and gain advice and approval from key stakeholders; acquire data regarding the community or population, both quantitative and qualitative; identify, analyze, and comprehend the areas of greatest need or impact; and research literature or current trends that potentially can offer solutions to the community's needs.[10,23] Data can be gathered through mechanisms such as surveys, interviews, and/or focus groups.

Type of Program

Once a clear vision has been created and a health needs assessment performed, the next step is to determine what type of telehealth program or service would offer the greatest number of benefits to the population of interest. There are different types of telehealth services that can be developed, including live videoconferencing (synchronous), store-and-forward technology (asynchronous), teleconsultation (asynchronous vs synchronous), telemonitoring, RPM, mobile health (mHealth), and tele-education. Based on the desired service, equipment and technology needs will vary. An important concept to remember is that telehealth does not change standard of care; therefore, providing care via telehealth should be the same as providing care in person. It should offer quality care that is patient centered and evidence based.

Live videoconferencing, or synchronous telehealth, is performed in real time between patient and provider and can include medical peripherals to perform an exam. This telehealth program most closely resembles an in-person clinical visit whereby the provider can perform cardiac, pulmonary, tympanic membrane, funduscopic, oropharynx, dental, and dermatologic exams using medical peripherals. The nurse, patient, or caregiver at the patient site will use the peripherals to obtain patient information while the provider will interpret the findings at the distant site. Synchronous telehealth visits have been found to help reduce health care costs by diverting minor acute complaints from more costly health care options, such as the emergency department.[24] When choosing synchronous televisits, the APRN must consider the following:

- Types of telehealth equipment and peripherals needed at the originating site
- Compatible equipment for the hub or distant sites
- Web-based encounter management portal
- Service agreement for the equipment

- Telehealth-knowledgeable information technology (IT) staff
- Type of vendor
- Knowledge, skills, and training/licensure of both sites
- Assessment of originating site regarding internet availability and room for the equipment

Cost is a huge factor for this telehealth service and can range from hundreds to thousands of dollars for initial setup, contractual service agreements, and links to electronic health records.

Store-and-forward, or asynchronous telehealth, uses stored images, videos, medical histories, laboratory results, and pathological reports that are sent to the provider or specialist to be viewed at a later time. Because real-time audiovisual transmission is not a requirement, cost for this telehealth service is small compared with synchronous telehealth and is based on the type of health care services. For example, assessment of diabetic retinopathy requires a capture device at the originating site and the ability to securely transmit the photos to the specialist at the hub site. Only a device that can read the image and return a secure report is needed at the hub site. There is currently no standard for type of camera or protocol, but the potential of diagnosing diabetic retinopathy early and preserving vision is promising using telehealth.[25] The direct-to-consumer or e-visit platform is the most common type of asynchronous telehealth and is dominated by for-profit organizations.[26] Consumers log on to a portal and answer a series of questions that are guided by algorithms using evidence-based guidelines. These answers are then sent to a provider for review, who will either diagnose and treat the patient or request a synchronous or in-person visit. Typically, the e-visit platform is only used for low acuity complaints and for patients aged 2 years or older. These e-visits can be used in an emergency department or primary care setting to decrease patient overflow while still maintaining quality health care and a provider-patient relationship.

Teleconsultation can use both synchronous and asynchronous modalities. Visits where live videoconferencing is needed, such as telemental health or specialist consultation, can be performed using the synchronous telehealth service. Telemental health can be used with various types of patients, such as adolescents, veterans, and older adults, and various types of diagnoses, such as post-traumatic stress disorder, victimization, domestic violence, and depression. Asynchronous visits can also be used to address health care concerns, such as consultation on a particular type of rash by a dermatologist where the primary care provider takes a picture of the rash and sends the image for review. Teleconsultation can be integrated into a primary or acute care setting to expand services that are offered to the patient population.

Telemonitoring and RPM both allow the provider to monitor patients remotely and closely observe for any changes that may warrant a call or visit (either in person or via telehealth). The difference between them is that telemonitoring is more often used to monitor patients within the inpatient setting, such as an intensive care unit, where a team of providers administer care.[27] RPM, also known as *home health monitoring*, occurs when health monitors and biosensors are used to send information to the provider or case manager. An example of the use of RPM is daily monitoring of weight, oxygen saturations, heart rate, and blood pressure for recently discharged patients with CHF. One nurse practitioner–led clinic used RPM devices, including a blood pressure cuff, pulse oximeters, and scales, to collect data, which were then transmitted to the nurse practitioner daily for review.[5] When any of the parameters fell outside of acceptable limits, the nurse practitioner would call the patients to discuss symptoms and any concerns, and an in-person nurse practitioner visit was made if warranted. The 4-month pilot study demonstrated a 9% 30-day readmission rate for patients with CHF, well below the 23% national average for Medicare patients.[5] RPM has also been used for monitoring HbA1c of diabetic patients,[20] electrocardiogram snapshots for patients with implantable cardiac monitors,[28] and vital signs and subjective feelings of health in older adults.[29]

mHealth is the use of technology, such as smartphones, smart watches, and tablets, to provide health care and preventive services to patients. Approximately 83% of physicians already use mHealth technologies for their patients.[30] A recent survey showed that 81% of Americans have smartphones and approximately 50% own tablets.[31] Another survey showed that 30% of US consumers own some type of fitness band, and, of those, 44% used it daily to track their biometric data (eg, number of steps, heart rate, sleep cycle).[32] According to the literature, in 2018 there were approximately 318,000 health apps available to consumers via an app store.[33] However, both providers and patients need to be cautious when using or recommending mHealth apps because few are developed by medical teams or regulated by the US Food and Drug Administration and may actually be inaccurate and ineffective, resulting in lack of expected outcomes and possible provider liability (see Chapter 5).[34]

Tele-education is an excellent modality for providing education and support for self-efficacy to providers, caregivers, and families. Project Extension for Community Health Outcomes, known as Project ECHO, uses the tele-education modality to provide education to remote or rural health care providers by specialists of academic medical centers using a hub-and-spoke model.[35] Specialists (hub site) meet with primary care providers (spoke sites) to review cases and discuss such things as differential diagnoses and plans of care. Project ECHO has been shown to be effective in educating rural providers and increasing access to care for their patient populations.[36] Continuing education credits can also be provided to providers, staff, or organizations using synchronous (eg, webinars) or asynchronous (eg, on-demand videos) modalities. Caregivers, families, and patients can also benefit from tele-education and should be considered when developing a telehealth program. Research has shown increased patient heath care outcomes with the use of tele-education. For example, one pilot study used a computer-based system to provide education and guidance to caregivers of patients with dementia. Results suggested that the program was beneficial in reducing caregiver burden.[37] Another study illustrated that videoconferencing using a mobile phone, also known as mHealth coaching, throughout a weight loss program resulted in greater weight loss as compared with videoconferencing at the beginning and end of the program.[38]

Stakeholders

Gaining cooperation and approval from stakeholders for a telehealth project is necessary, but who exactly are the stakeholders? This depends on the type of telehealth service to be developed and implemented, what population will be served, and how the telehealth services will be provided, as well as the community at the prospective site (Table 6-1). Regardless of who the stakeholders are, they should be involved in all phases of program development, implementation, and outcomes assessment. Core stakeholders for any type of telehealth program will include the clinical team, administrative and support staff, IT and legal teams, patients or patient groups (eg, in prisons or skilled nursing facilities), and other health care providers (eg, hospitals, local providers, specialty practices).

Identifying Telehealth Skills

As with any new technology, identifying and obtaining training on the proper use of telehealth equipment is important (see Chapter 3). Once a telehealth service, platform, and equipment are chosen, the next step is training and should include all those who will participate in the telehealth program. In addition to training on the mechanics of telehealth, participants must also be trained on telehealth etiquette and professionalism.

Telehealth equipment training will depend on the telehealth program and what telehealth services will be offered. Typically, equipment training is provided by the vendor. This training is often limited to installing and using the equipment. It often does not address the use from the provider's clinical perspective. It is important to have an IT team who will become intimately knowledgeable about the equipment in order to effectively troubleshoot any technical issues. The role of telehealth participants also needs to be defined, and they must also receive appropriate training to function in roles such as teleprovider, teleconsultant, or telepresenter. All roles should include training on

TABLE 6-1

POTENTIAL STAKEHOLDERS BASED ON TELEMEDICINE SERVICE

TELECONSULTATION	SCHOOL-BASED CLINIC	REMOTE PATIENT MONITORING	TELE-EDUCATION
Specialist Telepresenter IT support team Support staff (eg, scheduler, nurse, billing) Legal team (consents) Patients Families Primary care provider	School officials School nurse or telepresenter (or school nurse liaison) Primary care provider IT support team Legal team (consents) Scheduler Patients Caregivers Community	Biometric sensor or mHealth developer IT support team Case manager Support staff Data collection staff	Expert Administrative staff Support staff IT support team Distant/local participating providers

technical skills, such as how to prepare a room for an originating or distant site, how to check and prepare the equipment, proper use of the telehealth platform, proper use of telehealth equipment and its peripherals (if used), and proper medical training of the telepresenter if virtual physical exams will be performed.

Telehealth education can be provided using consultants, websites/webinars, modules, and certification programs. South Carolina's Area Health Education Center offers several telehealth-related on-demand webinars, such as "Foundations of Telehealth" and "Telehealth Billing and Reimbursement Bootcamp," as well as a telepresenter certification course. These courses are usually available gratis for those who register on their site.

To ensure that the telehealth team practices within the scope of practice as outlined by the profession, the team members should be aware of strategies specific to this modality of care. The American Telemedicine Association offers guidelines for various types of providers and types of telehealth services on their website, including core operations for provider-patient interactions, tele–intensive care unit operations, operation procedures for pediatric telehealth, telestroke, and pediatric telemental health.

Telehealth etiquette and professionalism are also important skills for providers to be familiar with. As mentioned earlier in the chapter, telehealth does not change care or scope of practice; it is simply a different way of providing care. There has been criticism that this modality of care has the potential to negatively impact the provider-patient relationship.[39] Therefore, when performing a televisit, the provider should maintain a good "webside" manner via good communications skills, which is expressed not only in the words that are used but how those words are delivered via tone of voice and body language.[40] Performing a synchronous visit should not project the perception of disinterest by the provider for the patient, but rather providers should be active listeners and empathetic. Telehealth etiquette includes such things as being well positioned in front of the camera so the patient can clearly view the provider's face, wearing solid-colored or muted-patterned clothing, having a neutral background, looking at the camera during communication to give the impression of direct eye contact, and minimizing any kind of disruptions (see Chapter 8).

Technology and Resources Needed

When setting up a telehealth program, technology and resources will be needed, including personnel, equipment, network, funding, and expertise. Organizations can be used as a resource for gathering data, identifying needs, and providing support for telehealth ventures. Several organizations exist that provide information related to telehealth, including the following:

- American Telemedicine Association
- Center for Connected Health Policy
- National Consortium of Telehealth Resource Centers
- Center for Telehealth and e-Health Law
- Healthcare Information and Management Systems Society

Personnel

Setting up a telehealth team is an important ingredient for success. The team members need individualized special skill sets in order to accomplish the goals of the program. Skills are needed in the areas of administration, IT, finance, legal, and clinical care.[41] The administration team's responsibilities include managing contracts, identifying telehealth regulations specific to the desired program, communicating between all members, and scheduling. The IT team should be responsible for installing and updating the equipment, assessing broadband availability for both the originating and distant sites, installing dedicated telehealth circuits at the originating sites, and troubleshooting technical problems. Evaluation of telehealth reimbursement and formulation of a business plan to include payment systems will be the responsibility of the financial team. Legal advisors will be used for regulatory issues related to the telehealth program, as well as review of processes and any type of consent development. Finally, the clinical team assists with the development of protocols and workflows, identification of training needs for staff, and evaluation outcomes for both the program and the patients.

Equipment

Equipment needs will be dependent on the type of telehealth program created and should be carefully considered before purchasing. Available telehealth equipment consists of hardware (eg, computer, laptop, handheld device), audiovisual equipment (eg, camera, display monitor, headphones, microphone, speakers), power supply at originating and distant sites, networking routers, devices (eg, house sensors, biosensors, implantable medical devices, wearables, health monitors), and telepresence robots.[27] A needs assessment for the program would be beneficial, identifying and correlating the goals (short and long term) with the technology that will satisfy them.[41] Vendors can be found online, through recommendations from similar programs or via networking, and during conferences where telehealth is a topic. It is encouraged that the APRNs visit sites where the prospective equipment is being used. They should inquire about provider, practice, and patient satisfaction with the equipment and vendors; benefits to its use; barriers they have encountered and how they have been overcome; support from suppliers/vendors; how the equipment is being used; and resources needed. The APRN should be comfortable with the vendor and receive reasonable follow-up before purchasing the equipment. It will also be important for the APRN to identify potential added costs, such as platform and maintenance fees. Many sites have found that they can operate videoconferencing session by using existing programs such as Zoom. This enables the cost to be minimal; however, the platform must be Health Insurance Portability and Accountability Act (HIPAA) secure.

Network

The purpose of most care provided via telehealth is to reduce health care barriers for rural and remote communities. If the population to be served is in a rural or remote area, then an assessment of broadband connectivity within these communities must be assessed. An optimal business plan can be developed for a telehealth program, but it cannot be realized if there is no way to connect with the population of interest. According to the Pew Research Center, only 63% of the rural population have broadband connectivity in their homes, and this access is typically slower than urban areas.[42] The Federal Communications Commission is attempting to overcome this digital divide through its Connect America Fund Phase II and will allocate funds in order to provide fixed broadband services to certain eligible areas across the United States.[43] Some telehealth vendors attempt to overcome this lack of broadband connectivity by providing connectivity through cellular networks; therefore, this may be an option for the telehealth program if broadband availability is an issue.

Funding

The telehealth program business plan should include a detailed budget, including overhead expenses, staff salary and benefits, and telehealth equipment cost. Depending on the telehealth program, equipment can be expensive and can include initial cost of the equipment and its annual maintenance/platform fees. Instead of using personal monies to fund the telehealth program, attempts should be made to find funding that aligns with the program's mission and goals. This funding can be through investments, collaborative relationships, patient encounters, and grants. The Health Resources and Services Administration, National Institutes of Health, and Rural Health Information Hub provide information on various grant opportunities.

Experts

The final type of resource that should be sought during the planning phase of the telehealth program is relationships with experts in the field. These collaborators can be a wealth of information, providing information regarding how their programs are successful, and may help identify and address potential barriers. Experts can be found at conferences, organizations, or meetings that provide telehealth components; via word of mouth; and through literature searches to identify those authors who report on pilot programs that are similar to the proposed one.

FOR REFLECTION 1:

Implementing a Telehealth Program

 You have been asked to start a telehealth program in order to better meet the needs of the patients served by your practice. The practice has noticed that those patients who have to travel a long distance tend to miss appointments and only return when they are in crisis. Choose a patient population and describe the steps you would take in order to get the program started. Focus on the type of program that will be used, the stakeholders, the skills needed, the technology and resources required, and the barriers to overcome.

Legal and Regulatory Issues/Reimbursement

During planning of a telehealth program, APRNs must be cognizant of telehealth laws and policies of their state. APRNs must seek this information within the state where they practice, as well as where the patient resides. There are some professions that are allowed to practice over state lines, whereas others are restricted from other states. Telehealth laws and policies vary between states[44] and can include such topics as licensure, credentialing and privileges, reimbursement, malpractice insurance, fraud and abuse, and patient privacy and security.[45] See Chapter 5 for more details.

Licensing

Receiving approval for a nurse practitioner license means that a person has completed requirements in order to practice within his or her state of employment. Those nurse practitioners who do not use the telehealth modality typically will only need to be licensed in the state in which they practice. However, telehealth has given nurse practitioners the ability to cross state lines to provide telehealth services to a greater number of people. Nurse practitioners cannot, however, use their home state's license to practice across state lines; therefore, they need to obtain licenses both within the state where they reside and in state(s) where their patients live. Obtaining licenses within multiple states can be cumbersome and expensive, so limiting the telehealth program to a single or few states would be most economical. The National Council of State Boards of Nursing has spearhead the creation of an APRN Compact, similar to the current Nursing Licensure Compact, which will allow APRNs the ability to practice in multiple states.[46] In order for the APRN Compact to go into effect, 10 states need to enact the legislation; to date, only 3 states—Idaho, Wyoming, and North Dakota—have done so.[46]

Credentialing and Privileging

Credentialing is the process of evaluating an APRN's ability to practice and includes verification of education, licensure, and certification. The process can take several months and is initiated by the employer. Once credentialed, the APRN can bill government agencies (eg, Medicaid, Medicare) and insurance companies for services provided. Following credentialing, an APRN's scope is further defined in a process called *privileging*, which involves evaluation of the APRN's education, credentials, experience, and performance. Both credentialing and privileging can be slightly altered in regard to practicing telehealth. In order to provide telehealth services, the APRN must be credentialed at both the originating and distant sites. This credentialing can be achieved by a full credentialing process at both locations or credentialing by proxy at the originating site.

Credentialing by proxy was created in response to the Medicare Conditions of Participation's knowledge of the difference between providing care in person vs virtually and created a streamline process of credentialing providers that aligned with the guidelines but that was not as extensive as the traditional method.[47] Certain conditions have to be met in order to use credentialing by proxy, including that the distant site must be a Medicare-participating hospital or a telehealth entity, and that there must be establishment of a written agreement between the originating and distant sites.[47] This written agreement must show the following[47]:

- The provider is credentialed and privileged through a program that exceeds Medicare standards.
- The provider is credentialed and privileged at the distant site.
- The distant site has provided the originating site with a copy of the current privileges of the provider.
- The provider is licensed to practice in the state where the originating site is located.
- There has been a review of the services provided by telehealth providers to the distant site.
- The distant site is a contractor of telehealth services to the originating site (this allows the originating site to comply with the Conditions of Participation).

Although credentialing by proxy offers time and cost saving benefits over the full credentialing process for hospitals, the Foley & Lardner 2017 Telemedicine and Digital Health Survey showed that only 33% of hospitals that responded used credentialing by proxy regarding telehealth services.[47]

Reimbursement

Businesses are driven by the profit margin, and health care is no different. Health care receives most of its funding from insurance reimbursements made by both government and private payers. This holds true for telehealth reimbursements as well; however, legal policy is a major influence. Medicare and Medicaid reimbursement of telehealth services is very complex and can be difficult to interpret.

Telehealth services covered by Medicare have several restrictions, including originating site location, types of originating site facility, types of codes used, and telehealth modality used. The patient's location (originating site) at the time of service has to be in a Health Professional Shortage Area or in a county outside of any Metropolitan Statistical Area.[48] Medicare made some exceptions to this geographical restriction in 2019 to include the treatment of substance use disorder or a co-occurring mental health disorder; diagnosis, evaluation, and treatment of an acute stroke; and treatment in renal dialysis centers for the end-stage renal disease services.[49] In addition to the location of the originating site, the type of originating site is limited by Medicare as well and includes provider offices, hospitals (including critical access), rural health clinics, Federally Qualified Health Centers (FQHCs), skilled nursing facilities, community mental health centers, and renal dialysis centers (hospital based or critical access hospital based).[48]

In addition to the location and type of telehealth services, reimbursement is dependent on Current Procedural Terminology (CPT) or Healthcare Common Procedure Coding System (HCPCS) codes.[48] These codes are based on the types of services provided to patients and can change annually. Finally, Medicare will only cover services rendered via synchronous telehealth, except for specific programs located in Alaska and Hawaii, or with some RPM servies.[48] It is also important to note that Medicare lists specific types of providers who are able to perform telehealth services. These include physicians, APRNs, physician assistants, nurse midwives, clinical nurse specialists, certified registered nurse anesthetists, clinical psychologist, and registered dietitians.[48] These Medicare rules can be confusing; therefore, the Health Resources and Services Administration created a tool to help providers determine whether an address is qualified for Medicare telehealth reimbursement.

Telehealth visits also require proper patient documentation, similar to what is required for in-person visits. The visit should include chief complaint, history, review of systems, exam findings, diagnosis, and plan of care. It is recommended that the virtual visit should also include a statement that services were provided via telehealth, whether the visit was synchronous or asynchronous, location of the patient, location of the provider, time of initiation and completion, and names and roles of all participants (eg, provider, support staff, originating site telepresenter).[50]

To file a Medicare claim, providers must use proper documentation, including approved CPT and HCPCS codes and Place of Service 02 code, which indicates a telehealth service.[50] Originating sites can also submit a Medicare claim and receive payment for a facility fee intended for the telehealth service using the code Q3014.[50] This fee is the lesser of the amount that equals 80% of the actual charge or 80% of the originating site facility fee.[50]

Medicaid has control at the state level regarding telehealth reimbursement within their programs, as well as having significant influence over private payer laws. Because states have flexibility in covering and reimbursing telehealth services, the reimbursement can vary across state lines (Table 6-2).[51] Key findings from the Center for Connected Health Policy's most recent report (May 2019) on telehealth laws and reimbursement policies include the following[52]:

- 50 states and Washington DC reimburse for some types of synchronous visits
- 11 states reimburse for asynchronous visits

TABLE 6-2

LISTING OF PARITY LAWS BY STATE AS OF 2018 AND SERVICES COVERED BY MEDICAID

TELEMEDICINE PARITY LAW

- Arizona[S,A,R]
- Arkansas[S]
- California[S,A]
- Colorado[S,R,H]
- Connecticut[S,A]
- Delaware[S,H]
- District of Columbia[S,A*,R*]
- Georgia[S,A]
- Hawaii[S,A*,G]
- Indiana[S,R]
- Iowa[S]
- Kansas[S,R]

- Louisiana[S,R]
- Maryland[S,A,R,G,H]
- Mssachusetts[S]
- Michigan[S,H]
- Minnesota[S,A,R,G,H]
- Mississippi[S,A*]
- Missouri[S,R]
- Montana[S,H]
- Nebraska[S,R]
- Nevada[S,A,H]
- New Hampshire[G,H]
- New Jersey[S,A*]

- New Mexico[S]
- New York[S,A*,H]
- New Mexico[S]
- Oklahoma[S]
- Oregon[S,R]
- South Dakota[S,G]
- Tennessee[S]
- Texas[S,R,H]
- Vermont[S,R,H]
- Virginia[S,A,R]
- Washington[S,A,R,H]

PROPOSED PARITY BILL

- Alaska[S,A,R]
- Maine[S,R]
- Pennsylvania[S]
- Rhode Island[S]
- South Dakota[S]

NO PARITY LEGISLATIVE ACTIVITY

- Alabama[S,R]
- Florida[S]
- Idaho[S]
- Illinois[S,R]
- North Carolina[S]
- Ohio[S]

- South Carolina[S,R,H]
- Utah[S,R]
- West Virginia[S]
- Wisconsin[S]
- Wyoming[S,H]

A, asynchronous visits; G, geographic restrictions; H, home allowed as originating site; R, remote patient monitoring, S, synchronous visits; *, law in place but no supporting policy or not written into budget yet.

Adapted from Center for Connected Health Policy. State telehealth laws & reimbursement policies. https://www.telehealthpolicy.us/sites/default/files/2019-05/cchp_report_MASTER_spring_2019_FINAL.pdf. Published Spring 2019. Accessed February 21, 2020 and American Telemedicine Association. State policy resource center. http://legacy.americantelemed.org/main/policy-page/state-policy-resource-center. Accessed February 21, 2020.

- 23 states place restrictions on the facility type of the originating site
- 34 states offer telehealth facility fee for the originating site
- 39 states and Washington DC have parity laws in place that oversee private payer telehealth reimbursements
- 14 states allow the home to be designated as an originating site but specify that no facility fee charge is permitted

This reimbursement information applies to Medicare/Medicaid and may or may not be applicable to private payers. It is therefore important for an APRN to be familiar with telehealth parity, which means that telehealth visits are covered by health plans the same as an in-person visit is. Not all states have parity laws (see Table 6-2). This can affect reimburse payments because individual private payers can dictate how much they will pay for a telehealth visit.

Malpractice

There is limited information available for providers regarding telehealth-specific malpractice insurance. This stems from the fact that telehealth is a rapidly growing health care modality and there is not enough information to perform a telehealth risk assessment adequately enough to develop coverage.[53] Center for Telehealth and e-Health Law reviewed a significant number of telehealth-related malpractice claims and discovered that the majority stemmed from the provider prescribing across state lines without previously examining the patient.[54] APRNs need to be familiar with the Ryan Haight Online Pharmacy Consumer Protection Act, which prohibits the prescribing of controlled substances online; however, telehealth providers have an exception that states that they must examine the patient at least once in person.[55] APRNs must also be knowledgeable about their state laws regarding telehealth visits and online prescribing. The best advice to preventing malpractice claims is to ensure that the scope of practice does not differ between virtual and in-person visits and that state practice guidelines are being followed. However, APRNs should consider telehealth-specific malpractice coverage and should consult with individual medical insurance companies to investigate possible telehealth coverage, whether it will incur an additional cost or rider, and whether it will extend across state lines.[45]

If a program is being developed as part of an FQHC, the Federal Tort Claims Act may not offer telehealth malpractice coverage. Three conditions must be met in order to be eligible for Federal Tort Claims Act: (a) the provider must work full-time (≥ 32.5 hours/week) unless practicing family medicine, general internal medicine, general pediatrics, obstetrics, or gynecology; (b) a contract must exist between the FQHC and the provider, not the provider's employer; and (c) compensation for telehealth-related services must be paid directly by the FQHC to the provider, not the provider's employer, and must include a 1099 form to the provider.[56] Essentially, the business relationship must be between the FQHC and the telehealth provider directly, and should not involve a secondary employer.

Fraud and Abuse

When setting up a telehealth program, the provider needs to ensure that the practice does not violate any type of state or federal laws, such as the federal Anti-Kickback Statute and Stark Law. The Anti-Kickback Statute prohibits any type of reward for any type of referrals for any type of items or services that are covered by the federal health care program and is intended to prevent increased cost and overuse, which may result in poor quality of health care and negative patient outcomes.[45] The Stark Law (ie, the Federal Physician Self-Referral Law) prevents providers and their families from referring patients to entities that are owned by the provider or immediate family members for the purpose of financial gain.[45]

Patient Privacy and Security

Protecting patient privacy should be of utmost importance when setting up a telehealth program and involves multiple aspects, including protection of identifiable health information, protection of patients' privacy, and limitation of potential security threats.[57] Telehealth platforms should be HIPAA compliant and ensure that the patients' protected health information is not compromised, as well as ensuring compliance with state privacy, confidentiality, and medical retention rules. In addition to protecting the patients' protected health information, the patients' privacy risks must be assessed. Telehealth comes with some inherent risks, but these risks must be minimized.

One such privacy or security risk involves RPM, where the collected information from home or biomedical sensors can be hacked by third parties. This information can be used to put a patient at risk (eg, room sensors that are intended to monitor movement and potential falls of an older adult can be used to relay information regarding the patient's daily routine and provide knowledge of when the patient is not at home).[57] These security threats should be minimized by using encrypted data, as well as restricting third-party advertisers from collecting and using patients' personal data.[57] Patient privacy should be ensured during a synchronous visit by providing limited access to nonessential personnel at both the originating and distant sites. Telehealth visits should not be performed in a public area, such as a hospital cafeteria or grocery store, because information can be overheard, violating HIPAA rules. Steps must be taken to maintain security when documenting in the electronic health record as part of the visit.

Barriers to Overcome

As with any new technology, barriers exist for the implementation and growth of the care provided by telehealth. Barriers reported through a systematic review of literature included cost, reimbursement, legal liability, privacy and confidentiality, security, effectiveness, efficiency, workflow, rural setting, profit margin, organizational size, implementation models, bandwidth, poor design, technology-hesitant staff for the telehealth team, demographics (ie, age, gender, geographical location, education level, socioeconomic status), resistance to change, lack of awareness, technology illiteracy.[58] Alghantani[59] performed a similar review of telehealth barriers and had similar results, including cost and reimbursement; privacy, security, and confidentiality of the patient; and resistance to change. Some of these barriers are inherent to the technology and will improve with greater use and broadband availability. Others require a restructuring of the workflows and protocols to better streamline the televisits. Policy changes are required for challenges related to profit margin and reimbursement. To increase telehealth adoption by technology-hesitant stakeholders, education and continuous support are key in reducing fear or resistance to change.

FOR REFLECTION 2:

Advanced Practice Registered Nurses as Leaders in Telehealth

Your practice would like to start a telehealth program. It has been agreed that you, as an APRN, would be the best person to lead and champion the program. You want to be sure that you are working within your scope of practice. What steps would you take to make sure you could legally carry, develop, and implement the telehealth programs? What areas would you need to explore?

IMPLEMENTING THE PROGRAM

Once a firm business plan has been created, the next step is to implement the program. The Telehealth Service Implementation Model (TSIM) was created by the Medical University of South Carolina (MUSC) Center for Telehealth, which is 1 of 2 Telehealth Centers of Excellence in the nation. The tool has 4 phases: strategy, design, transition, and operations (Figure 6-1).[60] This chapter has already discussed the development of the strategy and design; therefore, the focus of this section will be on transition and operations.

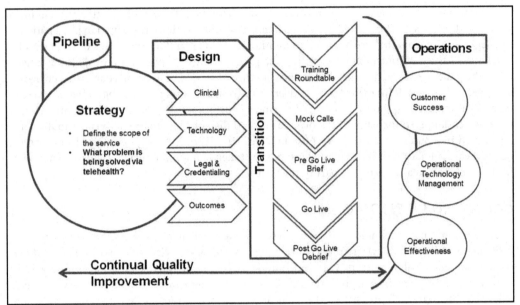

Figure 6-1. Algorithm for planning and implementing a telehealth program. (Reprinted with permission from Center for Connected Health Policy.)

Before going live with the telehealth program, it must first be thoroughly tested in order to identify and rectify any potential problems. Using a synchronous platform as an example, steps to transition should include the following:

- Train providers and support staff on equipment and workflow.
- Initiate several mock calls. It may be beneficial to have a telehealth champion located at both the originating site and the distant site to troubleshoot any technical problems and offer support and encouragement to the telepresenter and teleprovider. Communication between the telehealth team is extremely important during this phase of implementation.
- Set the go-live date.

Once the transition phase has resulted in multiple successful mock calls, the next step is operations. During the operations phase, the telehealth program's goals and business plan are revisited to ensure that the strategies developed are achievable and in alignment with meeting the needs of the patients. Input and buy-in from all stakeholders is key for successful implementation. Those stakeholders who have reservations or are technology hesitant may require extended support and education during the early phase of operations, but their input and recommendations should be valued during the reevaluation of the program's goals. Moreover, although problems were addressed during the transition phase, unpredicted events may occur during the televisits; therefore, a team needs to be in place to address these as soon as possible, which is the process of repeated evaluation and adjustments within a continual quality improvement cycle.[60]

Initially, the number of sites should be limited in order to recognize unplanned events and develop strategies to address them. Expansion of services should be gradual, using the continual quality improvement cycle. During expansion, marketing strategies should be used to bring attention to the new service and address any misconceptions or fears that usually accompany new technology.

PROGRAM EXAMPLE

South Carolina is a mostly rural state, and data show that rural residents have a higher rate of premature death, smoking, obesity, child poverty, and teen births when compared with residents of urban areas.[61,62] South Carolina is currently ranked 36th in the nation in overall health-related metrics.[63] Additionally, children in rural counties in South Carolina have been shown to be less likely to access well-child care and more likely to use tertiary care than those who reside in urban areas. The results of this health care needs assessment led to the expansion of existing brick-and-mortar school-based health clinics (SBHCs) to rural areas through school-based telehealth clinics (tSBHC), with the hope that connecting rural school nurses' offices to APRNs and pediatricians would prove to be both effective and cost-efficient. The pilot program was initiated with the knowledge that a diversity of funders would be necessary and full expansion into every school in one rural county was achieved through a private grant. The private grant allowed the purchase of telehealth equipment.

Internet access can be a huge barrier to successfully implementing a tSBHC, which continues to be a problem for South Carolina residents. Approximately 26% of those people who live in rural areas of South Carolina still do not have adequate internet access.[64,65] However, in 2018, the South Carolina House of Representatives passed a bill that would increase broadband connectivity across the state, supporting the telehealth initiative and increasing health care access to rural communities.[66] Assessment of the broadband connectivity of the chosen area was assessed and was discovered to be minimal; therefore, modular telehealth carts that used low bandwidth were purchased for the purpose of performing synchronous telehealth acute care visits. MUSC's IT team installed dedicated telehealth circuits and carts within the pilot schools. A web-based encounter-management portal or telehealth platform was chosen to ensure a live audiovisual interaction while maintaining patient privacy and HIPAA compliance.

Once the broadband connectivity and the telehealth carts were in place, the school nurses who would be the telepresenters were trained on the equipment and protocols. Workflow procedures and consents were developed. School nurses were also empowered with assessment tools and lab tests to assess for strep throat, urinary infections, and other ailments. Patient consents were reviewed by the legal team at MUSC to ensure that both the patients and the institutions were protected. Mock calls were performed to assess the synchronous communication and troubleshoot any potential problems once the school nurses were comfortable with the process. Go-live dates were set once the school nurses and providers were proficient with the equipment and protocols.

Before the go-live date, members from the tSBHC team and the school nurses, who were integrated fully into the community, attended several back-to-school events to broadcast the news about the school-based telehealth programs. Consents were given to parents to complete during these events and in back-to-school packets. If a child came into the school nurse's office with an acute complaint and she deemed it necessary that the child be seen by a provider, then the parent was notified and a written consent obtained (if one was not obtained at the beginning of the school year) before the televisit occurred. Throughout the pilot program, the protocols, workflows, and consents were modified to better streamline the visits.

By 2013, South Carolina, in search of innovative solutions to combat health care disparities, began appropriating funds to form a centralized Center for Telehealth and a consortium of health care systems and stakeholders to promote the development of telehealth programs. As this support became a recurring item in the state budget, the tSBHC program and others were expected to rapidly expand to meet the needs of the population. The steps toward this rapid program development and expansion mirror those of the TSIM process described here.

Although the strategy and design phases had begun in the pilot, the team, which included an APRN, was tasked with focusing on a value proposition and exploring the 4 aspects of the design phase in more detail. The value of school-based health would first be realized for the state of South Carolina through decreasing health care disparities with longer-term goals of decreasing high-cost use patterns in the most rural areas, which is a combination of the access to care and cost savings models. This helped to focus the expansion effort to areas of highest tertiary care use, with a particular focus on asthma as one of the most common and costly chronic diseases of childhood. Stakeholders at all levels of the socioecological framework were engaged, from state legislators and the State Superintendent and Department of Education, to local school districts, families, and health care providers. The formation of a statewide workgroup and local advisory boards helped with the development of statewide strategy balanced by locally tailored initiatives. Technology choices were guided by the need for low-broadband solutions with high clinical reliability. As the demand for expansion continued, the interest of local providers also likely increased. Simultaneously, it became clear that efficiency was key to engaging busy school nurses. An open access endpoint management system was developed to create a tiered, locally focused call pool, allowing for a rapid response to a school nurse's request for a visit that was first routed to local providers and then to those at increasing distance. Continuity of the medical home was maintained through communication with the primary care provider with every visit.

Successful expansion of the program has also become dependent upon the team's ability to continuously replicate the transition phase with each new school district and eventually to guide local provider groups to do the same. To date, the program has expanded to cover many of the rural areas in the state, with outcomes including high patient satisfaction, achievement of quality metrics, and reduced use of the emergency department in the longest-standing programs (publications pending). APRNs have played various pivotal roles in administration and clinical care throughout the lifespan of the tSBHC program. A lead APRN role was established to help coordinate the clinical providers, lead trainings, and engage school nurses. Additionally, when legal issues arose regarding the South Carolina Nurse Practice Act, the advocacy of large nurse practitioner groups was crucial to the passage of Bill S345, which increased the scope of practice for APRNs and specifically included language to address the use of telehealth. At a macro view, the development of this program mirrors that of many telehealth programs, with the APRN playing a central role as a knowledgeable leader in the care team.

GROUP EXERCISE

Consider the South Carolina school-based telehealth program example and envision the roles of the APRN. How do these roles translate to other telehealth programs? For this activity, divide into 2 groups. Each group should describe and outline a type of telehealth program that addresses a specific outcome: access to care, cost savings, or access to market. Delineate the roles that the APRN can fill in this program.

CONCLUSION

For the APRN to develop a telehealth practice, a systematic process, such as the TSIM model, must to be followed for successful implementation. The first step in this project is analyzing why telehealth would be appropriate for the identified problem and then performing a health care needs assessment to assist in the development of the specific type of telehealth practice that is required to meet the population's needs. Once this is attained, then the APRN should develop a solid business plan, to include creating a detailed telehealth design, gathering stakeholders, researching telehealth laws and billing, and assessing funding options. Pilot testing of the telehealth design is ideal and should include multiple mock calls to recognize and address any technical or staff difficulties. Repeated quality checks are required once the program goes live in order to address and resolve unpredicted events, allowing for slow but steady expansion. It is vital for success that a strategic method is followed.

THOUGHTFUL QUESTIONS

1. Evaluate the current telehealth rules/regulations regarding Medicare/Medicaid and private insurers in your area. What is the feasibility that you, as an independent APRN, will be able to incorporate telehealth within your practice? What possible limitations will you face? Will this impact your ability to provide telehealth services? Why or why not?

2. You currently practice with another APRN in an urban primary care clinic. The APRN has heard of how the telehealth modality can overcome barriers and increase access to care for those living in rural areas. This APRN approaches you with the idea of extending primary care services to a very remote area just outside of the state and believes it can greatly increase the clinic's revenue. What should you and the APRN consider regarding licensure and billing? Should profit be a major factor in incorporating telehealth in your existing practice? Why or why not?

3. You are a new DNP graduate from a school of nursing that has a reputation for successful integration of telehealth education within the program. The interviewer is aware of your telehealth knowledge and believes that you would be an ideal candidate to assist in implementing a school-based telehealth program into 25 schools within the next 6 months. Currently there are a few brick-and-mortar school-based clinics associated with the hospital, but no telehealth. What advice would you provide this organization regarding developing a sustainable telehealth program?

4. You are part of a telehealth team developing a telehealth program between various specialists from the local hospital and the 2 rural primary care clinics. The program is in the transition phase and is currently performing mock calls. Your team encounters some resistance from the staff at one rural primary care clinic, but the other rural clinic is doing well. What are some potential barriers that are occurring, and how can you resolve them? What are some measures that can be implemented if the resistance persists after the go-live date?

CASE STUDY

A new DNP graduate, Brooke, who grew up in a very rural town, understands the complexity of chronic care management because an older sibling died at a young age related to complications from type 1 diabetes. The barriers to care for this family included lack of reliable transportation, gaps in health care literacy, lack of pediatric type 1 diabetes knowledge by the local provider, and a large distance to a pediatric endocrinology clinic (120 miles). Brooke had some exposure to telehealth in graduate school and believes that she can decrease health care barriers in her home town, where she plans to practice primary care with the local physician, who has been practicing in the same office for almost 40 years. To address the various barriers, Brooke develops a plan to develop a telehealth program in the clinic and establish a relationship with cardiology, endocrinology, pulmonology, and dermatology specialists with an academic medical center about 200 miles away, as well as register with Project ECHO to learn more about diabetes management across the lifespan.

(continued)

CASE STUDY (CONTINUED)

Brooke establishes a relationship with the Center for Telehealth in the academic medical center, who has agreed to assist her with the development of her program by assessing the bandwidth availability and installing/maintaining the telehealth cart at the originating site. Brooke is awarded a $100,000 grant for integration of telehealth into a rural community and purchases a telehealth cart with peripherals, as well as some iPads and RPM equipment (blood pressure, glucose, and oxygen saturation monitors). The physician and nurse are a little concerned about how the new program may impact the practice and patients. Brooke realizes that she needs to consider their concerns as she continues with development of her plan because she knows the need is there and the telehealth access to care model would meet the health care necessities of this community.

The clinic is located in a remodeled house that is very old. Extensive wiring is needed in order to install the needed jack and enable broadband connectivity. The telehealth cart and other equipment is delivered and placed in Brooke's office; however, she is unable to set the cart up until she can connect to the internet.

Questions

1. What steps did Brooke take to develop the telehealth program?
2. What barriers did she encounter?
3. What could she have done in order to make this program more easily implemented?
4. How could she enlist the help of the nurse in implementing the program?

REFERENCES

1. Cunningham N, Marshal C, Glazer E. Telemedicine in pediatric primary care: favorable experience in nurse-staffed inner-city clinic. *JAMA.* 1978:240(25):2749-2751.
2. Rau K. NP news. Expanding the NP's role through telemedicine. *Nurse Pract.* 2000:25(4):105-108.
3. Reed K. Telemedicine: benefits to advanced practice nursing and the communities they serve. *J Am Acad Nurse Pract.* 2005;17(5):176-180.
4. Foster PH, Whitworth JM. The role of nurses in telemedicine and child abuse. *Comput Inform Nurs.* 2005;23(3):127-131.
5. Moore JA. Evaluation of the efficacy of a nurse practitioner-led home-based congestive heart failure clinical pathway. *Home Health Care Serv Q.* 2016;35(1):39-51.
6. Veit ST, Chisholm CA, Novicoff WM, Rheuban K, Cohn W. Perinatologists and advanced practice nurses collaborate to provide high-risk prenatal care in rural Virginia communities. *J Obstet Gynecol Neonatal Nurs.* 2014;43(1):s26-s27.
7. Rutledge CM, Haney T, Bordelon M, Renaud M, Fowler C. Telehealth: preparing advanced practice nurses to address healthcare needs in rural and underserved populations. *Int J Nurs Educ Scholarsh.* 2014;11.
8. Henderson K, Davis TC, Smith M, King M. Nurse practitioners in telehealth: bridging the gaps in healthcare delivery. *J Nurs Pract.* 2014;10(10):845-850.
9. Fathi JT, Modin HE, Scott JD. Nurses advancing telehealth services in the era of healthcare reform. *Online J Issues Nurs.* 2017;22(2). doi: 10.3912/OJIN.Vol22No02Man02
10. AlDossary S, Martin-Khan MG, Bradford NK, Armfield NR, Smith AC. The development of a telemedicine planning framework based on needs assessment. *J Med Syst.* 2017;41(5):74.
11. Vanderwerf M. *10 critical steps for a successful telemedicine program.* AMD Global Telemedicine. https://www.amdtelemedicine.com/downloads/10_steps.pdf. Accessed February 21, 2020.
12. Kamenca A. *Telemedicine: A Practical Guide for Professionals.* Phoenix, AZ: MindView Press; 2017.
13. Senanayake B, Wickramasinghe SI, Eriksson L, Smith AC, Edirippulige S. Telemedicine in the correctional setting: a scoping review. *J Telemed Telecare.* 2018;24(10):669-675.
14. Chess D, Whitman JJ, Croll D, Stefanacci R. Impact of after-hours telemedicine on hospitalizations in a skilled nursing facility. *Am J Manag Care.* 2018;24(8):385-388.

15. Hooshmand M, Yao K. Challenges facing children with special healthcare needs and their families: telemedicine as a bridge to care. *Telemed J E Health.* 2017;23(1):18-24.

16. McConnochie KM, Wood NE, Herendeen NE, ten Hoopen CB, Roghmann KJ. Telemedicine in urban and suburban childcare and elementary schools lightens family burdens. *Telemed J E Health.* 2010;16(5):533-542.

17. Zhai YK, Zhu WJ, Cai YL, Sun DX, Zhao J. Clinical- and cost-effectiveness of telemedicine in type 2 diabetes mellitus: a systematic review and meta-analysis. *Medicine (Baltimore).* 2014;93(28):e312.

18. Ramchandani N. Virtual coaching to enhance diabetes care. *Diabetes Technol Ther.* 2019;21(S2):S248-S251.

19. Rodríguez-Fortúnez P, Franch-Nadal J, Fornos-Pérez JA, Martínez-Martínez F, de Paz HD, Orera-Peña ML. Cross-sectional study about the use of telemedicine for type 2 diabetes mellitus management in Span: patient's perspective. The EnREDa2 study. *BMJ Open.* 2019;9(6):e028467.

20. Su D, Michaud TL, Estabrooks P, et al. Diabetes management through remote patient monitoring: the importance of patient activation and engagement with the technology. *Telemed J E Health.* 2019;25(10):952-959.

21. Tye ML, Honey M, Day K. School-based telemedicine: perceptions about a telemedicine model of care. *Stud Health Technol Inform.* 2017;245:1239.

22. Halterman JS, Fagnano M, Tajon RS, et al. Effect of the school-based telemedicine enhanced asthma management (SB-TEAM) program on asthma morbidity: a randomized clinical trial. *JAMA Pediatr.* 2018;172(3):e174938.

23. Wright J, Williams R, Wilkinson JR. Development and importance of health needs assessment. *BMJ.* 1998;316(7140):1310-1313.

24. Nord G, Rising KL, Band RA, Carr BG, Hollander JE. On-demand synchronous audio video telemedicine visits are cost effective. *Am J Emerg Med.* 2019;37(5):890-894.

25. Horton MB, Silvia PS, Cavallerano JD, Aiello LP. (2016). Clinical components of telemedicine programs for diabetic retinopathy. *Cur Diabet Report.* 2016;16(12), 1-10.

26. Elliot T, Shih J. Direct to consumer telemedicine. *Curr Allergy Asthma Rep.* 2019;19(1):1.

27. Bhattacharyya SB. *A DIY Guide to Telemedicine for Clinicians.* Gateway East, Singapore: Springer Nature; 2018.

28. Versteeg H, Timmermans I, Widdershoven J, et al. Effect of remote monitoring on patient-reported outcomes in European heart failure patients with an implantable-cardioverter-defibrillator: primary results of the REMOTE-CIED randomized trial. *EP Euorpace.* 2019;21(9):1360-1368.

29. Hamilton T, Johnson L, Quinn BT, et al. Telehealth intervention programs for seniors: an observational study of a community-embedded health monitoring initiative [published online ahead of print April 17, 2019]. *Telemed J E Heath.*

30. Athenahealth. What is mobile technology? https://www.athenahealth.com/knowledge-hub/healthcare-technology/what-is-mobile-health-technology/healthcare. Accessed February 21, 2020.

31. Pew Research Center. Mobile fact sheet. https://www.pewinternet.org/fact-sheet/mobile/. Published June 12, 2019. Accessed February 21, 2020.

32. Liu S. Fitness & activity tracker – statistics & facts. https://www.statista.com/topics/4393/fitness-and-activity-tracker/. Published May 22, 2019. Accessed February 21, 2020.

33. Liquid State. The rise of mHealth apps: a market snapshot. https://liquid-state.com/mhealth-apps-market-snapshot/. Published March 26, 2018. Accessed February 21, 2020.

34. Larson RS. A path to better-quality mHealth apps. *JMIR Mhealth Uhealth.* 2018;6(7):e10414.

35. University of Mexico. Project ECHO. https://echo.unm.edu/. Accessed February 21, 2020.

36. Zhou C, Crawford A, Serhal E, Kurdyak P, Sockalingam S. The impact of Project ECHO on participants and patient outcomes: a systematic review. *Acad Med.* 2016;91(10):1439-1461.

37. Gustafson DH, Gustafson DH, Cody OJ, Chin MY, Johnston DC, Asthana S. Pilot test of a computer-based system to help family caregivers of dementia patients. *J Alzheimers Dis.* 2019;70(2):541-552.

38. Alencar MK, Johnson K, Mullur R, Gracy V, Gutierrez E, Korosteleva O. The efficacy of a telemedicine-based weight loss program with video conference health coaching support. *J Telemed Telecare.* 2019;25(3):151-157.

39. Terry C, Cain J. The emerging issue of digital empathy. *Am J Pharm Educ.* 2016;80(4):58.

40. McCormick M. What makes a good telemedicine physician? Three essential qualities. https://www.eagletelemedicine.com/what-makes-a-good-telemedicine-physician-three-essential-qualities. Eagle Telemedicine. Published July 23, 2018. Accessed February 21, 2020.

41. American Academy of Pediatrics. Getting started in telehealth. https://www.aap.org/en-us/professional-resources/practice-transformation/telehealth/Pages/Getting-Started-in-Telehealth.aspx. Accessed February 21, 2020.

42. Perrin A. Digital gap between rural and nonrural America persists. Pew Research Center. https://www.pewresearch.org/fact-tank/2019/05/31/digital-gap-between-rural-and-nonrural-america-persists/. Published May 31, 2019. Accessed February 21, 2020.

43. Federal Communications Commission. Connect America fund phase II auction (auction 903). https://www.fcc.gov/auction/903. Updated February 20, 2020. Accessed February 21, 2020.

44. Garber KM, Chike-Harris KE. Nurse practitioners and virtual care: a 50-state review of APRN telehealth law and policy. *Telehealth and Medicine Today.* 2019;4:1-8.

45. Balestra M. Telehealth and legal implications for nurse practitioners. *J Nurse Pract.* 2018;14(1):33-39.

46. National Council of State Boards of Nursing. APRN Compact. https://www.ncsbn.org/aprn-compact.htm. Accessed February 21, 2020.

47. Lacktman NM. Telemedicine credentialing by proxy: what hospitals and telehealth companies need to know. https://www.foley.com/en/insights/publications/2018/02/telemedicine-credentialing-by-proxy-what-hospitals. Published February 19, 2018. Accessed February 21, 2020.

48. Center for Connected Health Policy. National policy: telehealth and Medicare. https://www.cchpca.org/telehealth-policy/telehealth-and-medicare. Accessed February 21, 2020.

49. Centers for Medicare & Medicaid Services. Telehealth services. MGMA. https://www.cms.gov/outreach-and-education/medicare-learning-network-mln/mlnproducts/downloads/telehealthsrvcsfctsht.pdf. Published January 2019. Accessed February 21, 2020.

50. Lunt S. Navigating telehealth billing requirements. https://www.mgma.com/resources/financial-management/navigating-telehealth-billing-requirements. Accessed February 21, 2020.

51. Centers for Medicare & Medicaid Services. Telemedicine. https://www.medicaid.gov/medicaid/benefits/telemed/index.html. Accessed February 21, 2020.

52. Center for Connected Health Policy. State telehealth laws and reimbursement policies. https://www.telehealthpolicy.us/sites/default/files/2019-05/cchp_report_MASTER_spring_2019_FINAL.pdf. Published Spring 2019. Accessed February 21, 2020.

53. American Telemedicine Association. State policy resource center. http://legacy.americantelemed.org/main/policy-page/state-policy-resource-center. Accessed February 21, 2020.

54. Matray M. Telemedicine malpractice insurance. Cunningham Group. https://www.cunninghamgroupins.com/telemedicine/. Accessed February 21, 2020.

55. Natoli CM. Summary of findings: malpractice and telemedicine. Center for Telehealth and e-Health Law. http://www.ctel.org/research/Summary%20of%20Findings%20Malpractice%20and%20Telemedicine.pdf. Published December 2009. Accessed February 21, 2020.

56. Lacktman NM, Ferrante TB. Congress proposes change to Ryan Haight Act to allow telemedicine prescribing of controlled substances. https://www.foley.com/en/insights/publications/2018/03/congress-proposes-change-to-ryan-haight-act-to-all. Published March 5, 2018. Accessed February 21, 2020.

57. Hall JL, McGraw D. For telehealth to succeed, privacy and security risks must be identified and addressed. *Health Aff (Millwood)*. 2014;33(2):216-221.

58. Scott Kruse C, Karem P, Shifflett K, Vegi L, Ravi K, Brooks M. Evaluating barriers to adopting telemedicine worldwide: a systematic review. *J Telemed Telecare*. 2018;24(1):4-12.

59. Alghatani KM. Telemedicine implementation: barriers and recommendations. *Journal of Scientific Research and Studies*. 2016;3(7):140-145.

60. Medical University of South Carolina. Telehealth Service Implementation Model (TSIM): a framework for telehealth service development, implementation, and sustainability. https://muschealth.org/-/sm/health/telehealth/f/tsim-summary.ashx?la=en. Accessed February 21, 2020.

61. South Carolina Institute of Medicine and Public Health. New rankings shed light on where South Carolina counties could improve health. http://imph.org/2016countyhealthrankingssc/. Accessed February 21, 2020.

62. *US News and World Report*. Best states: South Carolina. https://www.usnews.com/news/best-states/south-carolina. Accessed February 21, 2020.

63. South Carolina Institute of Medicine and Public Health. South Carolina rural health report. http://imph.org/wp-content/uploads/2011/08/rural-health-report.pdf. Accessed February 21, 2020.

64. Wildeman MK. SC continues to invest in telehealth, but internet connections lag. *The Post and Courier*. https://www.postandcourier.com/business/sc-continues-to-invest-in-telehealth-but-internet-connections-lag/article_231c8572-349f-11e9-b4e9-ef122b41ecb2.html. Published March 3, 2019. Accessed February 21, 2020.

65. Barton T. SC House passes bill to expand high-speed internet access in rural areas that need it. *The State*. https://www.thestate.com/news/politics-government/article228793939.html. Published April 5, 2019. Accessed February 21, 2020.

66. Advanced practice registered nurses, scope and standards of practice. S.345, 122nd Sess, 2017-2018 (SC 2018).

7

Advanced Practice Registered Nurse Telehealth Practice Modalities

Patty Alane Schweickert, DNP, FNP-C
Lynn Wiles, PhD, RN
Katherine E. Chike-Harris, DNP, APRN, CPNP-PC, NE
R. Lee Tyson, DNP, PMHNP-BC, ANP-BC
Tonya L. Hensley, DNP, FNP
Kathryn B. Reid, PhD, FNP-C
Rosalyn Perkins, MNSc, CNP, WHNP-BC
Rebecca A. Bates, DNP, FNP-C
S. Craig Thomas, MSN, NP, ACNP-BC, ACNS-BC, CHFN
Teresa Gardner Tyson, DNP, FNP-BC
Brian Myers, MBA, MTS
Allison Kirkner, MSN, RN, ACNP-BC

CHAPTER OBJECTIVES

Upon review of this chapter, the reader will be able to:

1. Compare how the traditional scope of nursing practice and nursing competencies align with telehealth nursing practice.
2. Identify how telehealth can provide relief for the provider shortage and extend provider capacity.
3. Examine how patient satisfaction affects traditional care and telehealth care.
4. Describe how the advanced practice registered nurse (APRN) actualizes telehealth nursing through telehealth use cases.

Schweickert PA, Rutledge CM, eds.
Telehealth Essentials for Advanced Practice Nursing (pp 141-169).
© 2020 Taylor & Francis Group.

As APRNs embrace telehealth technology, it must align with traditional scope of practice and nursing competencies. As nurses use and experience telehealth, they will identify aspects that are meaningful for enhancing the telehealth patient care experience. Patient satisfaction measurements began as a way to measure quality of care by quantifying satisfaction, creating a new arena for health care. Patient satisfaction is now tied to the Centers for Medicare and Medicaid Services (CMS) Value-Based Purchasing Program and Private Payor Initiatives.[1] Patient satisfaction data denote perceptions of quality care and quality patient care experiences, all of which are meaningful for evaluating care and implementing change. Engaging with the technology is only part of the telehealth experience because the meaning of care is derived from the outcomes. Patient-centered care is key to improved outcomes, and establishing patient relationships is key to patient-centered care. Because patient satisfaction is a fundamental indicator of how well technology meets patient expectations, it is important that nurses be able to identify and express indicators of the quality patient experience within meaningful telehealth programs and projects.

ALIGNMENT OF TELEHEALTH AND TRADITIONAL PRACTICES IN ADVANCED PRACTICE NURSING

The APRN scope of practice and nursing competencies are fundamental to advanced nursing education, regardless of the educational delivery format and practice training environments. Fulfilling these core aspects of APRN education is achieved whether the education is delivered through a traditional in-person format, in the virtual care environment, or through real-time distance learning using telehealth. In addition, clinical competency development is likewise achieved through a variety of educational formats, including traditional in-person clinical, simulation (in-person or virtual), and real-time distance learning using telehealth. All nursing programs must "design and utilize innovative nursing practices to prepare graduates for contemporary health care delivery and must have clinical learning experiences using diverse teaching methods."[2(p843)] This is more important today than ever before. Resources pertaining to APRN scope of practice and professional practice competencies abound, as do educational approaches and technologies to facilitate advancing APRN education and practice. Imbedding telehealth as both an educational strategy and an essential clinical competency is an increasingly essential component of APRN education.

Additionally, in the *Consensus Model for APRN Regulation: Licensure, Accreditation, Certification & Education*,[3] APRN education must meet specific requirements. The APRN education requirements can be met through a variety of delivery formats, and the use of telehealth as a distance learning and educational delivery vehicle aligns with the Consensus Model. From a competency standpoint, the Consensus Model provides the basis for the framework for APRN competency. Because nurse practitioners comprise the largest segment of the APRN workforce, the National Organization of Nurse Practitioner Faculties provides a robust set of documents explicating standards for nurse practitioner competency. Professional organizations for clinical nurse specialists (CNSs), certified nurse midwives, and certified registered nurse anesthetists (CRNAs) build on the work of the Consensus Model and National Organization of Nurse Practitioner Faculties guidelines to provide additional role and population specific guidance.

Scope of Practice

The nursing scope of practice is the conceptual framework for the practice of nursing in the context of nursing regulation and authority that specifies what actions, procedures, and care the nurse is authorized to perform. The APRN scope of practice is mandated by individual state nurse practice acts from state boards of nursing and medicine that outline the role, behaviors, functions, and responsibilities aligning with the educational preparation and competencies for the designated nursing position. States regulate collaborative practice agreements that provide the framework for practice privileges and how practice can occur. Prescriptive authority is also controlled under the umbrella of scope of practice. There is practice authority variability across states; there is also variability in the prescriptive authority of APRNs across states.

One of the most significant contributions of the APRN role is in improving access to care to rural, underserved, and vulnerable populations. This is also where telehealth can have the most impact. APRNs working under full practice authority have led to increased rural patient access to care.[4] Allowing full scope of APRN practice in primary care has also led to improved outcomes of chronic diseases among vulnerable populations.[5,6] Care provided by primary care APRNs has been shown to be comparable to primary care physicians' care, with state provisions for full practice authority being supported by the evidence in improved management of symptoms and improved outcomes.[7,8] APRNs need full scope of practice authority in all states to exponentially affect rural and underserved care through telehealth nursing practice. However, full practice authority has been granted to APRNs in less than half of US states as of this writing. The nursing scope of practice in each state affects health care delivery by affecting the APRN workforce, care delivery, access to care, use of health care resources, and cost of care.[4] Reducing the regulatory restrictions on the APRN scope of practice can increase capacity of APRNs to provide much needed care while reducing costs, particularly in states with large rural and medically underserved populations.[4,9]

Degree of autonomy for the APRN is controlled by the state, not only related to scope of practice but also to educational preparation for entry level of practice and competency assessments for practice and licensure. The Consensus Model, as developed by the National Council of State Boards of Nursing, was designed to be a national standard for guidance for consistent APRN educational requirements, licensure, certification, and accreditation to enhance the ability of APRNs to practice to the full scope of educational preparation and licensure.[3] The Consensus Model supports APRN telehealth practice because the scope of practice in telehealth nursing aligns with the traditional scope of practice, although there are additional considerations, including credentialing, licensure, and practice across state lines (see Chapter 5). Included in the Consensus Model is a provision to allow for advanced practice nursing via the APRN Compact.

The APRN Compact has important connection with the Consensus Model, which would enable states to align regulation of APRN roles. This would provide more uniformity in practice across states, facilitating development of cross-state telehealth nursing practice standards. APRNs will be well positioned for embracing telehealth as an essential tool in nursing with enactment of the Compact because the Compact would provide cross-state licensure, enabling interstate telehealth practice. The ability to practice in multiple states offers APRNs the opportunity to practice in expanded geographical regions and would put nurses in a position to begin widespread telehealth nursing practice. Additionally, nursing must explore how the scope of practice will be affected by practice in the virtual care environment so that the art and science of nursing can be actualized through nursing presence.[10]

Competencies

Competencies in nursing are defined for each APRN specialty as the standard level of proficiency that must be achieved for practice. Nursing competencies establish the guidelines for APRN educational programs of study to enable full scope of practice to be granted to licensees. The behavior for the APRN in each specialty track is subsequently outlined here and is consistent with the care provided to the specific patient population focus and arena for both in-person and telehealth care.

Nurse Practitioner Competencies

Regarding alignment with nurse practitioner competencies,[11] because nurse practitioner core competencies are acquired through mentored patient care experiences, telehealth mentoring experiences are important to incorporate in the curriculum so that nurses can develop skill in using telehealth to provide direct care to patients and in evaluating and providing evidence-based care using telehealth. The nurse practitioner critically evaluates and translates telehealth research, integrating this new knowledge into nursing science to develop new models and approaches to nursing care and care delivery systems. Leadership competencies enable nursing leaders to advocate and advance incorporating telehealth into nursing practice to affect population health. This can lead the way to working collaboratively with a variety of stakeholders to provide improved access, quality, and decreased cost of health care using new models of care developed using telehealth technologies and through creation of innovative partnerships. The nurse practitioner can incorporate telehealth technology best evidence for care into practice to continuously improve quality of clinical practice with emphasis on improving access, cost, quality, safety, and patient satisfaction with health care. The nurse practitioner should be knowledgeable regarding telehealth organizational design, financing, and legal and regulatory policy related to telehealth. Practice inquiry competencies provide leadership in the translation of new telehealth knowledge into practice and are able to use telehealth in practice to generate knowledge and improve outcomes. Nursing telehealth education will allow nurses to lead telehealth practice inquiry, analyze clinical telehealth guidelines and apply these to practice, and disseminate this evidence to improve nursing practice and patient care outcomes.

Technology and information literacy competencies can contribute to the integration and design of telehealth models and systems of care, demonstrating improved access, cost, quality, and satisfaction and showing command of information literacy in telehealth. With telehealth knowledge, the nurse can guide patients and families in using telehealth for care and care delivery and provide patient and family education using telehealth. Policy competencies contribute to the development of ethical policy development toward telehealth and advocate policies that promote access, equity, quality, and cost. Telehealth delivery system competencies will enable the nurse to be knowledgeable of telehealth organizational practices and the interactions of systems used in telehealth to improve health care delivery while facilitating widespread standard use of telehealth models of care. Telehealth education will enable the nurses to evaluate the effect this delivery system has on patients, providers, and the system at large across the continuum of care.

Telehealth is a new tool for many nurses, and investigating the ethical principles in decision making regarding use of telehealth and applying these principles to telehealth as it relates to individuals, populations, and these new systems of care will be important to the discipline of nursing and to nursing practice. Independent practice competencies enable the nurse practitioner to function as a licensed independent practitioner when practicing independently using telehealth in the management of patients and patient populations, and involvement with regulatory agencies going forward will be essential to allow nursing to define the nurse's role in telehealth practices and health care of the future. Telehealth education will also allow the nurse to use telehealth in primary care, including health promotion, disease prevention, and patient education and counseling, as well as for disease management and palliative and end-of-life care. Finally, telehealth education aligns with the nurse practitioner competencies by use in patient-centered, culturally competent care because telehealth can replicate the in-person visit and connect health care providers in a variety of settings. These 9 nurse practitioner competencies are required of nurse practitioner students, and nursing programs must incorporate advanced technologies into education and practice in order to prepare graduates for today's changing health care delivery practice environment.[2]

Clinical Nurse Specialist Competencies

The CNS competencies were refined in the *Statement on Clinical Nurse Specialist Practice and Education: Third Edition* and are linked to the three spheres of influence: patient direct care, nursing and nursing practice, and organization and systems. These competencies align with a technology-infused environment of practice.[12] Regarding alignment with telehealth practice, providing direct care and engaging with patients and families in a holistic manner to advance nursing management of the patient health arena is embodied in the educational preparation of the CNS, according to state and federal Nursing Practice Acts, because telehealth practice is within the scope of nursing practice and telehealth nursing practice. The direct care behavior competencies dictate that the CNS develop innovative program delivery, provide patient-centered care, and show leadership in taking evidence forward in care planning. These behaviors completely translate to the telehealth practice arena because they can be accomplished using telehealth as a tool.

The CNS is charged with being competent in determining individual vs systems-level approaches. This can be an important aspect of the contribution of the CNS in telehealth as well. CNS consultation is facilitated in telehealth using advanced technology to connect the CNS with others to provide consultation related to systems and resource availability and use. Due to ease of communications using technology, the CNS will have more opportunity to lend this aspect of leadership to health care. The systems leadership competency is core to the CNS role, and just as in the traditional environment, in the virtual care environment, the CNS can work to effect real change in the clinical and political arena inside and across systems to improve care. The CNS collaborates as part of the role to improve clinical outcomes, and telehealth enhances the CNS's ability to collaborate, lending to increased access and equivalent outcomes as compared with traditional care settings.

Telehealth provides new opportunities for the CNS to engage with patients and families on an individual and systems level to find innovative ways to improve population health. Using mobile devices, applications (apps), and home monitoring, the CNS has new reach and connection to the patient. Because the CNS is also a frontline care provider, he or she can use telehealth to achieve the coaching competency by using technology to connect with and educate patients, families, and colleagues about how to use telehealth to support and improve care and care practices. Clinical research conducted by the CNS will be important to provide the foundation of practice in the virtual care environment for CNS systems integration and clinical practice concerns and to provide evidence for continuous quality improvement as health care changes due to the influx of advanced technologies in the health care arena. The CNS will also assess how technology affects the art of nursing, to include nursing presence and relationships with systems and individuals in the virtual care environment. Finally, the CNS will use skills in traditional practice to quantify and qualify ethical virtual care environment practice at all levels of service, including patients, families, providers, health care systems, and the community at large, to ensure moral components of care.

Certified Registered Nurse Anesthetist Competencies

Currently, the competencies for CRNA practice is in development via the American Association of Nurse Anesthetists by way of the Full Scope of Practice Competence Task Force.[13] However, the draft CRNA professional competencies reflects alignment with use of telehealth in CRNA practice. The specifically designed draft technology and informatics competency expresses support and connection for the CRNA to use technology to improve care and systems of care, and through transformational leadership, the CRNA can actualize improved care outcomes. Telehealth can be used by the CRNA in practice to actualize many of the intended draft competencies, including independent decision making, because telehealth will allow enhanced collaboration for improved practice. Cultural competency is inherent in all traditional CRNA practices and is imbedded in telehealth practices as well. The ability to care for culturally diverse patients over a wide geographical area using telehealth requires that the CRNA be culturally competent and use skills, behaviors, and attitudes that lend to respect and a positive learning environment, just as in traditional practice.

Telehealth is an interprofessional endeavor, and the proposed interprofessional competency lends well both to telehealth practice and to traditional practice in the environment of patient-centered care. Continuous learning and professional engagement to promote the CRNA profession are fully supported in telehealth practice because it enables remote connections for learning opportunities and enables distance-learning opportunities via live videoconferencing, online classes, collaborations, group discussions, and webinars. Using telehealth to connect to others for team-based care, mutual goal achievement, and support is possible using telehealth in practice.

Additionally, the CRNA can contribute to the further development and assimilation of technology into nursing practice through producing evidence for CRNA telehealth practice. This research is vitally important for nursing to conduct and produce new evidence as to how the CRNA practices the art and science of nursing in using telehealth. Positive experiences using telehealth will be enabled by the CRNA as he or she transmits a positive attitude in care delivery, just as he or she does in person, although practice in the virtual care environment requires technology etiquette skills and enhanced skills in receiving and transferring presence that must be gained for a successful encounter. In the operating room, the CRNA must work within constricted time frames, and telehealth could improve productivity and timeliness of care through extension of patient oversight and expertise using telehealth. The CRNA can also contribute to improved wellness of self and patients through use of telehealth to prevent lifestyle diseases and contribute to wellness.

Nurse Midwifery Competencies

There are 9 nurse midwifery competencies that align to application of telehealth technologies to practice.[14] Just as nurse midwives contribute to traditional evidence discovery through applying expert knowledge to best practices evidence to evaluate outcomes, so too can they make this contribution to evaluate telehealth nursing practice outcomes. The nurse midwife can identify gaps in practice, and creative solutions to address such issues can be explored. Telehealth can be used as a tool to resolve these complex and sometimes long-standing problems to improve care for mothers and newborn infants.

It is important for nurses to be knowledgeable, active, and prominent in the policy arena so that nursing perspectives and concerns are adequately addressed and nurse midwives have a voice. Team-based midwifery care can be enhanced by advanced communications technologies, and telehealth can be used in the creation of programs to address disparity in care using a team approach. As APRN nursing telehealth practice grows, it is important to explore and research nursing theory that aligns to telehealth practice and to develop telehealth nursing models and theory that support nursing telehealth practice. Competency in using health information systems and advanced technologies to improve outcomes through safety and quality care assessments is a requirement of the environment of care today. The more confidence nurse midwives have using technology, the better equipped they will be to provide care in this digital age and connect improvements in care with the internet of things going forward. Reimbursement and resource management are essential to nurse midwife practice, and telehealth can help increase provider capacity and efficiency. Finally, nurse midwives are called upon to develop and produce evidence for midwifery telehealth nursing practice and for improving patient care outcomes.

PROVIDER SHORTAGES AND SOLUTIONS
TO CHALLENGES OF PROVIDING CARE

The provider shortages characteristic of our health care system have been present and growing in complexity for at least the past 20 years. There are increasing challenges to meet care needs due to several factors, including the general aging of the US population, the pervasiveness of multi-chronic illnesses and lifestyle diseases, the aging of the health care workforce, and the limited capacity of educational programs to significantly increase the numbers of new practice ready graduates. A 2014 survey reinforces the severity of the provider shortage; over 80% of physicians were found to be at or over capacity, with inability to care for additional patients.[15] As of June 2016, over 40% of the United States had insufficient primary care services.[15] The provider shortage is expected to continue, and by 2030 an estimated shortage of up to 120,000 primary and specialty care physicians is projected.[16] Coupled with the US population's continual growth by 11% and estimates that 50% of the population will be over 65 years old by 2030, there is urgent need for strategies that enable the health care system to be able to provide care to all who need and request care.[16]

The 2018 American Association of Medical Colleges report found that if uninsured, nonmetropolitan, underserved populations had the ability to utilize care at the same rates as populations without such barriers, 31,000 more physicians would have been needed in 2016; if all US citizens were compared, the need would have been 95,000.[16] A recent study indicates need for up to 2.3 million additional health care professionals by 2025 to be able to provide care for our aging communities.[17] APRNs can help fill this gap by increasing the number of practice-ready new graduates. Progress is steady, as evidenced by the increase in nurse practitioners by 22,000 from March 2018 to January 2019, for a total workforce of 270,000.[18]

Linked to the provider shortage is the nursing preceptor shortage, predominantly in rural areas, due in part to lack of available APRNs in rural clinical practices and a lack of preceptor training programs to adequately prepare APRNs to fill the preceptor role. There is also competition from other nursing programs and from students in other disciplines for these preceptors and practice sites. Additionally, many APRNs have not been trained as preceptors, and there is little incentive for nurses to serve as preceptors due to busy patient loads with short staffing patterns. Decreased availability of clinicians to precept due to their own technologic learning needs is also becoming more of a factor.[2] Additionally, the model that has been used for precepting APRN students, which is traditionally a one preceptor to one student ratio, further limits the precepting opportunities for students. This apprentice model, where a student is directly under a volunteer preceptor and is overseen by a member of the nursing faculty, limits the number of APRN students able to come through the pipeline to rural communities. Obviously, new strategies are needed to increase the numbers of practice-ready APRN graduates so that APRNs can increase workforce numbers and significantly fill the provider shortage gap.

Health care policy affects the nursing shortage in a variety of ways, and a significant factor is the Affordable Care Act because it enables millions of people to obtain health insurance and seek primary care services. Therefore, more people are requesting care in this environment of provider shortages, especially in rural and underserved areas.[19] Many rural areas lack sufficient ability to provide important care services for primary, dental, and mental health care and are identified as a Health Professional Shortage Area (HPSA). The HPSAs correlate to the degree of health of the community.[19] In order to recognize where physician provider shortages occur, the US Department of Health and Human Services designates geographic areas, groups, or populations and decides whether they are an HPSA or a Medically Underserved Area (MUA).[20] The US Department of Health and Human Services defines an HPSA as having 1 physician or less for every 3500 or more people, or 1 for 3000 if the community has higher identified needs.[16] MUAs are defined as not having enough primary care providers (PCPs) to care for the population, having high infant mortality, high poverty, and/or a high elderly population.[21] The Health Resources & Services

Administration and state Primary Care Offices collaborate and base designations on relevant data to establish whether a shortage qualifies as an HPSA.[22] Scores are assigned corresponding to a 0 to 25 scale based on the population-to-provider ratio, the percentage of the population below 100% of the federal poverty level, and the travel time to the nearest source of care outside of the HPSA designation.[23] Shortages affect patients by denying care availability, requiring long-distance travel, and incurring long wait times to see a provider, resulting in poor satisfaction and decreased outcomes.[24] A designation as an HPSA or MUA enables access to special government funding, programs, and other opportunities to provide assistance to develop programs and allocate innovative resources to these populations and facilities.

Telehealth technology can connect providers with their society of patients and use technology as an avenue to create innovative ways to provide care in the setting of provider shortages. Telehealth can increase provider capacity and support and enhance team-based care.[25] Telehealth has enabled an increased nurse-to-patient ratio of 15:1, as compared with the traditional ratio of 11:1.[26] Telehealth provides an opportunity to increase provider capacity without decreasing quality because telehealth visits are comparable to traditional visits.[27,28] Rural practices may benefit most from this extended APRN capacity because they have some of the greatest provider shortages and a dearth of resources. Telehealth also provides rural and underserved patients access to specialty providers, which can improve patient care outcomes by providing diagnoses and care not otherwise available. Nurses are essentially isolated in geographically distant rural regions. Telehealth offers opportunity to connect patients with providers, as well as providers with providers, to support nursing practice. Nurses should be instrumental in developing care delivery innovations and building collaborative practice with interprofessional teams using telehealth. Nursing faculty who are able to use telehealth in student education will be able to extend their capacity as educators and more effectively communicate with students in the practicum setting. Increasing the number of APRNs is also cost effective; services that had a physician-to-nonphysician full-time employee ratio of 0.41 or higher resulted in greater earnings than those that did not.[29] This cost savings could be compounded with use of telehealth.

Achieving Healthy People 2020 goals, such as improving blood pressure and glucose control, lowering cholesterol, and decreasing smoking and obesity, could lower the need for health care providers as population health improves. However, it would be expected that as overall population health improved, more providers would be needed due to more people living longer.[24] There is no single solution to the provider shortage because many issues affect this problem. A multilayered approach with flexibility to adjust to changes and innovations is needed. However, telehealth is a universal application to the problem of provider shortages that can work on many different layers of this issue. Extending provider capacity, improving communications and collaborations between providers, and enabling specialty consults for isolated patients brings access to care. Improving frequency of care and monitoring via remote patient monitoring (RPM), improving chronic disease management, decreasing provider isolation, and enabling virtual classroom education is also possible using telehealth. Preceptors and faculty can help to increase the number of new graduates by using telehealth, spreading specialty expertise over wider geographic areas while decreasing barriers to providing care in geographic areas.

There are many societal pressures demanding action to seriously address these seemingly insurmountable problems to improving health, including the connected consumer and need to contain the ever-increasing health care costs. We are fortunate to have entered the digital information age, where scientific knowledge and technological innovations are partnering to enable never-before-imagined health care capabilities by being able to deliver care to patients without regard to barriers of time and geographic distance. The realization of a health care system that can adequately address these issues will rely on the ability to incorporate the scientific and technological achievements into standard health care practices while at the same time using these tools to improve primary prevention of disease through extending provider reach and improving the efficiency and ability to care for patients.

For Reflection 1:

Increasing Provider Capacity

Think about a rural clinical site you have experienced. Consider at least 4 ways that the clinic could use telehealth to increase provider capacity. What types of technology could be used?

Patient and Provider Satisfaction With Telehealth

In today's health care environment, patients expect quality service and convenience, producing a positive patient experience. Patient satisfaction correlates to the quality of care and is therefore an important indicator in health care.[30] It is also important to measure patient satisfaction in telehealth visits because telehealth is more than just the use of technology in health care; it also is part of the overall patient experience.

Patient satisfaction and its relationship to quality care has been an important quality indicator since the late 1970s, when a survey tool called the Patient Satisfaction Questionnaire measured physician and medical care attributes, including interpersonal skills, patient wait time, emergency care delivery, and the cost of care.[30,31] In 1985, Press Ganey began surveying patients and tracking hospital patient satisfaction, and over the next 15 years, the collective data enabled comparisons between hospitals.[32] In 2001, an Institute of Medicine report entitled "Crossing the Quality Chasm"[33] provided a roadmap for health care to organize and develop models of care focused on new performance indicators, including patient satisfaction metrics. In 2002, the US federal government began to use patient satisfaction data to evaluate quality of care; CMS and the Agency for Healthcare Research and Quality collaborated to implement the Hospital Consumer Assessment of Healthcare Providers and Systems (HCAHPS) Survey. HCAHPS is a national, standardized, publicly reported survey of patient perceptions of hospital care, which enables comparisons between local, regional, and national hospitals.[1] HCAHPS has 3 stated goals: to produce comparable data across facilities regarding patient perceptions of care, to use the transparency in reporting to encourage improvements in care, and to increase accountability for the quality of the hospital care.[1] The first publicly volunteered reporting of HCAHPS was in 2008. Then, as part of the Deficit Reduction Act of 2005, hospitals were eligible for payment if they voluntarily reported their HCAHPS satisfaction scores, and participation rose to 95%.[30] The Affordable Care Act also reflected financial incentives for voluntary reporting because reimbursement is influenced by comparative performance between facilities and improvement on HCAHPS satisfaction scores. Today, HCAHPS patient satisfaction results are part of the Patient Experience of Care domain in the Hospital Value-Based Purchasing Program, linking patient satisfaction results to hospital payment.[30]

Congruent with the in-person visit, the entire patient experience affects telehealth patient satisfaction. Patient satisfaction is multifaceted and is formed by patient perceptions and expectations, resulting in the patient experience. The patient experience involves relationships and communication in a patient-centered culture, and patient satisfaction is an important component of patient-centered care. Patient satisfaction surveys enable objective measurement of the patient's perspective of care that is meaningful to improved outcomes and has public comparisons for transparency of care and impetus for improvements. HCAHPS patient satisfaction surveys query the perception of interpersonal relations, technical quality, accessibility and convenience, finances, efficacy, outcomes, continuity, physical environment, and availability.[1] Identifying what makes up a satisfying experience for the patient and targeting those features for improvement can maximize the patient experience throughout the care continuum. The experience can be conceptualized through expectations of the patient by providing a culture of service that is empathetic to patient factors that affect satisfaction.[30] Satisfaction as a measure of contentment can only be measured as compared with the patient's perceptions and expectations.[30] Therefore, patient satisfaction should be measured in telehealth similarly to in traditional visits because the telehealth visit mirrors the in-person visit for the purpose of health care delivery. Therefore, it is important to measure and reflect upon how telehealth patient satisfaction mirrors the quality of care that is delivered.[30]

However, patient satisfaction indicators and variables specific to telehealth should also be studied and identified in order to understand patient perceptions and expectations regarding the telehealth visit. For example, assumptions that older, and therefore potentially less technologically savvy, patients are opposed to telehealth have not been supported in the literature. In fact, studies in Australia[34] and the United States[27,35,36] showed that older adults did not feel that telehealth led to a loss of privacy and that they were interested in the novel use of technology. Furthermore, many preferred telehealth visits as convenient, relatively inexpensive modes to receive care in the internal medicine, home rehabilitation, and emergency care settings.

Additionally, a significant overall satisfaction measure is quality of nursing communication, likely related to the amount of nursing empathy exchanged, because higher levels of empathy enable enhanced understanding of a patient's needs.[30] Empathy is an inherent part of nursing, and it is therefore important that nurses learn to transmit empathy to the patient in the virtual care environment. The patient's perception of empathy must also be measured to ensure that he or she perceives empathy in the nursing virtual care encounter to continue high satisfaction with nursing communication. Additionally, the nurse must be able to address emotional factors that can affect the telehealth patient experience, including anxiety and distress or trust and confidence, using effective nursing skills in the virtual care environment. Nursing must focus on building skills in transmitting empathy and nursing presence in the virtual environment so that nurses can connect with patients in a meaningful way, just as they do in a traditional visit. Patients often form conclusions about their health care experience related to achieving their intended goal for the visit. Therefore, measuring elements that are valued by the patient can help assess patient satisfaction in telehealth. Ease of scheduling, access to care, provider availability, wait times, length of time with the provider, communication quality, patient literacy of information, and understanding all affect telehealth visit satisfaction, just as they affect in-person visit satisfaction.[30,37] Additionally, with telehealth, the remote connection site and staff are part of the patient experience along with patient perceptions regarding the ease and proper functioning of the technology.

The telehealth patient experience is an important indicator to measure as telehealth practice grows to ensure high-quality care. Patient satisfaction is a significant gauge of how closely the virtual encounter equals patient expectations.[37] Factors affecting patient satisfaction include how much time the patient has invested in the visit, whether the patient was treated holistically, how skilled and confident the nurses were, and whether the patient understood what he or she was told.[30] There is growing evidence of patient satisfaction in telehealth and the virtual care environment. For example, a systematic review of telehealth in palliative care in rural regions to assess caregiver outcomes revealed equivalent quality-of-life reporting, decreased anxiety, decreased caregiver burden, improved family functioning, improved mood, decreased depression, and feelings of increased social support using telehealth interventions.[38] Rural rheumatology patients reported the perception of satisfactory care with high satisfaction scores and that avoiding long-distance travel improves satisfaction.[39] Patient and provider satisfaction in teledermatology was high, and providers found the ability to form interpersonal relationships using the videoconferencing technology a positive factor in telehealth live videoconferencing, as well as good image visualization and good visualization for patient assessments.[40]

A systematic literature review on telehealth found that patients viewed telehealth as effective and efficient and that it met patient expectations of ease of use, cost savings, improved outcomes, patient preference, better communication capacity with providers, and time saved in traveling to the facility.[37] In the review, an examination of how technologies are perceived, used, and related to satisfaction among patients and providers, found high satisfaction for both groups. Patients cited that not having to travel long distances was satisfying, and providers found confidence and ease in operating the technology highly satisfying. Additionally, a study comparing telehealth to routine in-person visits resulted in a 95% very satisfied rating of the telehealth care and a first visit rating as preferred or just as good as traditional care. Shorter wait times and improved access to care also scored high in reasons for satisfaction.[27]

FOR REFLECTION 2:

Telehealth Patient Satisfaction

What are some of the ways telehealth patient satisfaction data can be used to improve the patient experience? How can issues, attitudes, and assumptions specific to technology affect provider and patient telehealth satisfaction?

TELEHEALTH USE CASES

Many APRN innovators and early adopters have already assimilated into the world of telehealth and telehealth nursing and have developed programs of care to address complex patient problems that remained unresolved and are in need of new strategies. Several of these use cases are explored to demonstrate innovative APRN telehealth leadership and participation in telehealth programs.

The Health Wagon

The Health Wagon is a free nurse-managed health clinic in southwest Virginia. The mission of The Health Wagon is to provide compassionate, quality health care to the medically underserved people in the mountains of Appalachia. The Health Wagon is southwest Virginia's only dedicated safety net clinic and is the oldest known mobile clinic in the nation, formed by a nurse 40 years ago who traveled on rural mountain roads in her Volkswagen Beetle to deliver health care to individuals in the mountainous region of southwest Virginia. Since that time, The Health Wagon has evolved from a Volkswagen Beetle, to a used Winnebago, to a singlewide mobile home that served as a stationary clinic, to the thriving organization it is now. Today, The Health Wagon has a $2.6 million–dollar budget and provides care from 2 brick-and-mortar stationary clinics in Clintwood and Wise, Virginia, as well as 4 mobile units in medically underserved Lee, Scott, Wise, Dickenson, Buchanan, and Russell Counties.[41] The mobile units travel to 11 sites within the 6-county service area, where a licensed practical nurse (LPN) and nurse practitioner provide evidence-based quality care. The Health Wagon has grown from a 1-person staff to a staff of 20 with 5 Doctors of Nursing Practice/nurse practitioners, 1 registered nurse (RN), and 4 LPNs, plus ancillary staff, and has recorded 16,670 visits/encounters.

The underserved patients that The Health Wagon treats face extreme challenges to achieving better health and access to health care, including poverty, unemployment, low educational attainment and literacy, geographical barriers, limited public transportation systems, and food insecurity. Due to the organization's remote service area, in recent years The Health Wagon has become increasingly reliant on the use of telemedicine to provide the highest level of care to its thousands of patients. In partnership with the University of Virginia's (UVA's) College of Medicine, the Appalachian College of Pharmacy, and a host of other academic institutions and independent providers, The Health Wagon has become the highest user of telehealth services in Virginia. Providers from around the region donate their time to see patients virtually at one of The Health Wagon's stationary clinics to address health concerns that are outside the scope of PCPs. The Health Wagon currently hosts telehealth clinics, including, but not limited to, the following specialties:

- Endocrinology
- Colposcopy
- Cystoscopy
- Wound care
- Cardiology
- Psychiatry
- Behavioral health
- Gynecology
- Diabetes education
- Lipid management
- Dermatology
- Pain management
- Podiatry

The Health Wagon uses 3 telemedicine carts with medical peripherals to deliver most of its telehealth services. All Health Wagon providers have also been trained on mobile telehealth applications, which allows both providers and patients to use their computers or smartphones to see patients who are unable to make it to a stationary or mobile clinic site.

The Health Wagon, in partnership with UVA, has also developed the first telecystoscopy clinic (Figure 7-1). Residents of rural southwest Virginia have some of the worst health outcomes in the state, due in part to high smoking rates.[42-45] Not only does smoking increase the risk of cardiac and vascular problems, but it leads to high rates of cancer, including bladder cancer. Bladder cancer is of particular interest because it is the most expensive cancer to treat due to the intensity and technical nature of follow-up. Every 3 months for the first year after a diagnosis, bladder cancer survivors require cystoscopy. This novel telecystoscopy clinic provides an opportunity for patients to undergo an in-office cystoscopy procedure by an APRN where a video camera is passed into the bladder to inspect the bladder lining for tumors, while the remote physician observes and assesses the imaging (Figure 7-2). This procedure helps rural and often indigent patients avoid a long drive to a tertiary/specialty facility for a 15-minute procedure for bladder cancer surveillance. Access to this procedure also enables eligible residents of the central Appalachian region to receive lifesaving bladder cancer screenings that would otherwise be inaccessible. Family nurse practitioners with The Health Wagon perform monthly clinics where individuals who have been identified as having an increased likelihood for developing bladder cancer can undergo this revolutionary new procedure. Southwest and southside Virginia residents have limited access to urologists because there is a shortage of physicians in this rural area.[46] Further, a disproportionate number of these patients are underinsured, necessitating hundreds of miles of travel to an academic setting to receive safety-net care. This innovative project improves access for these patients to quality bladder cancer care. Additionally, the investigators intend to leverage the nationally renowned telemedicine infrastructure to overcome this barrier to bladder care by training RNs in rural locations to

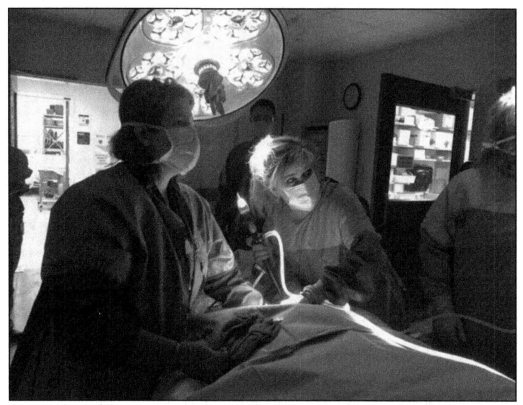

Figure 7-1. First APRN Telecystoscopy Clinic. (Reprinted with permission from The Health Wagon.)

perform flexible cystoscopy, interpreted virtually in real time by a board-certified urologist. This technology will allow instant feedback to both the RN and patient and obviates the need to travel many hours for care.

University of Virginia COVID-19 In-Home Remote Monitoring Program

The new coronavirus disease (or COVID-19) is emerging as one of the most devastating pandemics in modern history. This infection has rapidly spread across the globe, and to date, presents one of the most serious challenges to human health ever experienced in modern times. Community spread (also known as person-to-person contact) via aerosolization and fomite transmission has rapidly disseminated COVID-19 throughout the world. Symptoms range from mild and flu-like to acute respiratory distress syndrome and death. Asymptomatic spread has worsened the extremely contagious nature of this disease, overwhelming health care systems world-wide.

In the early stages of the COVID-19 pandemic, telehealth was identified as an important tool to help diagnose and treat patients virtually while limiting exposure to patients and health care providers. At the UVA Health System, institutional leaders and advanced practice providers (APPs) quickly recognized the role that telehealth could play in monitoring select patients with suspected or known diagnosis of COVID-19 that did not meet criteria for hospital admission but were at high risk for future deterioration and hospitalization. To address this need, an in-home remote monitoring (IHM) program for COVID-19 was quickly developed and deployed by the APPs, composed of nurse practitioners, physician assistants, and CRNAs from throughout the institution.

Figure 7-2. An APRN at The Health Wagon performing telecystoscopy. (Reprinted with permission from The Health Wagon.)

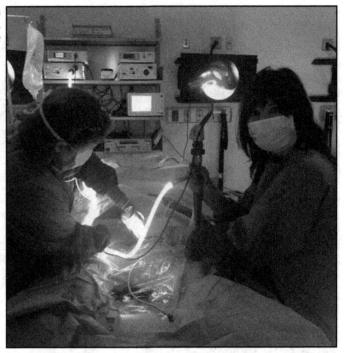

Figure 7-2. An APRN at The Health Wagon performing telecystoscopy. (Reprinted with permission from The Health Wagon.)

To develop the COVID-19 IHM program, APPs gathered an interprofessional team, including UVA institutional leaders and telehealth experts, as well as local remote monitoring experts from Locus Health. The program uses a variety of remote monitoring equipment. APPs working in the program were first identified on a volunteer basis, and later by availability, primarily by redistribution of inpatient APPs. These APPs were quickly mobilized and attended the training sessions developed for the program, focusing on the program goals, technology, workflow, and care of the patient using interactive remote monitoring.

The program works by initially identifying patients who present to their UVA PCP (either in-person or virtually) or the UVA emergency department who are positive for COVID-19 screening questions. These patients are then connected to an established in-person UVA COVID-19 clinic, where further workup and testing is performed. At the advent of the pandemic, testing took up to 7 days for results, so many patients were sent home with results pending. Now, there is a rapid test and results are available within 4 to 24 hours, depending upon which test is utilized. If the patient is stable enough to not require admission to the hospital, but is high risk for escalation of the disease due to comorbidities, such as advanced age, hypertension, diabetes, and lung disease, the patient is invited to be monitored in the IHM program. Using a tailored remote monitoring platform from Locus Health, patients are delivered a tablet, and medical peripherals including an automatic blood pressure cuff, pulse oximetry, and thermometer. After delivery of the IHM equipment, the on-call APP contacts the patient to instruct them on how to use the equipment and the frequency of performing and documenting vital signs based on his or her clinical status: typically every 4 hours. APPs monitor the dashboard vital signs and communications from patients 24/7, contacting the patient via phone call for vital signs that are out of expected ranges or to address any concerns patients may communicate to the APP using the remote monitoring equipment. Medication orders related to patient condition, such as antiemetics or antihypertensives, are placed as necessary by the APP monitor. For patients that decompensate, the APP triages and decides whether to escalate one of two ways based on the symptoms and risk factors: (1) The patient is recommended to be seen again in-person in the COVID-19 clinic, or (2) the patient is recommended to present immediately to the emergency department. Transfer to the emergency department is coordinated with the first responders and the emergency department staff to ensure mitigation of exposure to others, enabling a vital link in the isolation and transfer of contagious patients. To ensure continuity of care, providers complete a detailed sign-out via secure email, detailing patient condition and any outstanding issues to be addressed. Patients who test positive are monitored for up to 30 days via IHM; those with negative tests are monitored for up to 7 days. After cessation of monitoring, patients are delivered prepaid return addressed packaging with which to return their IHM equipment. The role of the APP in leading, developing, training, and scaling this program is invaluable in mitigating the spread of this highly contagious disease, while providing the ability to provide care for COVID-19 patients at a distance. The program is ongoing and, to date, has evaluated 40 patients of which 30 tested positive for the COVID-19 virus.

School-Based Telehealth

School-based health centers (SBHCs) have long served to bring care to students at school, where they spend most of their time. School-based telehealth, or teleSBHC (tSBHC), is a way to provide school-based services in an efficient and innovative way. With the decreasing costs of telehealth technologies, tSBHCs can provide access to more students with lower overhead than traditional brick-and-mortar SBHCs. SBHCs and tSBHCs have been shown to increase health care access for rural children, increase student seat time, decrease student absences and emergency department visits, and improve academic performance.[47-49] tSBHC programs allow students to be seen by a PCP or specialist remotely, from their school, ultimately minimizing missed classes and long commutes. Quality SBHCs offer a variety of health care services, including acute care, chronic disease management, case management, specialty care, dental services, and behavioral health services.

A model tSBHC program is North Carolina's Health-e-Schools program. The purpose of the program is to increase access to health care, predominately in rural areas in western North Carolina, for students, faculty, and school staff members. The program has been shown to decrease barriers to student learning through improving attendance and improving health. tSBHCs also limits the days lost at work for parents and guardians.[50] When students are sick at school, the school nurse is usually the first point of contact. For many tSBHCs like the Health-e-Schools program, school nurses serve as telepresenters, operating the telehealth equipment and allowing their students to be diagnosed, referred, and prescribed, as appropriate, without leaving school. The National Association of School Nurses[51] believes that school nurses are in an ideal position to help increase access to care for their students. School nurses are often the only health care providers that students see. They can bridge the gap between education and health care. This position, combined with telehealth capabilities, enhances the nurse's ability to provide expanded, coordinated health care at school. The program uses high-definition videoconferencing technologies with medical peripherals for connecting the remote provider, such as the family practice nurse practitioner, to the school to provide primary care. In this program, the nurse practitioner provides primary care services to the entire Health-e-Schools system. Specialty providers are also able to connect remotely with the schools to provide consultations and care.

The program works by having the school nurse perform an initial assessment and triage of the student's needs. If the student requires further medical care, he or she is enrolled in the telehealth program, if not already enrolled. At participating schools, any student, faculty, or staff can use the services offered; minors require parent or guardian permission, which is requested at the beginning of each school year. The program accepts many insurances, has a sliding scale fee, and does not turn away anyone for lack of ability to pay. Once the nurse practitioner or physician is available at the remote site, the telehealth visit can begin by each site signing onto the videoconferencing site. Once the provider is virtually connected with the student, a history of present illness and review of systems is conducted. For the physical exam, the school nurse serves as the connecting provider's hands. Medical peripherals can be used to examine the student's heart and lung sounds, ears, nose, throat, and skin. Once the examination is complete, the provider can gather any additional history and discuss findings and the management plan with the student and parent/guardian. If the student needs further care or a prescription, care is scheduled or a prescription is ordered. A copy of the encounter summary is sent to the student's PCP for continuity.

Another example of a tSBHC is at the Medical University of South Carolina (MUSC). A local pediatrician, with a small grant, started the South Carolina SBHC program. Subsequently, South Carolina passed legislation in 2013 that provided state funding for the advancement of telehealth initiatives throughout the state. With grants to expand telemedicine services to the rural communities, the tSBHC program was implemented in 3 rural schools. The MUSC Center for Telehealth was recognized as 1 of 2 Telehealth Centers for Excellence by the Health Resources & Services Administration in 2017.[52] In addition to grants, the tSBHCs are supported through insurance reimbursement. Telemedicine visits are reimbursable via Medicaid and some private insurers in the state of South Carolina. However, South Carolina is one of the states that does not have a much-needed parity law.

tSBHCs serve the underserved pediatric population within Title I or rural schools and Head Start to high school in many South Carolina schools.[52] Schools interested in joining the tSBHC program can submit requests through the MUSC tSBHC office. Currently, tSBHCs are integrated into approximately 100 schools across the state of South Carolina, with the number expected to increase to approximately 140 by the beginning of the 2019-2020 school year. Approximately 8 schools in Charleston County provide both in-person and telemedicine services, with a provider (physician or APRN) physically present on school grounds at least 1 day a week. One of these clinics offers full-time services, where an APRN is on site 4 days a week. Within the tSBHCs, the APRN serves as a provider for the telemedicine visits. The lead APRN also has administrative duties, which include overseeing the education of school nurses regarding the use of the telemedicine equipment, being a liaison for school nurses with the MUSC Center for Telehealth, developing protocols related to tSBHCs, and encouraging the growth of tSBHCs across the state.

All the schools in the tSBHC have telehealth carts equipped with medical peripherals for live videoconferencing encounters. The school nurse is the key player in the tSBHC as the one who determines who gets seen by a tSBHC provider and who initiates the telemedicine visit. When a visit is needed, the school nurse or telepresenter will enter a request through the telehealth platform. This request then notifies the provider either via text message or email regarding the visit request. The responding provider logs into the system to connect to the school for the virtual visit. The provider interviews and assesses the patient using the medical peripherals. Once the visit is complete, the provider charts the visit in the facility's electronic health record (EHR). If the telepresenter was a school nurse, then the school nurse on the telehealth platform, which allows the school to bill insurance and receive a site fee for use of the school nurse's office for the visit, completes a form.

The lead APRN and tSBHC manager are responsible for organizing training for new staff. New staff receive both SBHC and telemedicine orientation, which typically lasts 1 week. The orientation consists of equipment training, protocols, etiquette, mock visits, and shadowing every established provider for a half day. Currently, the tSBHC has 4 physicians, 4 APRNs, and 3 telepresenters, as well as support staff. After training, the lead APRN is readily available for any questions or troubleshooting. MUSC's tSBHC also has an information technology department to help troubleshoot any equipment or connectivity issues. School nurses receive in-person training by the MUSC tSBHC staff.

Heart Failure

In an effort to reduce 30-day readmissions to UVA after heart failure admission, an innovative method using the Grand-Aide model was proposed. The Grand-Aide program concept uses specially trained nurse extenders under the supervision of an experienced APRN to make frequent home visits to patients to improve health and decrease hospital and clinic visits.[53] An experienced heart failure nurse practitioner was selected to provide program development and supervision,

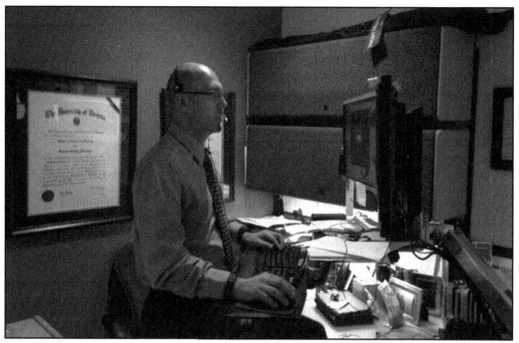

Figure 7-3. The heart failure APRN providing direct patient care through telehealth, using real-time interactive video-conferencing. (Reprinted with permission from S.C. Thomas.)

clinical care delivery, education curriculum, job descriptions, and the operational plan. The concept for this heart failure telehealth program was to use specialty-trained certified nurse's aides or LPNs to make home visits to patients living with heart failure, particularly after being discharged from the hospital after a heart failure exacerbation. These home visit staff would have intensive training on medications, signs, symptoms, and the dietary recommendations that were specific for the patient population. The staff would work under the close supervision of an experienced heart failure APRN using telehealth technologies.

Therefore, as an outreach to patients with heart failure, the UVA Heart Failure Clinic implemented the first chronic care heart failure Grand-Aide program.[53] This program was unique because the patient was able to interact directly, albeit remotely, with an APRN as technology bridged the distance gap between the patient's home and the APRN's location. In this program, the APRN can supervise from 3 to 5 home visit staff, thus leveraging that APRN up to a 5:1 ratio (Figure 7-3). The home visit staff covers approximately 100 patients per year, handling 15 to 30 patients at any given time, making between 4 and 6 home visits per day. This specific program covers a 60-mile radius of the main medical center campus, with 3 LPNs in the field and 1 remotely located acute care nurse practitioner. For 2 years, ending in 2015, 986 Medicare patients were discharged from UVA with the primary diagnosis of heart failure.[54] To enroll patients, team members approached patients and families in the hospital and obtained verbal consent or interest in the program. Approximately 130 patients met inclusion/exclusion criteria and were offered participation into the Grand-Aide program, with 108 participants accepting. Outcomes were obtained for the 108 Grand-Aide participants and 854 controls for all-cause readmissions and emergency department visits at 30 days and 6 months after hospital discharge.

Store-and-forward technology was used in this program, along with concurrent medical record review.[54] The APRN used either a desktop computer with audio and video capability or an iPad (Apple), and the home visit staff worked mainly from an iPad with cellular and Wi-Fi connectivity. The iPads were set up to access the medical center's EHR directly using a virtual private network secure connection. The iPads also had videoconferencing capabilities, thus allowing the virtual patient interactions to occur. Regarding the store-and-forward telehealth technology, the home visit staff recorded vital signs and patient symptom questionnaire information directly into the EHR so that both the supervising APRN and other members of the health care team could see the information obtained during the home visit. During a home visit, thorough and complete medication reconciliation also occurred, and edits were made in real time to the EHR. During the video or phone conversation, the APRN supervisor reviewed documentation obtained during the home visit as well as other pertinent medical history in the EHR, allowing for the best clinical decision making and providing the best information for patient care.

The home visit member saw the patient at home within 48 hours of discharge. The first procedure was medication reconciliation, and the home visit staff used a secure computer to access the EHR and compare medications in the system directly with the medication bottles at the patient's home. At every visit, the home visit staff obtained vital signs and completed a questionnaire about patient symptoms that was then placed into the EHR. The home visit staff then became the video operator, and the APRN reviewed the answers to the questionnaires, discussed findings, decided on education reinforcement needs, decided on therapy changes, and responded to any patient questions, all via live video with the patient, family, and home visit staff. Later visits used phone instead of video, if video was not needed. Home visit staff did not make clinical decisions, but rather reinforced the instructions of the APRN, as well as provided continued reinforcement for adherence with the medical regimen and teaching about danger signs and symptoms. A home visit staff member visited at least 3 times the first week, twice during weeks 2 and 3, once during week 4, and monthly thereafter. The duration of home visit staff support was individualized and could be as short as 2 weeks and as long as 5 years, depending on the needs of the patient. The frequency of visits could increase if symptoms worsened, or the home visit program could be discontinued if it was considered no longer necessary.

In the first year of the program, 30-day all-cause readmission for program participants was 9.5%, and over 2 years it was 11.8%.[54] This was a significant improvement and about 50% lower than the national average. Frequent home visits allowed for early identification and early intervention. Therefore, instead of patients worsening to the point of needing emergency care, slight changes were noticed and adjustments made while patients remained at home. A high percentage of heart failure patients presenting to the emergency department with shortness of breath are admitted, so keeping patients from having to seek emergency care greatly improves outcomes and costs. Overall, this program demonstrated an 82% reduction in heart failure 30-day all-cause readmissions and over a 40% reduction in emergency department visits for patients followed by this program over a 2-year period.[54] Additionally, the participants in this innovative program had higher severity scores and a greater number of comorbidities than in the control group, indicating that targeting interventions toward patients with higher severity can produce significant outcomes.

Antenatal and Neonatal Guidelines, Education and Learning Systems Program

APRNs have fueled the success of the University of Arkansas for Medical Sciences Institute for Digital Health & Innovation's perinatal telemedicine program, Antenatal and Neonatal Guidelines, Education and Learning Systems (ANGELS). ANGELS is a comprehensive system to improve access to high-risk obstetrical specialty care that uses APRNs as direct care providers, case managers, and second-level triage providers.[55] ANGELS's APRNs provide direct patient care both on-site and remotely through telemedicine, using real-time interactive video consultations (Figure 7-4). An example of how the practice works would be a rural woman with an abnormal pap smear who attends her county health unit for a telecolposcopy and connects with an APRN and gynecologist remotely through secure, interactive video. Real-time transmission of audio and video allows the APRN and specialist to guide the local nurse to biopsy the cervix and discuss

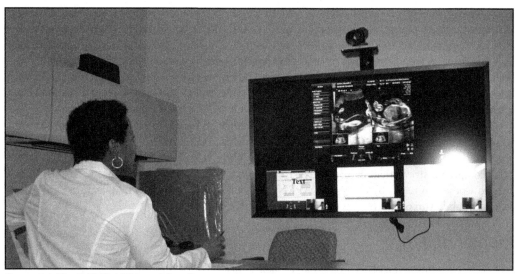

Figure 7-4. The ANGELS APRN providing direct patient care through telehealth, using real-time interactive videoconferencing. (Reprinted with permission from the University of Arkansas Medical Sciences Institute for Digital Health & Innovation.)

management options with the patient virtually. ANGELS's APRNs are consistently deployed within their full clinical scope to care for patients remotely through telemedicine. As case managers, APRNs initiate needed specialty referrals for high-risk pregnant women who require multiple visits with maternal-fetal medicine, genetic counselors, neonatologists, pediatric surgery teams, and other specialists. Offering telemedicine-aided case management allows management of at-risk pregnancies from any distance. APRNs arrange specialty visits at telemedicine clinics near the patient's home, including the patient's local obstetrical care provider. During a high-risk specialty visit, the APRN can facilitate consultations to multiple specialists for any patient, saving time and resources for the care team and connecting across numerous remote sites through a single, secure telemedicine visit. The second-level triage role of the APRN works in conjunction with ANGELS's 24/7 nurse call center who triages obstetrical patient phone calls to evaluate whether callers require emergency treatment, a next-day clinic visit, at-home self-care, and/or a follow-up evaluation.[56] Once a call center nurse has triaged the patient using a standardized protocol algorithm, an APRN will provide additional management instructions as needed.

APRNs embrace multiple technologies to provide telemedicine care. Real-time interactive video has been the leading technology used by ANGELS's APRNs to offer individualized consultation to their patients. This technology provides a live link to the remote patient and care team, giving APRNs live views of ultrasounds, instant patient interaction, and the ability to seamlessly collect patient data and offer clinical advice and support. Using this technology blurs the line between traditional in-person care and remote care because interactions are instantaneous. Emerging telehealth technologies include RPM and mobile health, which are ideal for tracking patient vitals and progress outside of regular clinical appointments and pushing education and reminders to patients for self-care. Social media is another telehealth tool that can engage and inform patients about how to care for high-risk pregnancies through an environment designed to share experiences or questions. APRNs can leverage all of these tools to improve the patient experience.

The infant mortality rate in Arkansas' Medicaid-covered population improved in the years since the implementation of ANGELS.[57] Preterm deliveries occurring in hospitals with neonatal intensive care units have shown a general increase since ANGELS began. In 2016, neonatal intensive care unit delivery levels increased to more than 70% for extremely preterm and more than 60% for moderately preterm babies.[57] The rate of postpartum complications in Medicaid deliveries decreased significantly 3 years following ANGELS's implementation, with any increases addressed through targeted education. Satisfaction surveys administered among ANGELS telemedicine patients demonstrated approximately 90% satisfaction ratings for ease in scheduling appointments and decreased demands on travel.[57] In 2018, ANGELS provided nearly 2000 high-risk obstetrical telemedicine consults with ultrasounds and over 2500 high-risk obstetrical case coordinations in Arkansas.[58] The nurse call center helped divert 429 unnecessary emergency department visits and over 2400 urgent care visits through advice provided by APRNs and call center nurses.[58]

In rural states like Arkansas, programs must capitalize on their best resources to improve access to high-risk obstetrical care. Where provider shortages are the norm, APRNs help fill the gaps where medical doctors and specialists are missing. With their specialty knowledge and ability to offer comprehensive patient care, APRNs are the ideal professionals to increase access to needed care to women in need. By equipping APRNs with telemedicine tools, any program can greatly extend its ability to reach into the hardest-to-reach places.

Mental Health

Lee Side Wellness (LSW) is a psychiatric-mental health nurse practitioner–owned and –operated private psychiatric practice. It is the largest independently held outpatient behavioral organization in the greater Cincinnati region and the largest nurse practitioner–owned outpatient mental health establishment in the state of Ohio (both based on the number of prescribers). The population serviced by LSW generally includes working professionals from an upper-middle class, suburban region of Cincinnati with mostly commercial insurance coverage and limited Medicare/Medicaid.

The role of the APRN is generally one of near autonomy, working to the fullest extent of their legal scopes of practice and consulting their physician collaborators as indicated, per Ohio law. The APRN provides psychiatric diagnostic services, prescribes and manages psychotropic medications, offers psychotherapy, and refers out as appropriate. Such referrals may include psychiatrists, psychotherapists, and other specialized internal services such as transcranial magnetic stimulation and pharmacogenomics counseling. When appropriate, the APRN may also refer out to such external services as laboratory studies, endocrinology, or neurology.

A critical role played by the APRN is the use of telehealth (more commonly known in the mental health industry as *telepsychiatry* or *telemental health*) to provide psychiatric services. APRNs use this innovative and alternative method to meet the needs of patients for whom in-person services are not practical or convenient, and in some cases telehealth is simply preferred. Examples of patients who take advantage of telehealth services include those who are physically incapacitated; those with inflexible work schedules; or those who are temporarily living elsewhere, such as college students. APRNs provide the same type and quality of services via this medium as that delivered with traditional, in-person encounters.

Unfortunately, as of this writing, telepsychiatry in Ohio is generally not reimbursable by most commercial insurances. Although there are occasional exceptions in select rural areas of the state, especially with certain Medicare/Medicaid products, this is undeniably a constraint for some who would otherwise benefit from this modality of service. At LSW, many patients will elect to pay out of pocket for this service because telepsychiatry is offered at an appreciably discounted rate when privately paid. When traveling expenses, time away from work, and other matters of sheer expediency are considered, many patients come out ahead by using telemental health.

LSW does not currently provide any specialized training to its clinicians who opt to deliver telehealth services. This is largely because many of its APRNs have prior experience in the teleconference field, and some newer graduates received a modest level of preparation in school. It should be noted that the chief clinical officer does provide informal tutelage and anecdotal tips to clinicians who express interest. It is also felt that most providers and patients are comfortable with a virtual platform because using videoconferencing services are becoming far more commonplace in society. This breaks down barriers in effectively engaging through a virtual medium.

Although there are many robust telehealth platforms available, the ones for telepsychiatry tend to go above and beyond the needed scope. It is often said that out of all medical disciplines, psychiatry lends itself most naturally to telehealth. This is because there is less acute need for physical examination of the patient, and labs and other conventionally hands-on methods of care are less compulsory. LSW currently uses a free app called Doxy.me, available for download to most smartphones and computers. It is quick, easy, and intuitive. It is often likened as being very similar to FaceTime (Apple), but Health Insurance Portability and Accountability Act compliant. There is a superior version of this app available for purchase with considerably more bells and whistles, although this is certainly not essential.

LSW uses an EHR that is specific for outpatient psychiatry. This lends itself nicely to a technology-driven practice that is equipped to provide telehealth services. Billing and eprescribing are also managed through this same system, allowing for a seamless delivery of virtual care. Patients access LSW telehealth services by setting up an appointment with the practice just as they would for a conventional session, specifying to staff that they wish their appointment to be via teleconference. They are then taught how to download the Doxy.me app to their device. At the time of their appointment, patients are cued in a virtual waiting room, where they wait briefly until the provider joins them. While they are in the waiting room, patients can continue to go about their day, whether at work or elsewhere. Patients can later communicate with their clinician by using the patient portal via the practice's EHR.

Clinical assessment through a telehealth platform does not differ greatly from assessment conducted during an in-person appointment. Although some elements are difficult to fully appreciate, such as body language and other forms of metacommunication, most elements of a standard mental status exam are assessed in the same manner. An added benefit is that providers are often able to perform a rudimentary assessment of a patient's environment, which cannot be accurately assessed in a face-to-face appointment. A limitation is that vital signs cannot be obtained in a telehealth appointment. In other environments where telehealth is used, such as in long-term care facilities, vital signs can be obtained by ancillary staff.

At LSW, telehealth appointments currently account for less than 5% of all appointments in the practice. However, telehealth has allowed the practice to expand its hours of services because providers are often willing to see patients at times when conventional office amenities would be unlikely, such as during evenings or weekends. Although specific data have not yet been gathered, it is surmised that offering telehealth services has allowed providers to retain patients who would otherwise not be able to attend face-to-face appointments during regular business hours.

TeleICU

The teleintensive care unit (teleICU) is a form of telehealth designed to enhance care delivery and patient safety for critically ill patients using remote monitoring and telepresence technologies and can bridge the gap in care regarding facilities where round-the-clock care is not present.[59] Studies show that critically ill patients who are treated by specially trained and certified providers have a decrease in ICU mortality of 40% compared with those who are not treated by specialists, yet only 47% of hospitals report having trained critical care providers 24/7 with a page response time of less than 5 minutes.[60] TeleICUs establish telepresence between the patient, the ICU staff, and the remote ICU monitoring staff. Technology includes 2-way videoconferencing with audio in the patient room. Using telehealth monitoring and command center staff, experienced critical care physicians, critical care APRNs, and RNs, real-time access to patient vital signs and data from the patient's monitor, radiology and lab reports, and EHR, including assessment findings and medications, is possible. Electronic surveillance equipment with an alert system identifies subtle changes in patient conditions. TeleICU consultation can be activated by the onsite staff members who are seeking assistance in patient care or by the remote staff who note trends on data that are analyzed in real time at the command center. If concerning trends are identified, teleICU staff members contact the onsite staff to gather more data. Conversely, if onsite staff nurses have questions or concerns about the patient's care, they can initiate a conference with the teleICU command center. In both cases, onsite staff nurses complete a patient assessment that is viewed by off-site providers. Collaboration between the onsite nurses and teleICU providers occurs, and recommendations about patient care and treatment orders are given.

Benefits of teleICU care include a reduction in alarm fatigue and improved adherence to best practices.[61] Monitoring of patients using a variety of technologies and remote experts can decrease the rates of alarms activated, and this added oversight can improve patient safety. Regarding best practices, evidence indicates that increased compliance with critical care best practices to prevent deep vein thrombosis, stress ulcers, ventilator-assisted pneumonias, and catheter-related blood stream infections.[62,63] For optimal patient outcomes, the ability for teleICU clinicians to be involved in a patient's care from admission to discharge, not only when emergencies occur, was paramount. Although virtual rounding at the teleICU command center occurs frequently, in order to increase the effectiveness of teleICU care, a best practice recommendation encourages the presence of teleICU providers at daily patient rounds.[6]

Hot-Spotting

Hot-spotting is a population health model to identify patients who may need higher-touch care. The name comes from a 2011 *New Yorker* article describing a model originating in Camden, New Jersey, where a physician named Jeffrey Brenner started the Camden Coalition of Healthcare Providers.[64] This model has demonstrated millions of dollars in savings by targeting the most vulnerable patients who account for the most hospitalizations and consequently the highest cost care. Working with these patients using a high-frequency contact model and helping them to best interact with the challenging health care arena, as well as providing social support navigation for needs such as affordable housing, helped to reduce the burden of disease and consequently the cost of care.

Hot-spotting is used by an APRN in a small free clinic in Virginia to improve care outcomes in a population with health care disparities. In this primary care setting, patients often live with chronic diseases that are not well controlled. The reasons for poor control are often rooted in challenges with one or more social determinants of health, such as unstable housing, inability to afford medications, low literacy, unreliable transportation, poverty, undiagnosed or uncontrolled mental health issues, or substance use. Creating a system that helps patients to address these health indicators, as well as chronic disease management, supports the individual to develop improved self-management skills and adherence to the agreed treatment plan.

The first step to hot-spotting is to create a patient registry to identify the highest-risk patients. Many EHRs have a population health function that can create a disease registry.[65] In a small clinic with an EHR that does not have this function, a Microsoft Excel spreadsheet with macros can be used to create a functional patient disease registry. Regularly running EHR reports helps identify patients whose chronic disease measures are out of range and who may benefit from higher-touch care.

High-quality chronic disease management requires partnering with the patient to improve self-management skills. Telehealth is used as a tool to connect with patients to provide patient education; review recent self-management skills, such as glucose or blood pressure readings; and screen for potential side effects from medications. The program uses the adaptive telehealth platform from a Virginia telehealth patient care teams program.

Telehealth can also be used to extend the reach of the PCP through home visits by visiting nurses who can provide an environmental assessment and patient education and then facilitate a telehealth connection with the provider during the home visit. During this telehealth visit with the APRN PCP, the patient may have a health assessment completed with the aid of the visiting nurse; medications can be ordered or changed; labs can be ordered; and patient goals can be established, reinforced, or celebrated when goals are attained. These telehealth visits help to decrease some of the barriers to care and improve patient engagement with their care team.

GROUP EXERCISE

Developing an Advanced Practice Registered Nurse Telehealth Program

Group 1 will develop an APRN-led primary care telehealth program focused on improving outcomes in diabetes. Group 2 will develop an RPM program for improving outcomes in chronic disease. Each group should outline the purpose, goals, specific targeted outcome, technology used, and role of the APRN, as well as how the program works.

RESEARCH EVIDENCE FOR IMPROVED OUTCOMES

Improving outcomes through exploring and measuring patient satisfaction is a way to capture elements of care that patients hold valuable. Patients are capable of determining what creates a positive patient experience, and their perceptions of quality care, respect for the person, and provision of patient-centered care resonate and align with high-quality care. Research to determine patient satisfaction with telehealth and to identify the issues relating to telehealth patient satisfaction has been conducted and reflect high overall satisfaction. Examples of this evidence include the following:

- A systematic review of telehealth in palliative care to assess caregiver outcomes identified 9 studies for inclusion, and 77.8% were scored as moderate quality and rigor as categorized by the Cochrane Collaboration tool.[38] This review focused on the effectiveness of using telehealth home-based palliative care with a variety of technologies, including videophones, regular telephones, and internet-based interventions. Although satisfaction was not a main point of investigation in the included studies, 5 reported caregiver satisfaction using telehealth. Other findings revealed equivalent quality-of-life reporting, decreased anxiety score in 2 studies, and a report of significantly decreased caregiver burden and another equivalency with traditional care. There is evidence of overall satisfaction with telehealth interventions; they were well received and suffered few technical problems. One study showed improved family functioning, and online programs reported improved mood, decreased depression, and feelings of increased social support using telehealth interventions. Of the 9 studies reviewed, 66.7% reported improvement in quality of life and decreased caregiver burden, anxiety, depression, or stress as a result of the telehealth intervention. Overall impressions are that telehealth in home-based palliative care improves quality-of-life indicators and lightens psychological caregiver stress, particularly for those living in rural and underserved areas.
- Patient satisfaction with rural rheumatology was evaluated in 107 patients in a rural region of Australia.[39] Patients reported the perception of receiving satisfactory care; satisfaction scores were close to 90%. Additionally, due to the burden of long-distance travel required to attend an in-person visit, many patients actually preferred the telehealth visit.

- A systematic review of the evidence for patient and provider satisfaction in teledermatology was conducted, with 40 studies meeting inclusion and exclusion criteria for evaluation.[40] The 2 technologies commonly used for teledermatology visits include store-and-forward and live-interactive videoconferencing. In this review, teledermatology store-and-forward visits revealed 96% patient satisfaction and 82% satisfaction in studies that measured satisfaction. Satisfaction was also high in the live intervention group, revealing 89% patient satisfaction and 100% provider satisfaction. The study reported that dermatologists liked the live visits because they included ability to form interpersonal relationships using the videoconferencing technology, and image and assessment visualization was good. However, with the store-and-forward method, there was less opportunity to engage in a patient-provider relationship, as well as longer wait times for appointments, and the communication and information receiving was rated as lower than the live videoconferencing visits.

- A telehealth systematic literature review of 44 articles from 2010 to 2017 focused on patient satisfaction, effectiveness, and efficiency of care and identified factors associated with telehealth patient satisfaction.[37] This review found that telehealth is viewed by patients as effective and efficient, and the technology was associated with high levels of patient satisfaction because patient expectations were able to be met using telehealth. They included ease of use, cost savings, improved outcomes, patient preference, better communication capacity with providers, and time saved in traveling to the facility. Twenty percent of factors of effectiveness were improved outcomes. Additionally, the researchers found that telehealth provides high-quality service as compared with traditional in-person service, with added benefits of increasing access to obtaining care and improving patient engagement, self-care awareness behaviors, and motivation to improve management of chronic disease. The health care community also benefits from telehealth because it can be used to improve provider knowledge through consultations and education, decrease missed patient appointments, and decrease wait times for appointments, and it has been influential in forming programs that decrease readmissions by improving self-care and medical management. Health care policy and regulations need continual adjustments and enhancements by way of parity of reimbursements because telehealth has been demonstrated to be a tool that can improve health.

- The University of Missouri Telehealth Network examined how technologies are perceived and used and how they relate to satisfaction among a survey of 286 patients, 21 providers, and 12 telehealth coordinators.[64] The survey found that patients and providers have high satisfaction and acceptance for telehealth, although their perceptions that make up their experiences are different. Patients found telehealth valuable for its ability to decrease the distance traveled to reach the care provider. Providers found that confidence with the technology quality for clinical care and ease in operating it for the encounter was high. Coordinators reported high confidence with the simplicity of using the technology and found that scheduling the appointments was efficient. Providers reported some technological challenges and noted that a lack of training decreased confidence and ability to use the technology. Overall, all 3 groups scored high in satisfaction as evaluated by a survey of perceptions and opinions of the users. Although patients liked the accessibility of the care, providers were confident they were able to deliver quality care, and coordinators felt it was highly satisfying to their role. Providers were skeptical of telehealth replacing hands-on care. It is possible that high telehealth satisfaction is translated to increased use of telehealth by request of patients.

- A cross-sectional survey of 3303 patients with 54% response rate at a CVS MinuteClinic evaluated satisfaction with telehealth visits as compared with routine in-person visits.[27] Ninety-five percent reported that they were very satisfied with the care and rated the visit as preferred or just as good as traditional care. Thirty-three percent preferred telehealth, and 57% liked telehealth as compared with traditional visits. A lack of medical insurance was associated with 21% increased odds of preferring telehealth. Being female was found to be a predictor of telehealth satisfaction, as was understanding about what telehealth is and receiving quality care at a convenient time and location. This survey also examined characteristics and attitudes of users to identify any variables pointing to preferences for using telehealth. Fifty percent of users focused responses favorably on the shorter wait times, linking motivation for use to satisfaction. Improved access to care was also associated to a higher reported satisfaction.

As more and more technology is merged with care, patient satisfaction with telehealth as part of the overall patient experience must be further explored. Additional technology-related factors, perception, and attitudes must also be discerned so that patient and provider attitudes and expectations for the virtual care encounter are met and accurately measured.

CONCLUSION

APRNs are poised to impart telehealth as a legitimate part of nursing practice as foundations of APRN practice align, support, encourage, and require that nurses be able to seamlessly incorporate telehealth into everyday nursing care. As APRNs explore how telehealth and traditional nursing practice align, they will gain confidence and fortitude in understanding the care concepts and working with the technology to improve access and outcomes, extend APRN provider capacity, and provide highly satisfying telehealth care experiences. APRNs can express this knowledge, creativity, and innovation through developing meaningful telehealth programs that address complex patient problems. With many states providing full scope of practice, this is the time for APRNs to fully immerse traditional and virtual practice and visualize how telehealth will change, support, enhance, and reshape nursing practice.

THOUGHTFUL QUESTIONS

1. In what ways could you connect nursing competencies for your APRN specialty to a telehealth practice that used remote monitoring?
2. Reflect on your current practice experiences and compare how you could affect more patients using telehealth to address the PCP shortage. What programs would you develop, and how would they work to extend provider capacity?
3. Does the HCAHPS satisfaction survey adequately capture satisfaction with telehealth and virtual care visits? Why or why not?
4. What would the advantages be regarding an APRN-led mobile primary care practice that incorporated telehealth as part of the services?

CASE STUDY

Samantha, a doctorally prepared nurse practitioner, owns and manages a family practice clinic that serves a large, underserved inner city and has a robust patient volume. Kitty is a CNS who works with Samantha and 4 other APRNs at the clinic. Many patients are over 65 years of age in this practice, and many are disadvantaged and have multiple chronic diseases, including diabetes, cardiovascular disease, pulmonary disease, and stroke. Stroke is prevalent in this community; it is in a part of the country called the Stroke Belt, known for high rates of stroke. This clinic also reports a high 30-day stroke readmission rate of 24%, much higher than the national average. A university medical center a short distance away has recently set up a home monitoring program for patients with strokes who are discharged from the hospital. However, under CMS guidelines, many patients with strokes in this practice are not eligible for this program. Samantha and Kitty want to address this gap in care by developing an RPM for the patients who fall through this gap. Toward that end, Kitty has contacted a local remote monitoring company, and they have decided to partner to develop a pilot program at no cost to the clinic. Samantha forms a stakeholder group of like-minded professionals to discuss development of such a program. She also wonders how the telehealth program could address other barriers the clinic faces, such as provider shortages.

Questions

1. When the group meets, what are some of the goals for such a program?
2. What would the purpose be, and how could it be accomplished to achieve a desired outcome?
3. What technology would be needed, and what data would it collect?
4. How would the data be used to improve outcomes?
5. Samantha is also concerned about whether such a program would be satisfying to her patients because she has such a strong relationship with them and wonders how that nursing presence could be translated using this program. How could this be measured to provide meaning to the program?

REFERENCES

1. Centers for Medicare and Medicaid Services. HCAHPS: patients' perspectives of care survey. https://www.cms .gov/medicare/quality-initiatives-patient-assessment-instruments/hospitalqualityinits/hospitalhcahps.html. Updated February 11, 2020. Accessed February 24, 2020.
2. Hawkins SY. Telehealth nurse practitioner student clinical experiences: an essential educational component for today's health care setting. *Nurse Educ Today*. 2012;32(8):842-845.
3. APRN Consensus Work Group & the National Council of State Boards of Nursing APRN Advisory Committee. Consensus model for APRN regulation: licensure, accreditation, certification & education. https://www.ncsbn .org/Consensus_Model_for_APRN_Regulation_July_2008.pdf. Published July 7, 2008. Accessed February 24, 2020.
4. Xue Y, Ye Z, Brewer C, Spetz J. Impact of state nurse practitioner scope-of-practice regulation on health care delivery: systematic review. *Nurs Outlook*. 2016;64(1):71-85.
5. Adashi EY, Geiger HJ, Fine MD. Health care reform and primary care—the growing importance of the community health center. *N Engl J Med*. 2010;362(22):2047-2050.
6. Landon BE, Hicks LS, O'Malley AJ, et al. Improving the management of chronic disease at community health centers. *N Engl J Med*. 2007;356(9):921-934.

7. Naylor MD, Kurtzman ET. The role of nurse practitioner in reinventing primary care. *Health Aff (Millwood)*. 2010;29(5):893-899.

8. Kaiser Family Foundation. Improving access to adult primary care in Medicaid: exploring the potential role of nurse practitioners and physician assistants. https://www.kff.org/medicaid/issue-brief/improving-access-to-adult-primary-care-in/. Published March 1, 2011. Accessed February 24, 2020.

9. Gadbois EA, Miller EA, Tyler D, Intrator O. Trends in state regulation of nurse practitioners and physician assistants, 2001 to 2010. *Med Care Res Rev*. 2015;72(2):200-219.

10. Fronczek AE. Nursing theory in virtual care. *Nurs Sci Q*. 2019;32(1):35-38.

11. Thomas A, Crabtree MK, Delaney K, et al. Nurse practitioner core competencies: April 2011. National Organization of Nurse Practitioner Faculties. https://www.pncb.org/sites/default/files/2017-02/NONPF_Core_Competencies.pdf. Published April 2011. Amended 2012. Accessed February 24, 2020.

12. National Association of Clinical Nurse Specialists. *Statement on Clinical Nurse Specialist Practice and Education: Third Edition*. https://portal.nacns.org/ItemDetail?iProductCode=STATEMENT_W&Category=WEB&WebsiteKey=cd0cefd9-bfa4-45cc-a6f8-1c4ea4450d93. Published 2019. Accessed April 28, 2020.

13. American Association of Nurse Anesthetists. Standards for Nurse Anesthesia Practice. https://www.aana.com/docs/default-source/practice-aana-com-web-documents-(all)/standards-for-nurse-anesthesia-practice.pdf. Revised February 2019. Accessed April 28, 2020.

14. American College of Nurse-Midwives. Definition of midwifery and scope of practice of certified nurse-midwives and certified midwives. https://www.midwife.org/acnm/files/ccLibraryFiles/Filename/000000007043/Definition-of-Midwifery-and-Scope-of-Practice-of-CNMs-and-CMs-Feb-2012.pdf. Updated February 6, 2012. Accessed February 26, 2020.

15. The Physician's Foundation. 2014 survey of America's physicians. https://physiciansfoundation.org/wp-content/uploads/2017/12/2014_Physicians_Foundation_Biennial_Physician_Survey_Report.pdf. Published 2014. Accessed February 26, 2020.

16. Kaiser Family Foundation. Primary Care Health Professional Shortage Areas (HPSAs). https://www.kff.org/other/state-indicator/primary-care-health-professional-shortage-areas-hpsas/?currentTimeframe=0&sortModel=%7B%22colId%22:%22Location%22,%22sort%22:%22asc%22%7D. Updated September 30, 2019. Accessed February 26, 2020.

17. Health Resources & Services Administration. Health Professional Shortage Areas (HPSAs). https://bhw.hrsa.gov/shortage-designation/hpsas. Updated May 2019. Accessed February 26, 2020.

18. American Association of Nurse Practitioners. Nurse practitioner role grows to more than 270,000. *AANP News*. https://www.aanp.org/news-feed/nurse-practitioner-role-continues-to-grow-to-meet-primary-care-provider-shortages-and-patient-demands. Published January 28, 2019. Accessed February 26, 2020.

19. Fathi JT, Modin HE, Scott JD. Nurses advancing telehealth services in the era of healthcare reform. *Online J Issues Nurs*. 2017;(22)2.

20. Health Resources & Services Administration. MUA Find. https://data.hrsa.gov/tools/shortage-area/mua-find. Accessed February 26, 2020.

21. Health Resources & Services Administration. Medically Underserved Areas and Populations (MUA/Ps). https://bhw.hrsa.gov/shortage-designation/muap. Updated June 2019. Accessed February 26, 2020.

22. Community Health Association of Mountain/Plains States. Understanding HPSAs and MUAs. http://champsonline.org/tools-products/rrresources/understanding-hpsas-and-muas. Accessed February 26, 2020.

23. Health Resources & Services Administration. Tools. https://bhw.hrsa.gov/shortage-designation/hpsas)-page-. Accessed June 25, 2019.

24. Heiser S. New findings confirm predictions on physician shortage. News release. Association of American Medical Colleges. April 23, 2019. https://news.aamc.org/press-releases/article/workforce_report_shortage_04112018/. Accessed February 26, 2020.

25. Kvedar J, Coye MJ, Everett W. Connected health: a review of technologies and strategies to improve patient care with telemedicine and telehealth. *Health Aff (Millwood)*. 2014;33(2):194-199.

26. Peck A. Changing the face of standard nursing practice through telehealth and telenursing. *Nurs Adm Q*. 2005;29(4):339-343.

27. Polinski JM, Barker T, Gagliano N, Sussman A, Brennan TA, Shrank WH. Patients' satisfaction with and preference for telehealth visits. *J Gen Intern Med*. 2016;31(3):269-275.

28. Nesbitt TS, Marcin JP, Daschbach MM, Cole SL. Perceptions of local health care quality in 7 rural communities with telemedicine. *J Rural Health*. 2005;21(1):79-85.

29. LaPointe J. Greater non-physician staffing helps healthcare revenue cycle. *RevCycle Intelligence*. https://revcycleintelligence.com/news/greater-non-physician-staffing-helps-healthcare-revenue-cycle. Published July 21, 2017. Accessed February 26, 2020.

30. Kash B, McKahan M. The evolution of measuring patient satisfaction. *J Primary Health Care Gen Practice*. 2017;1(1).

31. Ware JE Jr, Snyder MK, Wright WR, Davies AR. Defining and measuring patient satisfaction with medical care. *Eval Program Plann.* 1983;6(3-4):247-263.

32. Siegrist RB Jr. Patient satisfaction: history, myths, and misperceptions. *Virtual Mentor.* 2013;15(11):982-987.

33. Institute of Medicine. Crossing the quality chasm: a new health system for the 21st century. http://www .nationalacademies.org/hmd/~/media/Files/Report%20Files/2001/Crossing-the-Quality-Chasm/Quality%20 Chasm%202001%20%20report%20brief.pdf. Published March 2001. Accessed February 26, 2020.

34. Kaambwa B, Ratcliffe J, Shulver W, et al. Investigating the preferences of older people for telehealth as a new model of health care delivery service: a discrete choice experiment. *J Telemed Telecare.* 2017;23(2):301-313.

35. Greenwald P, Stern ME, Clark S, Sharma R. Older adults and technology: in telehealth, they may not be who you think they are. *Int J Emerg Med.* 2018;11(1):2.

36. Levy CE, Silverman E, Jia H, Geiss M, Omura D. Effects of physical therapy delivery via home video telerehabilitation on functional health and quality of life outcomes. *J Rehabil Res Dev.* 2015;52(3):361-370.

37. Kruse CS, Krowski N, Rodriguez B, Tran L, Vela J, Brooks M. Telehealth and patient satisfaction: a systematic review and narrative analysis. *BMJ Open.* 2017;7(8):e016242.

38. Zheng Y, Head BA, Schapmire TJ. A systematic review of telehealth in palliative care: caregiver outcomes. *Telemed J E Health.* 2016;22(4):288-294.

39. Poulsen KA, Millen CM, Lakshman UI, Buttner PG, Roberts LJ. Satisfaction with rural rheumatology telemedicine service. *Int J Rheum Dis.* 2015;18(3):304-314.

40. Mounessa JS, Chapman S, Braunberger T, et al. A systematic review of satisfaction with teledermatology. *J Telemed Telecare.* 2018;24(4):263-270.

41. The Health Wagon. https://thehealthwagon.org/hwwp/. Accessed February 26, 2020.

42. University of Wisconsin Population Health Institute. 2014 county health rankings key findings report. https://www.countyhealthrankings.org/sites/default/files/media/document/2014%20County%20Health%20 Rankings%20Key%20Findings.pdf. Published 2014. Accessed February 26, 2020.

43. Virginia Department of Health Professions Healthcare Workforce Data Center. 2008 Virginia physician workforce survey findings and recommendations. https://www.dhp.virginia.gov/media/dhpweb/docs/hwdc/medicine /2008PhysicianFindings8-6-2010.pdf. Published July 2010. Accessed February 26, 2020.

44. Bowman SW. Update: Virginia physician workforce shortage. Joint Commission on Healthcare. http:// jchc.virginia.gov/Final%20%20Physician%20Shortage%20color.pdf. Published September 17, 2013. Accessed February 26, 2020.

45. Virginia Department of Health. Behavioral risk factor surveillance survey: tobacco data. http://www.vdh .virginia.gov/brfss/data/#TOBACCO. Accessed February 26, 2020.

46. Pruthi RS, Neuwahl S, Nielsen ME, Fraher E. Recent trends in the urology workforce in the United States. *Urology.* 2013;82(5):987-993.

47. Children's Health Fund. 15 million kids in health care deserts: can telehealth make a difference? https://ms01 .childrenshealthfund.org/wp/wp-content/uploads/2016/04/White-Paper-4.4.2016.pdf. Published April 21, 2016. Accessed February 26, 2020.

48. Ollove M. Telemedicine in schools helps keep kids in the classroom. The PEW Charitable Trusts. https://www .pewtrusts.org/en/research-and-analysis/blogs/stateline/2017/01/04/telemedicine-in-schools-helps-keep-kids-in -the-classroom. Published January 4, 2017. Accessed February 26, 2020.

49. Reynolds CA, Maughan ED. Telehealth in the school setting: an integrative review. *J Sch Nurs.* 2015;31(1):44-53.

50. Center for Rural Health Innovation. Health-e-Schools. http://crhi.org/contact.html. Accessed February 26, 2020.

51. Buswell SA, Lechtenberg J, Hinkson E, et al. The role of the 21st century school nurse [position statement]. National Association of School Nurses. https://www.nasn.org/advocacy/professional-practice-documents /position-statements/ps-role. Published June 2016. Amended June 2018. Accessed February 26, 2020.

52. Medical University of South Carolina. Schools. https://muschealth.org/medical-services/telehealth/services /schools. Accessed February 26, 2020.

53. Grand-Aides USA. Grand-Aides USA summary. http://www.grand-aides.com/the-program/grand-aides -summary. Accessed February 26, 2020.

54. Thomas SC, Greevy RA Jr, Garson A Jr. Effect of Grand-Aides Nurse Extenders on readmissions and emergency department visits in Medicare patients with heart failure. *Am J Cardiol.* 2018;121(11):1336-1342.

55. Lowery C, Bronstein J, McGhee J, Ott R, Reece EA, Mays GP. ANGELS and University of Arkansas for Medical Sciences paradigm for distant obstetrical care delivery. *Am J Obstet Gynecol.* 2007;196(6):534.e1-9.

56. Rhoads SJ, Eswaran H, Lynch CE, Ounparseuth ST, Magann EF, Lowery CL. High-risk obstetrical call center: a model for regions with limited access to care. *J Matern Fetal Neonatal Med.* 2018;31(7):857-865.

57. Bronstein JM, Ounpraseuth S, Jonkman J, et al. Use of specialty OB consults during high-risk pregnancies in a Medicaid-covered population: initial impact of the Arkansas ANGELS intervention. *Med Care Res Rev.* 2012;69(6):699-720.

58. Benton T, Barringer S, Boulden B, et al. ANGELS Annual Report. 2017-2018. https://angels.uams.edu/wp- content/uploads/sites/81/2019/02/2018-Angels-annual-report-1901383a.pdf. Accessed April 28, 2020.

59. Sewell J. *Informatics and Nursing: Opportunities and Challenges.* Philadelphia, PA: Wolters Kluwer; 2016.

60. Castlight Health. Intensive care unit physician staffing. http://www.leapfroggroup.org/sites/default/files/Files/Castlight-Leapfrog-ICU-Physician-Staffing-Report-2016.pdf. Published 2016. Accessed February 26, 2020.

61. Healthcare Information and Management Systems Society. Reducing ICU length of stay: the effect of tele-ICU. https://www.himss.org/reducing-icu-length-stay-effect-tele-icu. Accessed June 25, 2019.

62. Lilly CM, Cody S, Zhao H, et al. Hospital mortality, length of stay, and preventable complications among critically ill patients before and after tele-ICU reengineering of critical care processes. *JAMA*. 2011;305(21):2175-2183.

63. Sadaka F, Palagiri A, Trottier S, et al. Telemedicine intervention improves ICU outcomes. *Crit Care Res Pract*. 2013;2013:456389.

64. Becevic M, Boren S, Mutrux R, Shah Z, Banerjee S. User satisfaction with telehealth: study of patients, providers, and coordinators. *Health Care Manag (Frederick)*. 2015;34(4):337-349.

65. Liaw ST, Taggart J, Yu H, Rahimi A. Electronic health records and disease registries to support integrated care in a health neighbourhood: an ontology-based methodology. *AMIA Jt Summits Transl Sci Proc*. 2014;2014:50-54.

8

Telehealth Competencies
Knowledge and Skills

Carolyn M. Rutledge, PhD, FNP-BC
Tina Gustin, DNP, CNS
Patty Alane Schweickert, DNP, FNP-C

CHAPTER OBJECTIVES

Upon review of this chapter, the reader will be able to:

1. Describe techniques that can be used as alternatives for many of the in-person assessment skills used by providers.
2. Describe the outline telehealth etiquette steps that must be considered when conducting a videoconferencing telehealth visit.
3. Discuss ethical issues that may affect the delivery of care through telehealth.
4. Describe competencies (knowledge and skills) that are required of the advanced practice registered nurse (APRN) in conducting a successful telehealth visit.

With the advancement of telehealth, APRNs are faced with developing new knowledge and skills or modifying their existing approaches to care in order to provide meaningful health care visits via telehealth. The competencies include interpersonal as well as technological and clinical skills. This can be very challenging because APRNs are faced with reconceptualizing the way they practice in a new or virtual environment. Telehealth-prepared APRNs must have excellent communication and organizational skills, as well as an understanding of technology. They must develop skills that enable the telehealth visit to be as seamless as possible. Specific emphasis in this chapter will be on the following:

- The virtual environment
- Ethical considerations
- Telehealth etiquette
- Required knowledge and skills

Schweickert PA, Rutledge CM, eds.
Telehealth Essentials for Advanced Practice Nursing (pp 171-191).
© 2020 Taylor & Francis Group.

Competencies specifically required for telehealth are grouped into the following:

- Interpersonal relationship
- Technological competencies
- Clinical competencies
- Implementation competencies

THE VIRTUAL ENVIRONMENT AND TELEPRESENCE

Nurses have historically practiced in the physical environment, where they are present in-person with their patients and with other providers. This environment allows nurses to form a relationship with patients through physical contact. It allows empathy to be demonstrated through touch. It enables providers to use their hands as they conduct their physical assessments. It provides the opportunity for nurses to use their senses as they diagnose their patients.

As technological advancements are being introduced into health care, a new virtual environment is being created. What exactly is a virtual environment? What does it mean to practice in a virtual environment? How do the nurse and patient enter the virtual environment? How does the nurse translate traditional, in-person nursing practice to this virtual environment? These are just some of the many questions to explore when thinking about how to care for the patient in the virtual environment.

As technology is applied to health care, creating this virtual environment, the APRN can connect and provide care to patients at a distance. Telehealth communication platforms using live videoconferencing enable providers and patients to see, hear, and interact with each other in real time, remotely. This format can be used to provide the patient with care, education, support, management, and monitoring virtually using technology.

Although new solutions, such as telehealth, are needed to address current health care challenges, including lack of access to care and health care provider shortages, new solutions to problems ultimately raise new issues and questions to consider. Accordingly, advances in communication technologies necessitate new ways of thinking about providing care in the virtual environment. Practicing in the virtual environment disrupts traditional practice:

> Technology has a major role in transforming the workplace, not only in terms of the machinery and equipment used but how we do things, how we organize ourselves as nurses, what we value, why we use technology and what influences our patterns of thinking.[1(p362)]

Exploring what a virtual environment is and how the provider and patient connect will set the foundation to assess similarities and differences of physically present practice vs virtual practice.

Health care has a history of adapting to new models of technology-driven care delivery. Sir Charles Wheatstone developed the first virtual reality technology in 1838 with the invention of the stereoscope.[2] A more modern version of the stereoscope, developed in 1939, was called the View Master.[3] Modern virtual reality technology has developed over the past 6 decades, resulting in wide virtualization technology applications in industry, disaster and emergency response training, automotive and flight simulation training, and medical and nursing education through simulation, including standardized patients, low- and high-fidelity mannequins, and virtual educational worlds.[4]

Virtual environments are defined in a variety of ways according to the specific use and discipline defining them, but all contain the sense of presence at their core. The computer gaming industry uses the terms *virtual environment* and *virtual worlds* somewhat interchangeably because they relate to technology for recreational use.[4,5] In computer gaming, a virtual world, sometimes termed a *virtual environment*, is a "synchronous, persistent network of people, represented by avatars, facilitated by networked computers."[6(p1)] Virtual environments are fundamentally technology-enhanced environments where participants "experience others as being there with them—and where they can interact with them"[7(p1)] and as a technology-enhanced, computer-generated display that "enables the people connected to feel present with one another."[7(p1)] This means that in the virtual environment, the user feels like he or she is present at the other site with the person he or she is connecting to. Users have a sense of presence in that remote environment.

Related themes of presence align to health care, as providers incorporate presence into therapeutic care. Heinrichs offers that when virtual environments are used for clinical purposes, they could be referred to as "immersive clinical environments or virtual clinical worlds"[4] because they have the features of presence, engagement, team-based activities, and real workplace settings. At their foundation, virtual environments are virtual spaces where people connect using technology, in real time, for realistic experiences to communicate with a sense of presence. Health care virtual environments use real-time videoconferencing technologies to connect users (provider and patient) to one another. In this way, users can see, hear, and interact with one another virtually as if they were physically present with one another.

This new environment of care presents new questions, such as when technology links the provider and patient together, enabling them to see and hear one another, does this constitute the virtual environment? In other words, does merely establishing the telecommunications technology link place the patient and provider in the virtual environment? The answer to this question is that the establishment of the telecommunications link enables the provider and the patient to communicate, creating a virtual space for their interaction. However, it is not until they communicate with a sense of presence that they are in the virtual environment. Connecting with the patient in the virtual environment requires establishing contact with the patient such that the patient recognizes your presence as a provider that is communicating with them. Therefore, while each person is in their own physical environment, they are also together in this new space that is formed using the technology to form a presence with one another. Therefore, to answer the question of whether providers can affect a sense of presence with the patient in the virtual environment, the answer is a resounding yes!

Presence

Nursing presence is traditionally accomplished through a combination of physical and psychological presence.[8] The physical presence becomes part of the experience when the provider touches a patient, such as in performing procedures, moving or assisting the patient, or using therapeutic touch. The psychological presence manifests through the use of mindfulness to produce meaningful communications with the patient. The dual characteristics of both touch and listening help the provider find significance in what the person is conveying so that these insights can be used to individualize improvements in patient health.[9]

> Healthy therapeutic relationships enhance wholeness and healing; they are the key to effective health promotion. Therapeutic nursing presence demonstrates caring, empathy, and connecting-qualities required to build rapport and trust between nurse and patient.[8(p1)]

However, practicing in the virtual environment raises questions as to whether a provider's presence can be accomplished without the element of physical presence and therapeutic touch. Additionally, can elements of psychological presence, including active listening and mindful connection, be achieved using technology?

In a study to assess quality of communications in teleconsultations using videophones in older adults, it was found that the interactions between the nurse and the patient felt as a momentary sense of being in one another's rooms and was experienced as nursing presence when security, familiarity, transparency, and focus on the patient was present.[10] Further, nurses used traditional nursing skills to develop nursing presence in the virtual environment, suggesting that traditional nursing skills of presence are transferable to the virtual environment. Nursing presence requires being present with one's whole self, and this aspect of nursing presence using traditional skills was demonstrated in a study involving regular telephones and non-video internet links. Participants described the feeling of nursing presence in their communications, suggesting that nursing presence can be communicated using common skills and non-video forms of communication technology.[11] Adding both audio and visual technologies increase the potential success of translating nursing presence to the virtual environment.

In physically present practice, providers use their senses to interact with and assess patients. The provider can also use these traditional skills to assess and interact with patients forming the provider-patient presence in the virtual environment, while "the technology offers additional transformational opportunities to be present with persons receiving nursing care as nurses center and are aware of the words, silences, and movements that are there and are not there."[12] Achieving authentic presence in the virtual environment requires presence to be developed without physical touch. Because the dimension of touch cannot be employed in the virtual environment, promoting and perceiving presence at a distance are important concepts to pursue for virtual practice.[8]

Promoting presence involves competencies necessary to enhance meaningful communication with the patient at a distance and involves maintaining a safe and secure space to engage with the patient, being experienced with the technology, being familiar with the patient, showing interest in the patient, and showing honesty and transparency. The sound of one's voice, inflections of speech, verbal interactions, and nonverbal body language play a greater role in the virtual environment. For example, facial expressions become more important as part of the listening and engaging process and can transmit valuable information to the patient.[13] An increased importance should be focused on promoting presence strategies as part of the development of telepresence competency.

ETHICS IN TELEHEALTH

Telehealth and the virtual environment bring unique ethical challenges to health care. Specific ethical situations of moral distress, moral conflict, and moral paradox are inherent in any practice, especially those using telehealth. Providers using telehealth must adhere to the same professional standards required during an in-person visit and be cognizant of and adhere to the laws as they apply to telehealth.[14] Conscience, commitment, compassion, confidence, competence, and comportment are foundational in forming the moral relationship.[15] The ethics of nursing practice are immersed in a holistic care approach through responsibility to another and alignment to the principles of respect, beneficence, nonmalfeasance, autonomy, and justice.[16-18] The ethical provider is seen as transparent, dependable, and trustworthy and ensures confidentiality.

Ethical care in the virtual environment mirrors ethical considerations in traditional, in-person care. However, new ethical concepts and issues arise in the virtual environment that lend consideration to technology design issues, equity of access, the provider-patient relationship, and therapeutic touch. Patients exposed to ethical encounters can trust that providers do all they can to optimize their health and welfare. They believe providers will be honest and provide them with competent care. They assume providers will respect their privacy and confidentiality. These perspectives can be challenged by the introduction of telehealth.[14] Common ethical concerns in traditional and virtual nursing ethics include the concern for maintaining patient privacy and security in all exchanges and data gleaned and transferred, as well as ensuring accuracy of information and confidentiality. Additionally, informed consent, autonomy of the patients, and empowerment are also essential ethical elements woven into the fabric of health care. The question of whether the same ethical standards and accountability apply to care in the virtual environment can be answered by examining practice in the virtual environment. Concepts such as ethical caring[16,17] and technological competency as caring[17] apply to the use of telehealth technology and support the concept of ethical caring in the virtual environment. Telehealth can affect the provider-patient interaction by removing the ability to touch and to see the environment. It is thus of utmost importance that the provider assures the patient that the platform being used is Health Insurance Portability and Accountability Act (HIPAA) secure and that doors have been closed, and then inform them of those who are in the room. It is also important to reassure the patient that he or she is not being recorded and that his or her information is secure and will not be shared unless agreed upon.

In order to maintain an ethical telehealth encounter, providers should take specific care to do the following[14]:

- Inform the patient/family of both the advantages and limitations to the telehealth services they receive.
- Ensure that the patient has access to care, especially in emergencies.
- Institute a back-up plan if he or she is unable to get the information needed during the telehealth encounter to make an appropriate diagnosis and develop the treatment plan.
- Confirm the patient's identity and the identity of those with the patient.
- Keep detailed records of the visit.
- Adhere to appropriate clinical guidelines/protocols.
- Obtain consent as needed.
- Introduce him- or herself and outline his or her credentials and then identify the others in the room, along with their credentials.
- Connect, collaborate, and communicate with any health professionals or family member that might be with the patient.
- Set up plan for continuity of care, referrals, and transmission of patient data.
- Select and use equipment that is secure and HIPAA compliant.
- Make sure he or she is in a private place when conducting the visit.
- Advocate and lobby for changes in laws and regulations that negatively affect the use of telehealth for patient care.

To identify the ethical aspects of telehealth nursing practice, nurses must be able to voice and identify the source of the ethical concern, using critical reflection to further specify the concern and discuss its consequences to the ethics of practice.[19] Telehealth must have a user-friendly design and patient-focused approach. Through knowledge of the traditional ethical issues that arise in practice, nurses can guide the use of technology in practice because respect for human dignity is important in the virtual environment just as it is in the traditional environment of practice.[20] Technology plays a role in ethical decision making by being part of the tools of care and communication in health care.

FOR REFLECTION 1:

Ethical Implications for Telehealth

You have a patient who needs to see a specialist. A specialist is available for consult via videoconferencing. What ethical concerns would you have? What steps would you take to make sure that no ethical issues were violated?

TELEHEALTH ETIQUETTE

Telemedicine requires professionals to develop the patient-provider relationship in a different and more deliberate manner.[21] One can be an excellent in-person provider but not a great telehealth provider. There is a different skill set required for this type of encounter.[22] Providers, regardless of profession, spend time learning how to demonstrate empathy, provide motivational interviewing, and read body language for in-person visits. They are not, however, trained in methods to translate these skills into a telehealth encounter. These skills do not intuitively transfer to a telehealth encounter. Despite the overwhelming use of social media for communication, this type of communication does not translate to telehealth. It has been suggested that the everyday use of technology has lessened individuals' abilities to empathize and pick up on nonverbal cues when using technology to communicate.[23] Research has shown that without proper training, even seasoned providers are unsuccessful in telemedicine visits.[24] The best technologies can fail without proper human interaction and preparation.

Although most providers have used social media platforms such as Skype (Microsoft), FaceTime (Apple), and Snapchat (Snap Inc) to communicate with friends and families, this informal approach often leads to lazy or unprofessional use of similar professional platforms. The casual nature of social platforms has led to disinhibited behaviors, such as diminished empathy and disinterested expressions.[23] This disinhibited behavior is diminished regardless of age, gender, or profession. It has even been speculated that everyday use of the internet has diminished individuals' ability to pick up on nonverbal cues. In order to optimize the provider's use of telehealth, the terms *telehealth etiquette* and *webside manner* have been coined.

Defining Telehealth Etiquette and Its Three Focus Areas

Telehealth etiquette can be thought of as the soft skills or *screenside etiquette* unique to the telehealth encounter. Telehealth etiquette includes both verbal and nonverbal expression from the provider. It includes the environment, the provider's performance, and privacy considerations unique to a telehealth encounter. This type of visit must be conducted in a different and deliberate manner from that of a traditional in-person visit. Many telehealth failures are not because of failed equipment, but because of poor etiquette and failed performance.[25] Telehealth technology is important, but without proper relationship building, telehealth is not going to work.[25] Patient satisfaction with health care encounters hinges on the communication with the provider, not necessarily the physical presence.[26]

When considering telehealth etiquette, there are 3 distinct categories that must be addressed: environment, performance, and privacy (Table 8-1). A telehealth encounter is optimized in situations where these 3 categories are addressed, enabling distractors to be removed. The provider should take time to address each of these issues prior to the encounter. He or she should also prepare the patient or caregiver to optimize the telehealth etiquette in his or her space.

Environment

The environment includes visual and auditory factors. Visual factors include the provider's appearance/actions, clothing choices, lighting, appearance of the room, and picture quality. Auditory factors include noises created by the provider, sounds in the background, and audio quality.

Visual Factors

Visual factors can enhance the telehealth encounter by enabling both the provider and the patient to focus on their relationship as opposed to being distracted by what they see in the environment. The provider's appearance must be considered when conducting a telehealth encounter. The transmission of a professional appearance is just as important in the telehealth encounter as

TABLE 8-1	
TELEHEALTH ETIQUETTE	
FACTORS	**EXAMPLES**
Environment	*Visual* • Provider appearance • Room appearance • Lighting • Picture quality *Auditory* • Provider noises • Background noise • Audio quality
Performance	Provider appearance/communication Use of equipment Provider preparation
Privacy	Privacy of sites Equipment privacy settings Consents

in an in-person visit. In person, the patient can see the provider's name badge located anywhere on the body. In a telehealth encounter, the provider should carefully place the badge within sight of the camera. Close-up shots should be used when possible because this fosters a sense of bonding between patient and provider. Along with a well-groomed professional appearance when conducting a telemedicine encounter, the provider must also consider clothing and jewelry choices. Dark colors and prints should be avoided.[27] Dark colors will wash out the appearance of the presenter, while shapes and patterns may blur on the screen, which may distract the patient.[28] Glittery, bright jewelry may divert attention away from the presenter. Movements that are not generally noticed or are annoying during the in-person visit are amplified on the screen.[28] An analogy is the difference between stage acting and television acting. The stage actor (in-person visit) uses larger movements and intonations. The television actor must practice subtle movements, gestures, and tone because they appear much larger on the screen.[29]

The appearance of the provider's room is equally important. The provider must make sure the room that is being televised is neat and professional in appearance. Clutter can be distracting to the patient and cause him or her to divert his or her attention from the provider. Food and drink left in view can be distracting to the patient, especially if the provider is eating or drinking while the session is being conducted.[30] The wall color should also be taken into consideration. Wallpaper with designs can distort the patient's view of the provider. The most desirable color for telehealth is a medium blue or gray in that it is soothing and least distracting. The wall paint should be flat-based paint to avoid any reflection from the wall. Objects in the background such as plants and pictures can also be a source of distraction. In one noteworthy encounter, a child being seen for oppositional defiant disorder and paranoia suddenly jumped up, threw his chair, and stormed out of the distant site. He screamed, "There is something growing out of your head!" In this case, the psychiatrist had not centered his head within the canvas, and he had a plant positioned on a shelf behind him. It appeared to the child that a plant was growing from his head. This mother was so distraught by her child's reaction she elected not to have a telehealth visit for her child again.

The lighting in the room should also be considered. Windows can cause shadows or cause the provider to become backlit, thus interfering with the visual quality of the interview. If the room is too dark or overly bright, it may be difficult to see the provider. The light source should be in front of the face, not behind. Any harsh lighting should be avoided. These considerations apply to both overhead and table lighting.

It is very important to make sure that the quality of the picture being shown on the screen is clear. It is disconcerting to have a loss of visual connectivity or picture distortion during a telehealth encounter. Equipment should be selected for videoconferencing encounters based on its picture quality. The equipment should be tested prior to the encounter to make sure the picture is easily seen by both the provider and patient.

Auditory Factors

The provider and patient/caregiver may be easily distracted by noises they hear, as well as by poor sound quality.[30,31] The provider should be cognizant of things he or she does that can produce distracting noises. For instance, the banging of bracelets, the clicking of a pen, the tapping of a keyboard, or the rustling of paper can be amplified over the audio connection. Chewing gum or eating can also produce distracting sounds and even make the provider's words unclear. Multiple providers in a visit must avoid any side conversations or taking phone calls.

Noises in the background can also produce a distraction. These include the voices or activities of people in the background, interruptions, traffic, construction, running equipment, ringing phones, or overhead announcements. In order to minimize external noises, the provider will want to shut the door, inform those at his or her site of the telehealth visit, put a sign on the door informing others that a telehealth visit is taking place, select a time for the interview when there is less activity, select a room that is removed from active areas, turn off or mute the phones, and mute announcements.

The telehealth equipment or connection may have an effect on the sound quality. Too often, there will be a buzzing sound when several people are connected to a visit or when a mobile phone is connected. This can be reduced by having the individuals on the session mute their microphones when they are not speaking. In order to keep the patient/caregiver from receiving unwarranted information, it will be important to turn the microphone off prior to the visit and once it is concluded. The provider should test the equipment prior to the session to make sure the microphone is connected, the sound works and is clear, and the connectivity is strong. A telehealth visit will fail if the audio is not functioning well.

One example of a problematic telehealth visit made worse by the provider's lack of awareness of the equipment resulted in an awkward situation for both the provider and patient. At the start of this visit, the provider asked the medical assistant who his next patient was. Upon realizing who he was seeing for the next virtual encounter, he commented to the medical assistant, "I don't know why they are even bothering with this visit. They never follow my directions and don't take or even fill their medication. This is a waste of all of our time." When the telehealth visit began and the provider asked how the patient was doing, the first comment was, "Not well. Apparently I do not follow directions and I am a bother to you. We will not be having this visit today." In this scenario, the microphone had not been muted on the computer, and the patient heard the conversation. The relationship between provider and patient was damaged to a degree that the patient ended the professional relationship with the provider.

Performance

The provider's performance can affect the telehealth visit as a result of unconscious expressions, poor ability to use the equipment, and not being prepared for the visit. Timing, pacing, and small talk must be purposefully considered. At the start of the encounter, the provider should introduce him- or herself and tell the patient a little about him- or herself. He or she should let the patient know what to expect from the telehealth visit. If this is not done at the start of the encounter, the whole appointment will feel distant and mechanical. The provider must make every effort to provide eye contact and create facial expressions that enhance the provider-patient relationship. It is distracting and conveys a sense of disinterest when the provider looks down, looks away, is half in the picture, or talks to another person while in a telehealth session. The camera on most computers is located at the top of the screen; however, the provider often tries to look directly at the patient, which makes them appear to be looking down and not visually connected to the patient. It is important for the provider to look at the camera and check the view the patient has in the small side screen. Some providers may portray a resting face that can be interpreted as disinterest or disagreement. The provider should be aware if he or she tends to develop a resting face and develop strategies to check him- or herself during the visit. The provider must maintain congruence between facial and verbal communication, realizing that body language demonstrated during an in-person visit is not seen on a telehealth screen. Silence, while appropriate in an in-person visit, is experienced as awkward, long periods of silence during a telehealth encounter. The provider should be sure to not interrupt the patient when he or she is talking. There is sometimes a video delay that could cause both the patient and provider to talk over each other. Because of this feature, the provider must practice active listening and repeat back what the patient has said so that the patient feels understood and validated.

The provider's performance with the telehealth equipment may be disruptive. For instance, if the provider is unsure how to use some of the telehealth settings, the provider may lose credibility and the patient may become less interested in participating in telehealth. It is thus important for the provider to practice with the equipment before the encounter and, if needed, have someone nearby that can address telehealth equipment issues if they occur. In a clinical encounter with a mother and child, the social worker began the consultation without first checking her equipment. This was the family's first encounter with telehealth. Unfortunately, at the start of the visit, the family could only hear the social worker, they could not see her. The telehealth platform had been working earlier in the day but had not been checked after lunch. After several minutes of confusion and frustration on both ends, the social worker realized that she had placed a sticky note over her computer's camera. In this situation, the family decided that a telehealth visit was not something that they would want to do again.

The provider must also come to the telehealth visit prepared with any necessary notes, test results, referral information, or care plans. It is disconcerting for a patient to feel as though the provider has no understanding of his or her health issues. Prior to a telehealth session, it is imperative for the provider to obtain the needed records, review them, and consult with other providers as indicated. This will allow the session to run smoother and the outcomes to be optimized. On the other hand, it is just as critical that the provider ends the telehealth encounter purposefully. The provider should not end the appointment abruptly by turning the camera off. He or she must be sure to leave time for questions and answers at the end of the session.

Privacy

With the introduction of telehealth technology, the provider may need to take extra steps to assure the patient that privacy and confidentiality are maintained during the visit. At the start of every encounter, the telemedicine presenter must first check to ensure that both the provider and patient are in secure, private settings. He or she may need to clarify and introduce those in the room on both the provider and patient side, get approval if the session will be taped, and inform the patient and caregiver of the privacy settings on the equipment. If possible, both the provider and patient should use the telemedicine camera to show one another the room. Most states now require that a consent for the telehealth encounter be signed prior to the visit; this should always be checked prior to the encounter.[32] Neither the provider nor the patient should record the session. Many telehealth consents now will state that recording will not occur and request that the patient does not record the session either. Some telehealth platforms do not have a recording feature. The provider should check for this feature when platforms are selected.

A compromise in privacy was identified during a telestroke encounter. A neurologist received a page in the middle of the night for a telestroke consult. He quickly got out of bed, turned on his computer located in his bedroom, and began the telestroke consult. During the initial assessment of the patient, he asked the provider from the remote hospital whether he could see how he was holding his hands outward to demonstrate what he wanted the patient to do. This is when the provider from the remote hospital quickly stated, "Yes, Doctor, we can see you and we can also the person in the bed behind you." This left the distant provider and patient frustrated that the neurologist was attempting to conduct a visit without providing patient privacy.

Even well-meaning providers who have been practicing for several years in the telehealth space have made errors due to a lack of training or understanding of the unique skill set and consideration necessary for a telehealth visit. It is of utmost importance that the provider keeps in mind telehealth etiquette issues that have the potential to derail a telehealth visit.

TELEHEALTH KNOWLEDGE AND SKILLS

The telehealth provider must develop or refine specific competencies to be effective in using telehealth to provide care. In general, the provider should be creative and able to solve problems as they arise during the visit. The provider must be a champion for telehealth and support the patient as he or she becomes accustomed to its use. It is helpful if he or she is open-minded to new technology/innovations and can see the benefits of its use. These telehealth advocates and providers will need to have specific knowledge and skills as they relate to the patient-provider relationship, use of technology, provision of clinical care, and implementation of telehealth. The provider must realize that even a provider with the most proficient skills can have a visit derailed if his or her telehealth etiquette fails.

Interpersonal Skills for Developing the Patient-Provider Relationship

As in the in-person visit, one of the hallmarks to providing care is to optimize the relationship between the provider and the patient. The most significant predictor of a successful encounter is the patient's perception of a positive provider-patient relationship. This not only improves the patient's satisfaction but can also greatly affect the health outcomes.[33] The patient's satisfaction is seen as so important that hospitals are now surveying patients who are discharged to determine their satisfaction with their providers while in the hospital. These Hospital Consumer Assessment of Healthcare Providers and Systems scores are used to assess communication with nurses and doctors, communication regarding medicine, staff responsiveness, and discharge information. The scores are provided to the public and can greatly affect reimbursement.

Without the ability to touch the patient, and with the introduction of the barrier created by technology, the provider-patient relationship can be affected negatively. It is thus vital that the provider make greater efforts to relate to the patient. This will require the refinement of interpersonal skills to overcome the barriers created with technology. These refined interpersonal skills will be needed to communicate effectively with the patient, provide empathy, and motivate the patient to participate in behavioral changes.

Communication Skills

The ability to communicate effectively in a virtual environment is a vital skill to successful telehealth encounters. Many of the skills learned for face-to-face communication are transferable to the telehealth encounter. The provider must be able to listen to the patient and ask appropriate follow-up questions. He or she must paraphrase and summarize what he or she hears to ensure that both the provider and patient have the same perspective. The provider must listen to the patient and portray feelings of empathy. It will be through effective communication that the provider will assist the patient in feeling that the patient is a valued member of the health care team and that the patient's input is essential to his or her health. This in turn will enhance the patient's satisfaction with the provider.[33]

However, because of the videoconferencing technology, the provider will not be able to rely on the ability to touch the patient or use certain body language techniques to connect with the patient. Rather than body language, the provider may need to rely more heavily on the words, tones, and facial expressions used to communicate. The provider must help the patient feel comfortable with the technology by verbally instructing and supporting the patient in its use. The provider will need to adapt readily to artifacts or a delay in sound that may affect the visit. The provider should develop a trusting provider-patient relationship that enables him or her to ask questions in order to understand the issues affecting the patient.

The provider will need to communicate effectively in order to assess the patient's condition, provide patient education, and impart medical guidance.[34] Specific techniques that are needed for effective communication include the following:

- Using a friendly tone
- Looking into the camera
- Having the patient teach back the information he or she has obtained
- Understanding and controlling biases
- Using translators or digital interpreters as needed to address language barriers
- Incorporating pictures or demonstrating techniques
- Including family members or friends in the encounter if acceptable to the patient
- Using open-ended questions
- Reflecting on what the patient says
- Summarizing information or the encounter

FOR REFLECTION 2:

Successful Communication

You have set up a telehealth encounter with Mrs. Jones to assess her understanding of the plan she was given upon discharge from the hospital. The session will be complicated by the fact that the patient is Hispanic and speaks broken English. What issues may affect the visit? What steps will you take to optimize your ability to communicate with the patient? What communication skills will you use?

Empathy

One of the hallmarks of nursing is the nurse's ability to convey feelings of empathy. By providing empathy, the provider connects with the patient and aids the patient in feeling understood and that the provider cares about him or her. The APRN strives to provide empathy as demonstrated by recognizing the patient's emotional needs at a distance and being able to respond appropriately. An empathetic provider can understand the situation the patient is in, relate to his or her feelings, and respond as needed. It has been shown that patients have a greater satisfaction if the provider demonstrates empathy even when the health outcomes are not favorable.[35] One study conducted at Massachusetts General Hospital suggested that patients undergoing surgery on their hands perceived their care as being high quality when the provider was believed to be empathetic.[35] It was found that 65% of satisfaction was correlated with feeling that the provider was empathetic.[36]

The ability to convey an understanding of a person's feelings is often demonstrated through touch, a technique that is not available in telehealth. It is thus imperative that the APRN learn to use other techniques in order to create empathy in the virtual environment. In telehealth, the provider will have to use words, facial expressions, and leaning in to demonstrate empathy. He or she must approach the patient with curiosity and in a nonjudgmental manner. The provider must listen and reflect on what he or she hears. The empathetic provider will seek to understand the patient's life and seek commonalities. The provider will recognize the emotions of the patient and be comfortable in trying to better understand them.

In using words, the provider may reflect on what he or she is hearing or seeing as he or she meets with the patient. For instance, if the provider hears the patient communicate sadness, or if the patient's expression portrays sadness, the provider can reflect by saying, "You seem to be sad" or "Are you feeling sad?" This will allow the patient to confirm or deny the feeling of sadness. The provider may also want to use words to portray what he or she would do if he or she were with the patient. For instance, the provider may say, "I would love to be able to just sit with you." These words can be as effective as the physical touch.

The provider may also use his or her expression to convey understanding of the patient. He or she can nod as the patient talks. The provider can be cognizant of his or her own expression and use it to mirror the patient's expression. Above all, the provider must look at the camera so that the patient feels as though the provider is attentive. By looking down or away from the screen, the provider may demonstrate a lack of interest in the patient and his or her feelings.

As an example of empathy, in a telehealth session with a teenager who had been diagnosed with cancer, the patient was tearful. The provider was not able to give the patient a hug or even a tissue for her tears. The provider used her words to convey empathy by saying, "I can imagine how difficult your situation is for you. I so wish I could give you a hug."

Another approach would be to state your own feelings, such as, "I am saddened that you are experiencing such a hard time. It makes sense that you would feel like that. How can I help you?" These responses open the door for the patient to express his or her concerns and feel that the provider is truly interested.

Motivational Interviewing

In today's society, so much of the health status of the population is based on behaviors. These health behaviors can range from preventive care activities to seeking care when needed and to the adherence to a plan of care or treatment regimen. Regardless of the reason for the behavior, the individual must be motivated to take the needed action. Preventive activities often include exercise, diet, and stress-relieving techniques such as yoga or meditation. In the area of seeking care, too often individuals either use the health care system when it is not needed or do not seek care when they should. In addition, often individuals do not follow the plan that has been established for care. This can be due to lack of understanding or confusion, social determinants of health (SDOH) affecting their ability to adhere, or their belief that the behavior is not needed or not important or they are incapable of change. As telehealth is introduced into health care, the provider may have an additional role in assessing the patient's willingness to use telehealth and then motivating the patient to use telehealth to receive support, education, and care. Regardless of the need, it is vital that the provider be equipped with motivational interviewing skills.

Stages of Motivational Interviewing

Motivational interviewing is a technique used to assist patients in creating the desire to participate in activities or behaviors that will benefit their health. Motivational interviewing is thus a skill that is necessary when using telehealth to interview and provide care to a patient. The provider

TABLE 8-2	
RULE MNEMONIC FOR MOTIVATIONAL INTERVIEWING	
RESIST	*Resist* the desire to tell the patient what they should do. Do not give suggestions or offer solutions.
UNDERSTAND	*Understand* what motivates the patient. Help the patient understand and verbalize what his or her motivation is to change behaviors. Put the patient in charge of clarifying or identifying benefits, barriers, and motivating factors.
LISTEN	*Listen* using empathy. Reflect on what the patient says to increase the mutual understanding of the patient's perspective. Use open-ended questions.
EMPOWER	*Empower* the patient to take action. Let the patient know that he or she is in charge of his or her actions and, in order to make behavioral changes, the patient must overcome his or her barriers and take the steps needed.

must realize that some patients are intrinsically motivated to participate in healthy behaviors. This is seen in those individuals that do not require encouragement to be actively involved in physical activities or diet on a regular basis. Then there are individuals who tend to need more extrinsic motivation or motivation from other sources to participate in health-promoting activities. It is the provider's responsibility to support those who are intrinsically motivated *and* those who are extrinsically motivated in overcoming barriers to needed behaviors. In doing so, the provider will be invested in providing the patients with education and determining their knowledge, understanding cultural issues and values related to the patients and their family, and incorporating family and friends as needed.

Providers use motivational interviewing to aid patients in overcoming barriers and developing the desire to participate in health-promoting behaviors. It is performed in conjunction with patients, where both providers and patients join forces to create the needed health-promoting behavior. It requires providers to include skills in communication and empathy as discussed previously. If patients are not actively involved in developing the plan, it will surely fail.

One of the more commonly used approaches to motivational interviewing is RULE (Table 8-2)[37]:

- **R** is resist: The provider must resist telling the patient what he or she should do. The patient should be the one who comes up with the idea or plan for what should be done.
- **U** is understand: The provider must seek to understand the patient's situation, needs, barriers, and motivating factors. Unless the provider understands the patient's situation, he or she will not be able to aid the patient in developing a meaningful or successful plan.
- **L** is listen: The provider must be an empathetic listener that hears and reflects on what the patient is saying. This will aid the provider in identifying what is important to the patient and guide the provider in supporting the patient as the plan is developed.
- **E** is empower: The provider must empower the patient to take action and work with family and friends to obtain support in making the needed behavioral changes.

RULE can be applied in the telehealth encounter as well as in in-person encounters.

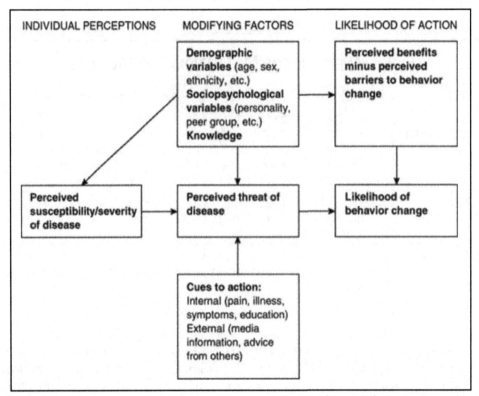

Figure 8-1. The Health Belief Model: Theoretical Framework for Identifying Beliefs that Impact Health-related Action

Barriers to Motivation

In order to motivate the patient to take action, the provider must assist the patient in identifying his or her barriers and develop a plan to overcome them. A common framework that can be used to address the barriers is the Health Belief Model (Figure 8-1).[38] The Health Belief Model states that the patient is likely to take action based on his or her perceived susceptibility to having trouble and his or her perceived seriousness of the problem. This leads to the patient's perceived threat of the disease. The threat is modified by factors such as his or her demographics, sociopsychological factors such as SDOH, and cues to action. The input from the provider is linked to the cues to action. The patient must also weigh the benefits to taking action against the barriers. Based on these constructs, the patient may or may not be likely to take action.[38] In conducting the motivational interview, the provider should keep each of these constructs in mind. This will help guide the interview and identify issues that will require a greater focus.

Recently, health care has begun to address the need to consider SDOH as barriers to health care. During motivational interviewing, the provider would be well served to address these barriers with the patient. Of specific concern are the barriers associated with access to health care (eg, transportation, collocation of providers, cost). This offers an opportunity for the provider to further emphasize the use of telehealth as a mechanism for overcoming access issues. Another SDOH that can be addressed through telehealth is the patient's health literacy. By following up with the patient through telehealth, the provider can better assess the patient's understanding of the plan of care. It is not uncommon for a patient to leave the office or hospital with confusion related to his or her plan of care. Using telehealth, the provider can assess patient concerns within 24 hours to determine the patient's understanding of the plan and what barriers he or she has encountered in implementing the plan. For instance, it is not uncommon for a patient to become confused regarding his or her medications following discharge from the hospital. The patient may not be able to obtain the medication due to cost or transportation, may be confused on which medication to take now vs the medication he or she was on prior to hospitalization, or may be unclear on why he or she needs to take the medication. A follow-up with the patient could eliminate potential problems and poor health outcomes.

Uses of Telehealth in Motivational Interviewing

Telehealth can be an asset in providing support for preventive behaviors, health-seeking behaviors, and adherence to the plan of care. The provider can use many telehealth tools to support the patient as he or she strives to participate in health-promoting activities. For instance, there are mobile applications (apps) that can be used to track patient outcomes. These apps allow the patient to keep track of information such as the foods he or she eats; his or her weight, heart rate, and blood sugar level; and the exercise he or she participates in. Many of these apps can be accessed through a patient's watch, phone, or tablet. The provider can greatly assist the patient by identifying useful apps and helping the patient to obtain and use them. Much of this information can be sent to the provider virtually, allowing for rapid intervention. It can also be used to assess the patient's adherence to the plan of care.

Telehealth can also be used to assist the patient in knowing when and when not to seek medical care. By providing the patient with telehealth options, the patient can contact and inform the provider about his or her concern prior to seeking care in the emergency department or provider office. For instance, it is not uncommon for new parents to become anxious regarding their new infant's health status. When parents have access to a provider via telehealth, they can obtain advice prior to making unnecessary trips. Telehealth can also help determine when a patient does need to seek care. A patient with congestive heart failure is a good example. If the provider can assess the patient's weight, oxygen saturation, and vital signs, he or she can determine whether the patient needs to be seen or can stay at home and be treated with a medication adjustment.

Follow-up visits via telehealth can allow the provider to assess the patient's adherence to the plan of care that was established. It can also increase the adherence by the patient, knowing that he or she will be participating in a follow-up visit. One traumatic example occurred when a patient was discharged following a diagnosis of cancer. The patient was provided a chemotherapy medication that was to be given once a week. The patient and spouse thought they understood the plan but became confused when they got home. As a result, the patient took the medication every day. The patient ended up dying. This may have been prevented if there had been follow-up to ensure that the patient and spouse understood the plan. Much of the recidivism to the hospital may be decreased with the use of telehealth as a follow-up mechanism.

Example of Motivational Interviewing

In one telehealth virtual encounter with a standardized patient, it became obvious that the interprofessional team of students was having difficulty motivating their older adult patient with multiple chronic conditions and depression. The group had become very focused on the patient's infection, which had already been treated in the emergency department. The students kept saying that the patient had to go back to the emergency department. The patient was getting defensive. During the break between the initial session and the continuation of the session, the students were given 3 suggestions: (1) Ask the patient what his typical day is like, (2) find out if he likes how it is, and (3) ask him what his day would be like if it was what he desired.

As the students asked these questions, the patient suddenly relaxed and started explaining what he desired. When the session was processed, the students asked the teachers if they had trained the patient to respond the way he did. The answer was no. The standardized patient expressed that he did not feel like the providers cared until they asked about his ideal day. It was only then that the patient felt the providers understood him and his situation. At that point, the patient was ready to work with the providers in identifying a solution to his health care issues.

GROUP EXERCISE

Transmitting Nursing Empathy and Demonstrating Motivational Interviewing

For this exercise, break the class into 2 groups. Group 1 will develop a short vignette to demonstrate how empathy can be transmitted using telehealth technology, and group 2 will develop a short vignette to demonstrate how motivational interviewing can be used in telehealth. When the groups are ready, have several members of each group demonstrate these skills for the class using their demonstration vignette.

Technological Skills

Nurses have long used technology to aid in care delivery by improving assessment, diagnosis, and treatment of patients and to facilitate communication with patients, specialists, and colleagues. Sandelowski[39] points out that the first nurses (1870s through 1930s) had 2 resources to provide care: their physical bodies, including their senses; and the use of inanimate objects, devices, and tools to facilitate care. Over time, more specialized devices and technologies allowed nurses to extend their ability to provide nursing care to patients using thermometers, hypodermic needles, and stethoscopes. There are now advanced telehealth technologies that allow nurses to be virtually transported to patients in remote sites to provide care.

Knowing the technology is an essential element in the telehealth paradigm. Therefore, technological competence is a requirement of telehealth practice. Additionally, technology can be a platform for helping the provider to know the patient through interactions within the virtual environment. One of the most common themes in nursing research on knowing the patient is time: time to talk with and conduct assessments and to provide education and nursing care.[40] Technology can increase the frequency and length of the time the patient interacts with the APRN, helping to increase the ability to know the patient. Personal knowledge of the technology relates to comfort and confidence among nurses using telehealth. As the patient is guided to engage in the virtual environment, the goal is for the technology to fade into the background allowing for the bond of presence to grow stronger between the nurse and patient.

Providers are consistently challenged by the different technologies that have become available, including electronic health records (EHRs). Rather than develop one system that communicates across varying practice sites, there are many EHR platforms, with most being unable to communicate with the others. This is frustrating to many providers when they encounter patients who have had health care visits at sites that use a different platform. For example, often patients have come to rely on the EHR to inform providers of the medications they are on. They have stopped bringing their medications to visits, assuming their latest medication changes have been documented in the EHR. However, this does not happen when patients are seen by providers using a different EHR platform. This can result in providers being constrained in knowing how to adjust medications to accommodate changes in the patients' conditions. With numerous vendors offering telehealth platforms, it is easy to become overwhelmed by the choices. Telehealth providers must be prepared to work with varying platforms and learn quickly. They must develop methods to augment continuity of care efforts when platforms do not communicate.

The ability to relate to the patient may be hindered by technical difficulties that interfere with communication. This can include poor reception, problems encountered with the connection, and provider or patient abilities. It is thus imperative that the provider develop the skills needed to navigate issues with the technology and support the patient in its use. Prior to an encounter, the provider must be prepared to select equipment; connect, start, and operate it; and clean and pack up the equipment. The provider should either be prepared to troubleshoot problems with the connection or have personnel available to manage the difficulties. If a problem persists, it might be better to discontinue the telehealth session and reschedule rather than continue and have a session that has a negative effect. The provider must develop the skills needed to identify when the session should be discontinued or when the issues can be addressed in a timely manner.

The provider should possess the skills needed to obtain buy-in from the patient and caregiver to participate in telehealth. The provider will need to assist the patient and caregiver in best understanding how to access the equipment, what equipment is needed, why it is needed, and how it will be used. During the session, the provider may need to instruct the patient on its use. One example is the use of a device that can be provided to patients for home assessments. The device can be bought in a retail store and used, for example, if a parent suspects that his or her child has an ear infection, the parent can contact the company maintaining the platform for an appointment with one of their providers licensed in the state. During the appointment, the provider can interact with the patient using the videoconferencing platform and through the peripherals (eg, stethoscope, otoscope, thermometer). The provider may request that the parent use the otoscope to show the child's eardrum. The device will provide a picture of how to connect the otoscope and do the ear exam. The provider can see the eardrum and instruct the parent on how to improve the view. Based on the information obtained, the provider can make a diagnosis and send a prescription to the patient's pharmacy if indicated.

Clinical Skills

The provider will need to be prepared with many of the same skills that are required for an in-person visit. It is still important to conduct a physical assessment using tools as well as observation skills. However, due to the lack of direct contact with the patient, the provider will require additional skills in using the telehealth equipment and peripherals to conduct the assessments. When observing the patient, new techniques may be needed. For instance, instead of having a post-stroke patient squeeze the provider's hand, the patient may be asked to grasp a book and lift it in front of the videoconferencing screen. He or she may be asked to draw on a sheet of paper and hold the picture up to the camera. In order to assess the patient's appearance and body language, the patient may need to move back from the camera, allowing for a more comprehensive view.

The provider will need to understand different platforms and the peripherals that can connect with each platform. For instance, in one situation, a provider who cared for palliative care patients was making trips to visit the patients once a month. She decided to incorporate telehealth in order to decrease her travel time and increase the patients' access to health care. In setting up the program, she sought a platform that would allow her to obtain the same information at a distance that she would seek during her home visits. This included being able to listen to heart and lung sounds; obtain oxygen saturation levels and weight; and receive information on the patients' pain levels, medication management, and well-being. In order to successfully implement the program, it was imperative that the provider learn to use the platform and peripherals to complete her assessment, obtain buy-in from the patients and caregivers, and ensure they were prepared to use the equipment.

Providers must bring specific clinical knowledge and skills to the telehealth encounter as they apply to the patient population and the medical issue addressed. Telehealth should be used to improve the ease, efficiency, effectiveness, and quality of the encounter. The provider must be equipped with the following knowledge and skills:

- Benefits of telehealth
- Clinical uses of telehealth
- Limitations of telehealth
- Deploying telehealth
- Collecting and managing patient data
- Applicable protocols

Implementation Skills

The provider has a vital role in implementing telehealth programs to optimize the health care of his or her patients. The responsibilities of this role can be divided into the following 4 categories:

1. Setting the stage
2. Preparing the environment
3. Conducting the telehealth visit
4. Managing the established plan

In order to set the stage for the visit, the provider must be sure the patient is receptive to the visit, participants for the visit are identified and notified, a time is scheduled for the visit, the patient and the provider have the needed equipment, and there is a place to conduct the telehealth visit. This will require the provider to make needed contacts and receive buy-in from those to be involved in the visit. The provider must understand the strengths of potential collaborators in order to select those who should be on the encounter. The provider will be required to schedule the patient, staff, equipment/platform, and space for the visit. Confirmation will be required so that the provider will know that all are on board. Follow-up notices will be needed at least 1 day before the session. Both the confirmation notice and the follow-up notice should include information on how to connect for the telehealth visit.

The telehealth provider will want to be sure the participants are prepared for the visit. Specific areas of focus include the following:

- Ensuring the patient understands what to expect during the visit
- Informing the patient that he or she may experience audiovisual delay
- Teaching the patient/caregiver how to use the equipment
- Providing the patient/caregiver with resources for technical assistance
- Having the patient/caregiver test the equipment before the session
- Helping the patient determine how to use the microphone and position the camera
- Informing the patient of potential exams that might occur and the appropriate attire to wear
- Ensuring the patient selects the participant(s) to be in the room with him or her and introducing all participants on the patient and provider side at the beginning of the session
- Ensuring that the patient/caregiver has developed comfort using the equipment
- Ensuring that the patient/caregiver knows that the session can be terminated at any time by either the provider or patient side[41]

The telehealth provider must prepare the environment for the visit. This will include making sure the needed information, equipment, and site are available and ready for use. Specific information may include medical information on the patient such as the history and physical, laboratory results, relevant notes, and any other diagnostic tests. The provider may also check to determine if a consent for the visit has been obtained. The telehealth provider should ensure that pertinent telehealth equipment is available, including peripherals. In some cases, there may be a need to include either equipment or personnel to assist with language or cultural barriers.[41] In preparing the environment, it will be important that telehealth etiquette be included as a framework for ensuring that the environment is ready for a successful telehealth encounter.

Once the environment is in order, it is time to conduct the telehealth encounter. The knowledge and skills as discussed previously will be required to maximize the effect of the visit. This must include the interpersonal, clinical, and technological skills. During the visit, the provider will need to have a way of collecting and documenting relevant data. He or she will also need to manage the time effectively and set priorities as needed. The provider will want to determine whether the telehealth visit was what the patient had expected and whether it had met the patient's needs. At the end of the visit, it is imperative that a plan be discussed and follow-up scheduled.

The role of the telehealth provider is not completed once the technology is turned off. The provider will be required to make sure the plan of action is implemented as discussed during the visit. This may include documenting the visit, scheduling follow-up visits, referring the patient to specialists or allied health professionals, scheduling needed tests, and providing the patient with information obtained following the visit. The provider may send the patient/caregiver a review of the visit along with the outlined plan. The telehealth provider may also need to provide a review of the visit to relevant colleagues, referring providers, or other individuals who may be involved with care coordination.[41]

CONCLUSION

In order to maximize the use of telehealth in the virtual environment, the provider must possess specific competencies (knowledge and skills). These competencies are used to develop meaningful therapeutic patient-provider relationships; appropriately use telehealth technologies; provide clinical assessments, diagnosis, and treatment plans; and conduct successful telehealth encounters. These competencies must provide for an ethical encounter and optimize the visit through telehealth etiquette.

Many of the competencies currently required for in-person patient visits can be used; however, modifications are required to work within the constraints imposed by technology. With the ultimate goal of the telehealth encounter being to create a sense of presence in the virtual environment, strategies to minimize the barriers created by the technology must be applied. It is only through a conscious understanding and awareness of how the telehealth encounter differs from the in-person visit that the provider will be able to create a sense of presence where the provider and patient feel they are present in the same virtual environment as if they are actually together. This as possible when the provider has the needed skills to create a seamless encounter with minimal distractors.

THOUGHTFUL QUESTIONS

1. How has the virtual environment changed how health care can be delivered? What does the provider strive for in the virtual environment?
2. Telehealth encounters can be compromised by etiquette that disrupts the encounter. How can poor telehealth etiquette affect the encounter? What steps would you take to optimize the telehealth encounter using telehealth etiquette?
3. The virtual environment restricts the use of many techniques used to connect with the patient during the in-person visit. What are some techniques that a provider can use in order to show empathy?
4. The telehealth provider must come to the telehealth encounter with skills specific to telehealth. What are the skills that are needed?

CASE STUDY

Ms. Smith is being released from the hospital following cardiac surgery. The procedure has been paid for through a bundle payment. She is entitled to follow-up care as part of the bundle payment. Your goal is to maximize her care and decrease her need for readmission. You have identified several issues that you feel need to be addressed to optimize her care. These include the following:

- Ensuring the patient understands her discharge instructions
- Seeing that the patient has follow-up
- Confirming that the patient is taking the correct medications
- Motivating the patient to make needed behavioral changes (eg, diet, activity)
- Setting up the patient and her caregiver with telehealth to monitor her health status and connect with providers

Questions

1. How will you use telehealth to assist this patient in optimizing her health outcomes?
2. What issues do you want to address with telehealth, and what equipment will be needed for the patient?
3. What skills will you use to provide for successful use of telehealth?
4. How will you optimize the patient's motivation to make behavioral changes using telehealth? What telehealth devices would help?

REFERENCES

1. Locsin RC, Purnell MJ, eds. *A Contemporary Nursing Process: The (Un)Bearable Weight of Knowing in Nursing.* New York, NY: Springer; 2009.
2. Wheatstone C. Contributions to the physiology of vision—part the first. On some remarkable, and hitherto unobserved, phenomena of binocular vision. *Philosophical Transactions of the Royal Society of London.* 1838;128:371-394. https://doi.org/10.1098/rstl.1838.0019
3. Sell MA, Sell W, Van Pelt C. *View-Master Memories.* Cincinnati, OH: Authors; 2007.
4. Heinrichs L, Dev P, Davies D. Virtual environments and virtual patients in healthcare. In: Nestel D, Kelly M, Jolly B, Watson M, eds. *Healthcare Simulation Education: Evidence, Theory, and Practice.* Oxford, United Kingdom: John Wiley & Sons; 2018:69-79.
5. Milgram P, Kishino F. A taxonomy of mixed reality visual displays. *IEICE Transactions on Information Systems.* 1994;E77-D(12):1321-1329.
6. Bell M. Toward a definition of "virtual worlds." *Journal of Virtual Worlds Research.* 2008;1(1).
7. Schroeder R. Defining virtual worlds and virtual research. *Journal of Virtual Worlds Research.* 2008;1(1).
8. Boeck PR. Presence: a concept analysis. *SAGE Open.* 2014;4(1):1-6.
9. Fredriksson L. Modes of relating in a caring conversation: a research synthesis on presence, touch and listening. *J Adv Nurs.* 1999;30(5):1167-1176.
10. Sävenstedt S, Zingmark K, Sandman PO. Being present in a distant room: aspects of teleconsultations with older people in a nursing home. *Qual Health Res.* 2004;14(8):1046-1057.
11. Tuxbury JS. The experience of presence among telehealth nurses. *J Nurs Res.* 2013;21(3):155-161.
12. Carroll K. Transforming the art of nursing: telehealth technologies. *Nurs Sci Q.* 2018;31(3):230-232.
13. Schmidt KL, Gentry A, Monin JK, Courtney KL. Demonstration of facial communication of emotion through telehospice videophone contact. *Telemed J E Health.* 2011;17(5):399-401.
14. American Medical Association. Ethical practice in telemedicine. https://www.ama-assn.org/delivering-care/ethics/ethical-practice-telemedicine. Accessed February 28, 2020.

15. Roach MS. *Caring, the Human Mode of Being: A Blueprint for the Health Professions.* 2nd rev ed. Ottawa, Canada: Canadian Healthcare Association Press; 2002.

16. Ray MA. Technological caring: a new model in critical care. *Dimens Crit Care Nurs.* 1987;6(3):166-173.

17. Ray M. Technological caring as a dynamic of complexity in nursing practice. In: Barnard A, Locsin R, eds. *Technology and Nursing: Practice, Concepts and Issues.* Basingstoke, United Kingdom: Palgrave McMillian; 2007:174-190.

18. Watson J. *Caring Science as Sacred Science.* Philadelphia, PA: FA Davis; 2005.

19. Rutenberg C, Oberle K. Ethics in telehealth nursing practice. *Home Health Care Manag Pract.* 2008;20(4):342-348.

20. Skär L, Söderberg S. The importance of ethical aspects when implementing eHealth services in healthcare: a discussion paper. *J Adv Nurs.* 2018;74(5):1043-1050.

21. Rienits H, Teuss G, Bonney A. Teaching telehealth consultation skills. *Clin Teach.* 2016;13(2):119-123.

22. Miller EA. The technical and interpersonal aspects of telemedicine: effects on doctor-patient communication. *J Telemed Telecare.* 2003;9(1):1-7.

23. Konrath SH, O'Brien EH, Hsing C. Changes in dispositional empathy in American college students over time: a meta-analysis. *Pers Soc Psychol Rev.* 2011;15(2):180-198.

24. Bulik RJ. Human factors in primary care telemedicine encounters. *J Telemed Telecare.* 2008;14(4):169-172.

25. Laff M. Telemedicine can build bridge to expand health care, say panelists. American Academy of Family Physicians. https://www.aafp.org/news/practice-professional-issues/20140205rgctelemedicineforum.html. Published February 5, 2014. Accessed February 28, 2020.

26. Heath S. What are patient preferences for technology, provider communication? *Xtelligent Healthcare Media.* https://patientengagementhit.com/news/what-are-patient-preferences-for-technology-provider-communication. Published March 12, 2019. Accessed February 28, 2020.

27. Polycom. *The Polycom Guide to Vidiquette.* https://www.polycom.com/content/dam/polycom/common/documents/guides/polycom-vidiquette-guide-enus.pdf. Published 2016. Accessed February 28, 2020.

28. Nulph RG. Just what should I wear? Videomaker. https://www.videomaker.com/article/c14/12990-just-what-should-i-wear. Accessed February 28, 2020.

29. Mirren H. Helen Mirren's top film acting tips. Masterclass. https://www.masterclass.com/articles/helen-mirrens-top-film-acting-tips?utm_source=Paid&utm_medium=Bing. Updated July 2, 2019. Accessed April 6, 2020.

30. Edelson C. Virtual bedside manner: connecting with telemedicine. Pediatric EHR Solutions. https://blog.pcc.com/virtual-bedside-manner-connecting-with-telemedicine. Accessed February 28, 2020.

31. Major J. Using telemediquette to make your telemedicine encounters effective. Arizona Telemedicine Program. https://telemedicine.arizona.edu/blog/using-telemediquette-make-your-telemedicine-encounters-effective. Published November 17, 2016. Accessed February 28, 2020.

32. Rheuban KS. Telemedicine: connect to specialists and facilitate better access to care for your patients. American Medical Association. https://edhub.ama-assn.org/steps-forward/module/2702689. Published October 7, 2015. Accessed February 28, 2020.

33. Heath S. 4 best practices for improving patient-provider communication. *Xtelligent Healthcare Media.* https://patientengagementhit.com/news/4-best-practices-for-improving-patient-provider-communication. Published March 18, 2016. Accessed February 28, 2020.

34. Heath S. 3 key traits of a positive patient-provider relationship. *Xtelligent Healthcare Media.* https://patientengagementhit.com/news/3-key-traits-of-a-positive-patient-provider-relationship. Published November 27, 2017. Accessed February 28, 2020.

35. American Academy of Orthopaedic Surgeons. Physician empathy a key driver of patient satisfaction. *PR Newswire.* https://www.prnewswire.com/news-releases/physician-empathy-a-key-driver-of-patient-satisfaction-300228070.html. Published March 1, 2016. Accessed February 28, 2020.

36. Heath S. Consumers say patient-provider relationship key to quality care. *Xtelligent Healthcare Media.* https://patientengagementhit.com/news/consumers-say-patient-provider-relationship-key-to-quality-care. Published November 15, 2017. Accessed February 28, 2020.

37. Hall K, Gibbie T, Lubman DI. Motivational interviewing techniques—facilitating behaviour change in the general practice setting. *Aust Fam Physician.* 2012;41(9):660-667.

38. Janz NK, Becker MH. The Health Belief Model: a decade later. *Health Educ Q.* 1984;11(1):1-47.

39. Sandelowski M. *Devices & Desires: Gender, Technology, and American Nursing.* Chapel Hill, NC: University of North Carolina Press; 2000.

40. Macdonald M. Technology and its effect on knowing the patient: a clinical issue analysis. *Clin Nurse Spec.* 2008;22(3):149-155.

41. Veterans Rural Health Resource Center–Eastern Region, Northeast Telehealth Resource Center. *Telehealth basics: curriculum for training CNAs on telehealth and telepresenting.* https://netrc.org/wp-content/uploads/2014/12/Telehealth-Curriculum-2013-with-cover.pdf. Published September 2013. Accessed February 28, 2020.

9

Telehealth and Interprofessional Collaboration

Carolyn M. Rutledge, PhD, FNP-BC
Tina Gustin, DNP, CNS

CHAPTER OBJECTIVES

Upon review of this chapter, the reader will be able to:

1. Describe interprofessional collaboration (IPC) and identify benefits and barriers to its use.
2. Outline ways telehealth can be used to allow for and enhance IPC.
3. Describe roles for the advanced practice registered nurse (APRN) in developing telehealth-enhanced IPC.
4. Discuss programs that have been developed to enable telehealth-supported IPC.

Effective communication across multiple health care professions is critical to ensure the delivery of safe and efficient care.[1] Most health care professionals enter their fields of practice with little training in interprofessional care, coordination, and communication. Even those who have received robust interprofessional training are re-enculturated to the traditional siloed approach when they begin practice. Current providers are siloed in practice not only because of the way they have been trained, but also due to geographic location. Telehealth is becoming a widely accepted approach for overcoming many geographic and access issues.

INTERPROFESSIONAL EDUCATION/COLLABORATION

In 2009, a partnership of leaders from 6 health professions' educational organizations (American Association of Colleges of Nursing [AACN], American Association of Colleges of Osteopathic Medicine, American Association of Colleges of Pharmacy, Association of American

Schweickert PA, Rutledge CM, eds.
Telehealth Essentials for Advanced Practice Nursing (pp 193-211).
© 2020 Taylor & Francis Group.

Medical Colleges, American Dental Education Association, and Association of Schools of Public Health) emerged as the Interprofessional Education Collaborative (IPEC).[2] This initial group filled an important national gap by identifying interprofessional competencies, frameworks, and strategies to inform curricular development around IPC. In 2011, the draft competencies were vetted and indorsed at a national meeting hosted by the Health Resources & Services Administration, Josiah Macy Jr. Foundation, Robert Wood Johnson Foundation, and American Board of Internal Medicine Foundation. The IPEC Institute was formed in 2012 and, for the first time, interprofessional faculty teams of 3 to 5 began attending training sessions with the intent of infusing the IPEC competencies into health care curricula.[2] In 2016, the IPEC document was updated with the reaffirmation of the value and effect of the 4 core competencies[3]:

1. Values and Ethics for Interprofessional Practice
2. Roles and Responsibilities
3. Interprofessional Communication
4. Teams and Teamwork

These competencies were further broadened to achieve the triple aim of improving the patient experience of care, improving the health of populations, and reducing the per capita cost of health care. The 2016 document reported on 60 additional organizations that have adopted the IPEC competencies and attended the IPEC Institute.[3]

Policies, as well as curricular and accreditation changes, have since strengthened the implementation of interprofessional education (IPE) in health professions' schools. The AACN's Essentials documents mandated that interprofessional curriculum content, competencies, and clinical opportunities be found in Baccalaureate, Master, and Doctor of Nursing Practice (DNP) programs.[4,5] Medicine, dentistry, pharmacy, public health, and schools of osteopathy also established expectations that the IPEC competencies be placed into curricula.[2] Faculty members from these professions have been integrating this content into already full and scripted curricular since. One problem with this mandate is the lack of multiple professions within certain programs of study. Many health professional programs are only able to add 1 or 2 professions to an interactive learning environment either in the classroom or in a clinical setting. Although this represents interprofessional learning, it does not mirror practice and the needs of patients. Incorporating telehealth into a curriculum to connect various professions is a means for expanding IPE and practice. Telehealth fits with the IPEC competencies in that it improves the value of health care; connects providers, thereby improving roles and enhancing responsibilities; allows for enhanced communication; and connects teams.

Benefits to Interprofessional Collaboration

Changes in health care resulting from the aging population, many with multiple chronic conditions, has increased the need for effective and efficient collaboration among health care professions.[6,7] Interprofessional teams that function well together "leverage information, experience, technology, and a culture of teamwork thus providing value for patients and families."[8(p129)] Interprofessional teams allow access to health care providers and allied health professionals who have developed the expertise to address specific patient issues. Well-functioning interprofessional teams can optimize the quality of care provided, increase access to needed treatment, and break down barriers to comprehensive care.

Barriers to Interprofessional Collaboration

Supper et al[9] conducted a review of 44 articles in the literature to better understand barriers to IPC. Barriers tended to vary according to profession. The most common issues included a lack of awareness of roles, encroachment by professions on each other, hierarchy, fragmentation of care, reimbursement, time, limited access to each other, geographical distance, unadaptable legislation, poor information systems, professional isolation, space, and lack of collocation. Many of these issues can be addressed with the use of telehealth. Issues that will need to be addressed include reimbursement models and legislation. These issues will vary significantly based on profession.

TELEHEALTH AND INTERPROFESSIONAL EDUCATION

Unlike the advancement of the IPEC competencies, telehealth education has not become a requirement for health professions' curricula. However, professional academic organizations mandate that programs incorporate technology as a requirement. Technology can be wide-ranging, to include electronic health records (EHRs), telehealth, and even robotic surgery. A review of the literature resulted in few programs that have integrated telehealth into curricular content.[7,10] A review of the literature in 2015 identified only 43 schools of nursing with telehealth content. In 2016, the American Medical Association (AMA)[11] endorsed telehealth in the classroom but recognized the barriers. Only 58% of medical schools in the United States offer telemedicine as either an elective or required course.[12] Although speech-language pathology, physical therapy, pharmacy, and dentistry are using telehealth, it is not a required part of the curriculum. Although formal academic preparation in telehealth is not mandated, society and many health care organizations are expecting graduates from health professional programs to understand telehealth delivery models, policy, billing, and use.

Key leaders from the AACN, American Nurses Association, and AMA agree that telehealth is important, but they are apprehensive about requiring that schools place this content into already-full curriculums. Given the growth of telehealth in health care settings, health care education has shifted to provide virtual learning experiences. Although elearning is evolving in individual programs, elearning as a strategy for IPE is less frequently reported.[1] It only makes sense that telehealth be placed inside the required interprofessional curriculum. Telehealth can then be used as the vehicle for interprofessional teamwork and communication.

Despite the documented value of IPE, barriers include geographic constraints and financial costs of bringing students together.[13] Telehealth can be used as a strategy to overcome these geographic barriers. Another goal of IPE is to flatten gradients to improve teamwork and ultimately improve patient outcomes.[14] All too often, when an interprofessional team of students comes together, a historical hierarchy is in place. This is a hierarchy where the medical student has been trained as the responsible team member for the patient, and the remaining team members take direction and orders from the medical student. Although good communication and teamwork is the essence of IPE, the hierarchical structure is often difficult to shift. Telehealth in this situation is the leveler of information. Each team member is learning the technology for the first time. Regardless of profession or degree level, each student is a beginner. The interprofessional team must navigate the new telehealth technology or platform as a novice team.

TELEHEALTH AND INTERPROFESSIONAL COLLABORATION

IPC is complicated, especially in rural areas where there is a shortage of providers and allied health professions.[15] To address this limitation in care, especially interprofessional care, telehealth is becoming a sought-after model. Telehealth can link interprofessional teams across landscapes that are geographically and economically diverse.

Many health care professions are beginning to embrace the role of telehealth as a care delivery model. The American Physical Therapy Association, American Speech-Language-Hearing Association, AMA, and American Occupational Therapy Association have developed position papers, policies, and some practice guidelines regarding telehealth delivery in their professions.[11,16,17]

Despite limited telehealth training, interprofessional teams have been using telehealth to improve access to care. Telehealth is becoming an optimal method for linking health care professions to each other, especially in remote, rural areas. All too often, the remote area has limited specialty and allied health care providers. This often results in the remote patient traveling long distances to receive care, the primary care provider (PCP) caring for conditions that would be better managed through specialty care, or the patient going without needed care. It is also beneficial in providing care in urban and suburban areas where there is a lack of collocation of various professions.

Telehealth allows the provider to consult with other professions regarding the management of various patient issues; connect the patient to providers not located in close proximity; reduce the isolation experienced by remote providers, often the nurse practitioner; and collaborate on care with other providers from various disciplines. Telehealth-enhanced IPC uses methodologies such as videoconferencing, eConsults, Project Extension for Community Healthcare Outcomes (ECHO), remote patient monitoring (RPM), and peripherals.

Telehealth and interprofessional care management is a newer strategy to manage chronic diseases. Multiple small studies have demonstrated that the use of telehealth by interprofessional teams is a feasible cost-effective delivery strategy that improves patient outcomes. One such study demonstrated how an interprofessional team (a nephrologist, nurse practitioner, nurses, clinical pharmacy specialist, psychologist, social worker, and dietician) effectively managed 451 patients with chronic kidney failure using telehealth devices that included peripherals.[18] The team effectively communicated with one another and the patient remotely. Although patient outcomes were not improved significantly in this study, the providers were able to meet collaboratively without having to drive to different locations to provide services, thereby increasing their productivity.

Care in remote areas is being further compromised by the closure of many critical access hospitals.[19] Even inner-city hospitals between 1970 and 2014 have had to close.[20] Telehealth is providing a new model of care that is now allowing many critical access hospitals to stay afloat. Telehealth is used to bring the expertise found in urban sites to rural hospitals via a telehealth platform. This allows critical access hospitals to keep more of their patients at their sites rather than transferring them to urban centers. Thus, rural sites can receive the revenue they had in the past. This is made possible through programs such as the tele–intensive care unit (ICU), tele–emergency department, and telestroke programs.

FOR REFLECTION 1:

Impact of Telehealth on Interprofessional Education

 Consider situations that you have been in with a patient who has multiple chronic illnesses. What professions would you want to collaborate with? How could you use telehealth to improve your ability to access the other professions? How would the patient benefit from collaboration with other providers?

ROLES FOR THE ADVANCED PRACTICE REGISTERED NURSE IN INTERPROFESSIONAL COLLABORATION

In order to provide telehealth-enhanced IPC, there are many roles that must be assumed. These roles fit into the scope of the APRN's practice. Specific roles include the following:

- Serving as the champion
- Identifying needed professions for the encounter

- Coordinating activities
- Identifying technology needs
- Planning for consent
- Understanding how reimbursement will be handled
- Being abreast of rules and regulations that may affect the visit

As in implementing other forms of telehealth, a telehealth champion is a must for telehealth-enhanced IPC. The APRN, by virtue of having worked closely with numerous professions, is well-prepared to serve as the champion. The role of the champion will be to advocate for the use of telehealth-enhanced IPC teams and see that the program is implemented. This may require the champion to research other telehealth-enhanced IPC programs to better understand barriers they encountered as well as benefits they have noted. By researching other teams, the champion may better understand the steps to implementing the program, equipment needs, funding required, reimbursement issues, and strategies for acquiring buy-in. The practice champion can use many of the strategies used by faculty, as discussed in Chapter 3.

As a clinician, the APRN will have insight into the patient/caregiver needs and be able to identify health care providers as well as allied health professionals that should compose the team. Professions that are often needed on the team include mental health providers, specialists, and physical therapists. In working with the patient and caregiver, issues may arise that might require the addition of other professions on the team. By keeping the patient/caregiver in the center of the team, the needs will become readily evident.

For the session to occur, there may be a need to coordinate the schedule of the selected professions with the schedule of the patient. This must be done well in advance and be accompanied by reminders. Be sure to send any links to the providers several days in advance as well as on the day of the session. If several professions will be at one site, space might need to be reserved where the equipment functions well. If the patient is present during the encounter, the APRN will need to make sure he or she is in a site that allows for reimbursement for the visit. The visit is rarely covered with the patient in the home. It will also be important for the APRN to make sure data that might be required for the visit are available and sent to those involved prior to the visit. The APRN may also need to have any consents completed prior to the visit.

The APRN may be responsible for selecting the telehealth platform that will be used for the visit. It will be important to choose a Health Insurance Portability and Accountability Act (HIPAA)–compliant platform that can be easily used by those engaged in the session. The APRN will also need to make sure all participants have access to the platform and know how to connect. Testing the connection prior to the session will be vital. Once the visit is complete, the APRN may need to schedule follow-up visits and make sure documentation is obtained. The APRN may also be responsible for overseeing the submission for reimbursement.

EXAMPLES IN PRACTICE

Virginia Mental Health Access Program

The Virginia Mental Health Access Program (VMAP), funded by the Health Resources & Services Administration under the Pediatric Mental Health Care Access Program, is an example of an interprofessional program in which the APRNs (family nurse practitioners and clinical nurse specialists) led telehealth integration. At the time the grant proposal was written, Virginia was ranked 47th in the nation regarding care for mental health issues in children younger than 18 years old.[21] In addition, Virginia ranked 42nd in the number of mental health providers per population.[21] Thus, the purpose of VMAP was to create a statewide program to address children with mental health issues in Virginia. Specifically, plans were to link PCPs of children (physicians

Figure 9-1. Diagram of VMAP telehealth program.

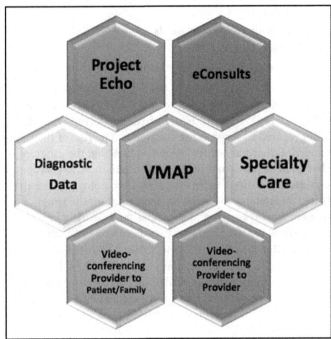

and nurse practitioners) with mental health providers using telehealth. A secondary goal was to use telehealth to further educate the PCPs. This program was set up to create connections using Project ECHO, eConsults, specialty care, and video consultation (Figure 9-1).

Project Extension for Community Healthcare Outcomes

A Project ECHO model[22] was established to provide education and training to PCPs who encountered children with mental health issues. The VMAP ECHO allows for case presentations similar to a grand rounds approach (providers can send in cases that they would like to receive assistance in managing). Any PCP can send in the case. The case is then reviewed by the VMAP ECHO team during a live HIPAA-compliant videoconferencing session (using a program such as Zoom). The review team includes mental health providers such as psychiatrists, psychologists, psych-mental health nurse practitioners, and social workers. During the VMAP ECHO, there can be didactic presentations, opportunities for discussions, and access to resources and links that might be helpful to the PCPs. In addition, screening tools and interventions may be provided. The sessions are recorded so that providers who miss the session can review them at their convenience.

The sessions last approximately 1 hour and focus on mental/behavioral topics that are common in children. After a didactic presentation, the chosen case is presented. The focus is on the 4 Rs: recognize, respond, refer, and resources. Every session includes peer-directed case formulations. Topics include anxiety, attention deficit hyperactivity disorder, autism spectrum disorder, mood disorders, early psychosis, suicide, substance use disorder, abuse, depression, and potential therapies.

The *hub* is the site where the mental health providers are located. The *spokes* are the PCPs who sign in for the session. The hub is equipped with large screens and monitors, cameras, microphones, and fiberoptic wiring that can link with 50 sites at the same time. The providers that make up the spokes use a computer with a monitor, camera, and microphone. Prior to the presentations, all protected health information is removed from the case to maintain confidentiality.

The cases focus on an interprofessional approach to care by including PCPs, nurse practitioners, psychiatrist, psychologists, and social workers. In addition, there is a focus on using community navigators and translators. The importance of including the patient and caregiver as part of the team is stressed.

eConsults

eConsults are an asynchronous way to connect providers to each other for consultation. A message is either emailed or texted from one provider to another, providing information on a case and requesting assistance related to assessment, treatment, or referral. No protected health information is transmitted with the case in order to protect the patient. This allows providers to connect without interrupting each other. The consulted provider can respond to the PCP by setting up a time to talk via a videoconferencing platform or telephone or to send a response via text or email.

In the VMAP program, the PCP can consult with a mental health provider through eConsults. This enables the PCP to receive information on how to care for the patient in the practice setting. This also helps the PCP understand when a referral is appropriate.

Videoconferencing Consultation

Videoconferencing allows for provider-patient interactions as well as provider-provider encounters. The mental health provider uses the videoconferencing platform to connect with the PCP in order to discuss patient cases. Many of the videoconferencing platforms allow for either participant to present materials on the patient and to present assessment tools/data so that both providers can view the same documents at the same time.

Videoconferencing is also used to connect the mental health provider with the patient for evaluation and treatment. Terms used for the mental health visit include *telepsychiatry*, *telepsychology*, or *telemental health*. The videoconferencing platform allows the patient and mental health provider to see each other while they are meeting. This allows for communication to be expressed through visual cues (eg, body language, affect, appearance).

Critical Access Hospitals

One of the most significant issues facing health care, especially in rural and underserved areas, is the closure of critical access hospitals. Many critical access hospitals have limitations in specialty care, decreasing their ability to treat critical patients. As a result, these patients are often transferred to more urban hospitals. This affects their patient census, often resulting in hospital closures. In order to keep some of these hospitals open, telehealth is being used to provide the critical access hospitals with some of the specialty and critical care management they are missing. Examples include companies such as Advanced ICU Care and their teleICU platform that has been used to provide support to the ICU from interprofessional teams of providers.[23] Telehealth allows the intensivist-led team consisting of nurses, physicians, respiratory therapists, and other allied health professionals to monitor and treat critical patients in the ICU. The APRNs in the hospital are supported by the ICU team. Support is provided to the ICU staff 24/7 using 2-way videoconferencing, thus allowing for real-time assessments and implementation of treatments before complications occur.

Readmissions

Patient readmission is another issue that is affecting hospitals and health care costs. Hospitals, through programs such as the Centers for Medicare & Medicaid Services' Hospital Readmission Reduction Program, are now penalizing hospitals for patient recidivism with diseases such as pneumonia, chronic obstructive pulmonary disease, and congestive heart failure.[24] Now, attempts are being made to use telehealth with interprofessional teams to decrease readmissions. Specific areas include monitoring patients after discharge and noting changes before a readmission is necessary. One study showed that by using an implantable monitor connected with a mobile application (app) to a tablet for patients with heart failure, the interprofessional team was able to respond to data quickly. This decreased the readmission rate from 19.3% to 5.2%.[25]

Other programs have used telepresence robots to conduct synchronous encounters between interprofessional teams and the patient/caregiver. This allows issues to be addressed in a timely manner.[26] This empowers the caregiver to provide care and support the patient. Levels of self-efficacy can rise significantly with the telehealth support, enabling the caregiver to feel comfortable in managing issues as they arise.

Specialty Consultation

APRNs are using asynchronous formats to obtain specialty consultation on many of their patients in primary care practices. In the DNP program at Old Dominion University (Norfolk, Virginia), one family nurse practitioner who was pursuing her DNP degree conducted a project where she collaborated with an optometrist on her patients with type 2 diabetes. She was finding that many patients with type 2 diabetes in occupational health were not following up with an ophthalmologist/optometrist to be assessed for diabetic retinopathy. She obtained an ophthalmoscope that was used on her iPhone (Apple). This allowed her to conduct fundoscopic examinations, take pictures, and forward them to an optometrist she was collaborating with. The optometrist was then able to assess the likelihood of the patient having diabetic retinopathy. The nurse practitioner was then able to contact the patient and relay the importance of seeing the ophthalmologist. This increased the number of patients who followed up with the ophthalmologist.

Another nurse practitioner in the DNP program who worked in a cardiology practice developed a collaborative relationship with the providers in the emergency department and primary care practices who frequently referred patients to the cardiology practice. He was concerned about the delay of providing care to patients with chest pain who had undiagnosed cardiac disease. Through his telehealth program, he connected with patients shortly after they were initially seen for chest pain through videoconferencing technologies. He was then able to order needed tests and follow-up on the results before the patients were able to get in for their initial cardiology visits. This enabled the patients to receive a diagnosis and needed care 2 to 3 weeks sooner than if they had waited to be seen in the cardiology practice.

FOR REFLECTION 2:

Telehealth Service Use

Consider that you would like to integrate a telehealth-supported connection with other professionals to address a complex patient population that you provide care to. What telehealth methodology would you select? How would you lead this initiative? Who would you involve? What barriers would you need to overcome?

TELEHEALTH AND ALLIED HEALTH PROFESSIONALS

Telehealth is not just for the primary care and specialty health care providers; it is equally important for the APRN to provide some care by working collaboratively with allied health professions. Telehealth is being embraced by physical therapy, speech-language pathology, dentistry, and pharmacy, to name a few. Regulations and scope of practice using telehealth varies by profession. Methods of use are as numerous as the number of health care professions. An example of a telehealth collaboration that might occur between APRNs and both specialists and allied health professionals can be seen in Figure 9-2 for a patient with cardiac disease.

In this situation, the APRN may collaborate with the physical therapist for cardiac rehabilitation, the respiratory therapist for optimizing the patient's oxygen status, the cardiologist to address cardiac

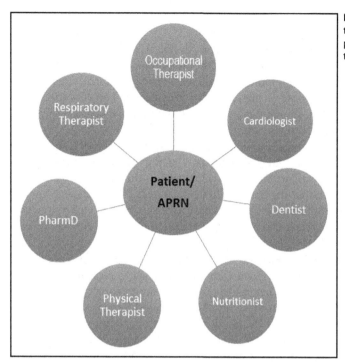

Figure 9-2. Diagram depicting a potential connection made between the patient/APRN dyad and other providers through telehealth.

function, the pharmacist regarding medication and side effects, the nutritionist on proper diet, and the dentist on the impact of periodontal disease and cardiac complications. These encounters can occur between the specialty providers/allied health professionals and the APRN or with the patient/caregiver involved. They may also occur between 2 professions or as a group. Data may be transmitted between providers/allied health professionals using either asynchronous/store-and-forward programs or synchronous videoconferencing and peripherals. However, in using such a model, it is important to be open and willing to embrace the varying uses of telehealth by each profession.

Respiratory Care

Respiratory therapists have used telehealth methodologies such as mobile apps to aid with diagnostic and treatment procedures. For instance, mechanical ventilation, such as airway pressure release ventilation, has been found to improve ventilation days and length of stay in the hospital. In order to overcome limitations in using airway pressure release ventilation, apps have been developed to support its use. Basics of Mechanical Ventilation (iMedical Apps) is one such app.[17,27]

Respiratory therapists have also used telehealth to acquire and transmit arterial blood gas data. With point-of-service analyzers, arterial blood gas data can be obtained and tested at the bed, allowing for more immediate response to the patient's oxygen and carbon monoxide levels. This can be a huge factor in the oversight of critical access hospitals for patients being mechanically ventilated. This allows the provider to respond quickly when the patient's respiratory status is compromised, allowing for better patient outcomes. This more rapid turnaround time often translates into faster intervention and better outcomes.[17,28]

Pulmonary rehabilitation can be enhanced with telerehabilitation. Telerehabilitation allows for the monitoring of patients using videoconferencing technology accompanied with monitoring devices and exercise equipment. This allows patients to receive telerehabilitation at a distance, thus reducing the travel and associated cost of an in-person visit. Interprofessional teams that include the respiratory therapist can collaborate and access the patient using this technology. Data have suggested that telerehabilitation outcomes are equivalent to in-person visits related to hospitalizations, costs, and reaching patients who might otherwise not receive care.[17,29]

Physical Therapy

Physical therapy is another field that has embraced telehealth. Physical therapists provide care in the home as well as in hospitals and clinics. However, they, like many other professions, can find it difficult to provide care to patients in remote or rural areas. Through patient-centered telehealth, more specifically through videoconferencing, they can provide care and education while they remain in their more clinical urban sites and patients are in their homes. Physical therapists can use motion sensors to monitor and treat patients at a distance.[17,30]

Physical therapists can also provide teleconsultation, allowing direct patient care to be carried out in hospitals that do not have access to physical therapists, such as critical access hospitals. Physical therapists can provide care to patients, such as burn patients, within hospitals from a central console at scheduled times, thus decreasing the need to track patients down. This has resulted in more efficient care with reduced health care costs. Stroke patients can be evaluated and treated by physical therapists using videoconferencing to meet with patients and providers and store-and-forward technologies to view images.[17,30,31]

Patients who are discharged needing long-term physical therapy can be provided care at home using videoconferencing platforms that are equipped with matrices used to measure and record range of motion and angulations. This is also helpful in providing care to patients with chronic diseases such as Parkinson's disease, seizure disorders, or other musculoskeletal issues.[31] Internet-based exercise programs can be used to enhance the physical mobility of patients who are in pain or postsurgery. Imaging allows physical data to be shared with other providers as well as the patient. This can increase the ability of interprofessional teams to develop treatment plans and to obtain patient buy-in.[17,32,33]

Nutrition

Registered dietitians have used telehealth to facilitate patient education regarding nutrition. For example, patients with diabetes can receive education and diet advice from registered dietitians by participating in a telehealth-supported diabetes self-management education (DSME) programs. Registered dietitians will lead the DSME program, enabling the patients with diabetes to better understand the effect of nutrition on their illness and make needed modifications to improve their health. The focus should be on blood glucose monitoring, exercise, medication, and other needed treatments. Effective management requires that patients understand and use appropriate technologies for blood glucose monitoring, medication compliance, and complex treatment strategies.[34-36] Studies have shown that DSME provided through telehealth that focuses on patient education and oversight has been effective in reducing blood pressure and HbA1c.[17,37]

Mobile apps have also been found to have a significant effect on optimizing patients' ability to improve their nutritional status. Registered dietitians have been able to enhance their effect on patients by introducing them to many of these mobile apps. One example is the use of an app that includes the transfer of blood glucose data automatically to the registered dietitians.[38] The registered dietitian is then able to respond to the patient via text messaging. Through the text messages, the registered dietitian can make changes in the patient's plan before complications occur.

The NUDGE Coaching mobile platform (nudgecoach.com) allows the registered dietitian to customize the mobile app in order to coach a patient regarding diet and collect data relevant to the patient and his or her health status. For instance, the registered dietitian can customize the app to collect data on blood sugar, weight, exercise, blood pressure, and other labs for the patient with diabetes. The registered dietitian can log on to the platform and have access to the data that the patient has entered, and can then make needed dietary corrections. The OnPoint Nutrition program in Philadelphia provides dietary counseling to patients all over the country using this platform.[39] In addition, it works with patients' providers to optimize patient outcomes. Patients and providers have learned about the online support program via their website (https://www.

onpoint-nutrition.com). Counseling is provided via a videoconferencing platform. Initial visits are conducted twice a week and then are spread out as needed. The initial goal is to involve patients in the program for a minimum of 10 weeks. Patients with diabetes, high blood pressure, obesity, and other dietary-related issues are managed through the program. The program works closely with bariatric surgeons by providing online counseling prior to bariatric surgery and then again starting 3 months after surgery. These are excellent mechanisms for collaboration with other health care professionals as they devise new care plans for patients.

Occupational Therapy

Occupational therapists have also found telehealth to be useful in their practices. Specific programs focus on improving activities of daily living and include mobile apps, videoconferencing, and robotics. Their goal is to improve the patients' ability to perform their activities of daily living by adapting their environment, teaching them skills and adaptive techniques, and addressing healthy habits/routines.[17,40]

RPM devices, such as self-monitoring, analysis, and reporting technology (SMART), allows the occupational therapist to track the activities and performance of the patient in his or her home. Based on the transmitted data, the occupational therapist can provide the patient with feedback and intervene as needed.[41] These approaches can be used for patients with declining health status, those with neuromuscular diseases, those sustaining injuries/trauma, as well as children with disabilities or developmental delays. Telehealth allows the occupational therapist to become an integral part of the interprofessional health care team addressing patient needs. Through telehealth, the occupational therapist is able to assess and transmit data to other professionals regarding the patient's changing health status. As a team, they can then develop appropriate plans of care.

Other Allied Health Professions

Telehealth is used by other allied health professions, such as lab science, audiology, and speech-language pathology.[17,40] Telemicrocopy allows lab technicians and/or specialists to identify cells and obtain specimens to diagnose illnesses.[41] The Health Wagon in southwest Virginia is run by 2 nurse practitioners with specialty support from the University of Virginia (UVA) Center for Telehealth. They can perform colposcopies with the gynecologist at UVA observing from 300 miles away. The gynecologist can view the procedure as it is happening and make requests for tissue samples from the most appropriate sites. Southwest Virginia also has many patients with bladder cancers as a result of the environment in coal mines. These same 2 nurse practitioners perform cystography and obtain specimens with the aid of the urologist at UVA (see Chapter 7). This approach has resulted in the patients receiving timely diagnoses and earlier management. Telemicrocopy has also been used to diagnose communicable diseases, such as malaria, parasites, and tuberculosis, in vulnerable populations, thus decreasing morbidity and mortality.[40]

Finally, in 2017, federal regulators approved remote management to fine-tune cochlear implants at a distance. This allowed for more timely management and a decreased need for office visits.[17]

CONSIDERATIONS REGARDING INTERPROFESSIONAL EDUCATION/COLLABORATION

Many of the issues inherent in interprofessional care also apply to the integration of telehealth. However, some of these issues may be further complicated by the use of telehealth and by provider/patient location. Currently, the rules and regulations vary by state and by insurance provider. Therefore, when developing an interprofessional telehealth program, 2 important issues must be considered: rules and regulations governing practice and the handling of reimbursement.

Rules and Regulations

Telehealth has only recently begun to be accepted for varying professions and by a diverse patient population. Thus, best practice is still being established. Organizations such as the American Telemedicine Association have developed some overall guidelines.[42,43] However, specialty organizations have been limited in their approach to telehealth guidelines by the professions they serve. State boards such as those in New York, North Carolina, and Pennsylvania have added the American Telemedicine Association practice guidelines.[17] Twelve regional Telehealth Resource Centers (TRCs) are now dispersed across the country to support evidence-based care models. The TRCs provide annual conferences as well as assistance and training for providers involved in health care from numerous professions. They are actively involved in informing providers of new regulations and connecting them with experts who can help facilitate the integration of telehealth within their practices and professions. It is not uncommon for providers from varying professions to meet at conferences provided by the TRCs and begin to develop collaborative relationships across professions.

With the increase in telehealth, there have been many federal and state bills introduced. In fact, telehealth has been one of very few bipartisan issues. Yet, they may vary significantly by state. As of the present time, there is no comprehensive federal legislation in place. These gaps in legislation may stifle the ability for telehealth to be fully operationalized. The policies that do exist often vary based on the providers' professions and states. The Creating Opportunities Now for Necessary and Effective Care Technologies (CONNECT) for Health Act is one law that has been enacted. The goal of CONNECT is to support platforms for telehealth in accountable care organizations and for Medicare providers to increase RPM by varying professions for those in rural areas and with chronic conditions.[44]

Some states, such as New Jersey and Minnesota, now have comprehensive legislation for telehealth that addresses content such as covering services, providing for reimbursement, consent, and practice standards. Policy support like the program in New Jersey has included allied health professionals, including speech-language pathologists, social workers, and nurses.[44] Professional boards have implemented telehealth policies in occupational therapy and physical therapy, which many states have followed with the enactment of laws. Although the policies for occupational therapy and physical therapy may be somewhat narrow, the resulting decrease in requirements may increase the use of these varying providers.

In order to mitigate resistance to telehealth, some states are using terms such as *telecommunications* and *electronic* rather than *telehealth* or *telemedicine* to refer to videoconferencing. This approach is similar to the approach used for the 2019 Medicare physician fee schedule, where the terms *telehealth* and *telemedicine* were avoided so that the services were not affected by the federal statutory limitations on telehealth being used in Medicare.[45] Future programs may limit the use of the telehealth terminology in order to receive needed support.

A 50-state survey assessed the laws and regulations of physical therapy and occupational therapy related to telehealth.[46] Twenty-seven states had created policies for occupational therapy connection with patients and/or providers via telehealth, and 28 for physical therapy. Occupational therapy and physical therapy providers in states that allow the use of telehealth could provide such care using their clinical judgment and practice guidelines to determine the services provided. They were not restricted based on geography. Often the policies used the term *telecommunication* to allow for the supervision of therapy assistance. The use of telehealth by occupational therapy and physical therapy varied based on what was allowed by the state. For instance, 14 states allowed videoconferencing in occupational therapy and 26 in physical therapy in order to either provide patient care or connect with a provider. Additional states allowed videoconferencing for supervision of the therapy assistant. Store-and-forward technology was allowed for occupational therapy and physical therapy in 12 states. Seven additional states included occupational therapy and physical therapy with policies for multiple professionals. RPM was allowed in only 4 states.[46]

As more professions receive legislative support for telehealth, barriers to interprofessional care will gradually be removed. It will become important for interprofessional programs to evaluate their outcomes to show not only cost benefits but also improved patient outcomes. Professions will need to continue to unite to lobby for needed changes in the rules and regulations that interfere with optimum telehealth-enhanced IPC.

Reimbursement for Interprofessional Telehealth

Reimbursement for IPC via telehealth varies based on provider, state, and service offered. Centers for Medicare & Medicaid Services began to address this issue in the 2019 Medicare physician fee schedule, in which they unbundled 4 Common Procedural Technology (CPT) codes and created 2 additional codes related to interprofessional consultation using the internet, EHRs, or phone.[47] These codes allow the patient's health care provider to be reimbursed for consults with another health care provider with specific specialty expertise on the patient's diagnosis and/or treatment. This reduces the need for the patient to meet with the specialty provider, thus decreasing cost, inconvenience, and time delay.

The new codes are presented in Table 9-1. These new codes outline how the care is reimbursed, with some codes benefitting the referring provider and others the consulting provider.

For reimbursement to occur, the following parameters must be met:

- The qualified health care provider (QHP) must be able to bill independently for evaluation and management services.
- A verbal consent for the consultation is obtained from the patient and documented in the patient's health records.
- The patient's consent confirms that the patient was made aware of any cost-sharing.
- Copayments must be collected for each service.
- The consultation is needed by the patient.

Other strategies used to reimburse in IPC models include bundled payment models. These models can be used to reimburse a set amount for the management of specific conditions. This approach is being used in surgery where the fee for the surgery includes the postoperative visits as well as skilled care provided at the practice site. For example, for patients undergoing orthopedic surgery, they may have one lump sum paid that will include the surgery, the postoperative visits, and physical therapy provided in the office. The follow-up may include telehealth visits. In an attempt to decrease the number of visits and improve the patients' recovery, support via telehealth is becoming an economical approach.

PATIENT/PROVIDER ISSUES

With the rapid increase in telehealth technologies, patients who are not adept at using technologies may be left behind in accessing specific care. As the gap broadens between the technology and the patient's competence in accessing and using it, the potential improvement in health care diminishes. Dalal et al[48] discovered that lack of knowledge in accessing and using telehealth platforms affected the patient's use of telehealth. This has been compounded by the varying technologies required for support by differing professions. It is possible for patients with chronic diseases to be monitored with RPM by their specialists, have weekly videoconferencing sessions with their mental health providers, and provide clinical data via their peripherals. As a result, patients may become overwhelmed by the numerous telehealth programs available to them and may resist telehealth all together. It is thus imperative that the patient be educated and supported as they use the needed technology.

Table 9-1

New Common Procedural Technology Codes for Collaboration via Telehealth

CPT CODE	REPORTS CONSULT	REPORT REQUIRED	ACTIVITY REQUIRED	TIME SPENT
99446	Consulted provider	An oral and written report to the requesting physician or QHP	Review and assessment of patient data Interprofessional review and consultations via phone or internet between consulting and referring provider	5-10 minutes
99447	Consulted provider	An oral and written report to the requesting physician or QHP	Review and assessment of patient data Interprofessional review and consultations via phone or internet between consulting and referring provider	11-20 minutes
99448	Consulted provider	An oral and written report to the requesting physician or QHP	Review and assessment of patient data Interprofessional review and consultations via phone or internet between consulting and referring provider	21-30 minutes
99449	Consulted provider	An oral and written report to the requesting physician or QHP	Review and assessment of patient data Interprofessional review and consultations via phone or internet between consulting and referring provider	31 or more minutes
99451	Consulted provider	A written report to the requesting physician or QHP	Interprofessional review of patient information and data/records via telephone/internet/EHRs More than 50% of the time may be in review	5 or more minutes review
99452	Requesting provider (QHP)	None	Time of the referring physician or QHP preparing for and participating in interprofessional consult	More than 16 minutes

Note: 50% of the time must be spent in consultation between providing and requesting provider for CPT codes 99446-99449.

Providers may be faced with some of the same issues regarding telehealth. Too often, providers do not receive adequate training in using telehealth.[49] In fact, they may not even be aware of the various technologies available for their patients. They may become overwhelmed and thus avoid the integration of telehealth within their practice. This may result in a disconnect between the varying providers involved in the care of the patient.

As interprofessional care increases, it is becoming important for providers to create an infrastructure where the data the patients collect can be transmitted to their different providers. The data and the providers' responses should also be accessible by the other providers involved in the patients' care. This will allow for more timely intervention by the appropriate health care professionals. In addition, it will minimize the overwhelm experienced by patients and allow for better coordinated care.

Another issue that has the potential to derail interprofessional care is the lack of infrastructure to support the telehealth platforms. This is especially an issue for those in remote, rural areas where the infrastructure is minimal and the broadband support is limited. At times, the patient may be located in an area known as a dead spot, where connectivity is nonexistent and the ability to use telehealth is null.[48] More states are setting the development of broadband as a high priority. For those that do have broadband access, the issue of HIPAA protection is high.[50]

Another issue affecting telehealth provision of IPC is the fact that too many of the platforms are not compatible with each other. This can create a further division between providers. In fact, Stevenson et al[51] found that even in the Veterans Health Administration, this incapability between systems greatly affected the ability to implement some telehealth programs.

GROUP EXERCISE

Collaborative Telehealth Programs

Reflect on the interaction and engagement of working collaboratively with allied health professionals using telehealth. For this exercise, divide into 2 groups. Group 1 will outline an interprofessional telehealth program for patients with strokes, focusing on the purpose, goals, providers, model, and technology to achieve targeted outcomes for the program. Group 2 will focus on outlining a strategy for enabling the providers to ensure reimbursement for an interprofessional telehealth program.

CONCLUSION

With the increase in patient living with multiple chronic conditions, the aging population, and the lack of providers and access to care in rural and underserved regions, it is becoming increasingly important for providers to collaborate interprofessionally using telehealth modalities. All too often, the APRN is the sole provider in providing care to the disadvantaged and rural populations, with very few specialists and allied health professionals located in their regions. This can greatly disadvantage the patient and overextend the role of the APRN. With the development of both synchronous and asynchronous telehealth programs, the APRN can now connect with other professions that are willing to collaborate at a distance. Through store-and-forward technologies, the APRN is better able to coordinate consultations with busy specialists and allied health professionals. Finally, by using videoconferencing technologies with peripherals and asynchronous data delivery, the APRN can schedule the patient with specialists and allied health professionals while he or she is in the office, thus decreasing the need for the patient and caregiver to travel great distances for care.

Telehealth modalities such as Project ECHO enable the APRN to receive input from other professionals who have expertise in the diagnosis and management of difficult cases. This grand rounds–type format allows the APRN to connect to a synchronous platform where he or she can hear how various professions address specific cases that have been submitted by providers in the community. The APRN is also able to submit patient cases that he or she would like input on managing. This has proved to be especially helpful in managing patients with chronic diseases, such as hepatitis and HIV. It has also aided the APRN in better understanding how to address the behavioral and mental health issues that may plague his or her patient populations.

RPM is another telehealth modality that can allow for IPC by collecting data on the patient remotely. These data can be obtained from RPM devices that are set up in the patient's home or through wearables. As the data are obtained, providers and allied health professionals can use platforms such as eConsults, videoconferencing technologies, and store-and-forward transmission of data to collaboratively address changes in the patient's condition. This can be an effective method for decreasing patient recidivism.

Telehealth has also been vital in keeping many critical access hospitals viable by providing the hospitals with the clinical expertise they lack. This is especially important for critical care and emergency departments. Advanced diagnostics can also be supported through the telehealth technologies allowing for patients to receive care by experts in specific fields. Patients can be better maintained near or in their homes where they can receive input and support from their families.

The use of telehealth to access interprofessional care is vital to both the provider and the patient. It provides a method of truly addressing the inequities found in health care, especially to rural and underserved populations. It allows providers to obtain the support so often lacking in rural regions. It decreases the limited access to providers that is so often inherent in rural and underserved communities. Telehealth has the potential to improve the health status of all populations regardless of location by providing access to specialty care and allied health that is too often overlooked or inaccessible.

THOUGHTFUL QUESTIONS

1. What barriers to care does telehealth-enhanced IPC overcome?
2. What professions can be connected using telehealth? What are some considerations that must be addressed in order to develop successful telehealth-enhanced interprofessional care?
3. There have been many telehealth-enhanced IPC models developed. What are some of the health care issues that can be addressed through the differing models? What are the purposes of the different models?
4. In developing telehealth-enhanced IPC for a patient population that you frequently see, what models would you use? What professions would you seek to collaborate with? What barriers would you need to overcome?

CASE STUDY

You have acquired many patients with type 2 diabetes in your practice. You do not have easy access to any provider other than the PCP in your practice. You are realizing that many of your patients have significant levels of uncontrolled diabetes and are experiencing sequelae that include depression, neuropathy, and kidney failure. They have trouble obtaining appointments with the ophthalmologist and podiatrist. You have decided that the practice needs to develop a program to better support the patients with type 2 diabetes.

Questions

1. What professionals should you collaborate with to address the issues your patients are facing?
2. What interprofessional models of care will you put in place?
3. Which models will be patient-provider focused, and how will they be implemented?
4. Which models will be provider-provider focused, and how will they be implemented?

REFERENCES

1. Abu-Rish E, Kim S, Choe L, et al. Current trends in interprofessional education of health sciences students: a literature review. *J Interprof Care*. 2012;26(6):444-451.
2. Interprofessional Education Collaborative Expert Panel. *Core competencies for interprofessional collaborative practice: report of an expert panel*. Washington, DC: Interprofessional Education Collaborative; 2011. https://nebula.wsimg.com/3ee8a4b5b5f7ab794c742b14601d5f23?AccessKeyId=DC06780E69ED19E2B3A5&disposition=0&alloworigin=1. Accessed February 29, 2020.
3. Interprofessional Education Collaborative Expert Panel. *Core competencies for interprofessional collaborative practice: 2016 update*. Washington, DC: Interprofessional Education Collaborative; 2016. https://nebula.wsimg.com/2f68a39520b03336b41038c370497473?AccessKeyId=DC06780E69ED19E2B3A5&disposition=0&alloworigin=1. Accessed February 29, 2020.
4. American Association of Colleges of Nursing. *The Essentials of Master's Education in Nursing*. http://www.aacnnursing.org/portals/42/publications/mastersessentials11.pdf. Published March 21, 2011. Accessed February 15, 2020.
5. American Association of Colleges of Nursing. *The Essentials of Doctoral Education for Advanced Nursing Practice*. https://www.aacnnursing.org/Portals/42/Publications/DNPEssentials.pdf. Published October 2006. Accessed February 15, 2020.
6. Healthy People 2020. Older adults. Office of Disease Prevention and Health Promotion. https://www.healthypeople.gov/2020/topics-objectives/topic/older-adults. Accessed February 29, 2020.
7. Rutledge CM, Kott K, Schweickert PA, Poston R, Fowler C, Haney TS. Telehealth and eHealth in nurse practitioner training: current perspectives. *Adv Med Educ Pract*. 2017;8:399-409.
8. Nester J. The importance of interprofessional practice and education in the era of accountable care. *N C Med J*. 2016;77(2):128-132.
9. Supper I, Catala O, Lustman M, Chemla C, Bourgueil Y, Letrilliart L. Interprofessional collaboration in primary health care: a review of facilitators and barriers perceived by involved actors. *J Public Health (Oxf)*. 2015;37(4):716-727.
10. Erickson CE, Fauchald S, Ideker M. Integrating telehealth into graduate nursing curriculum. *J Nurse Pract*. 2014;11(1):e1-e5.
11. AMA encourages telemedicine training for medical students, residents. Press release. American Medical Association. https://www.ama-assn.org/press-center/press-releases/ama-encourages-telemedicine-training-medical-students-residents. Published June 15, 2016. Accessed April 6, 2020.
12. Greiwe M. Medical schools and telehealth: learning webside manner. *OrthoLive*. https://www.ortholive.com/blog/medical-schools-and-telehealth-learning-webside-manner. Published September 20, 2018. Accessed April 6, 2020.
13. De Voest M, Meny L, VanLangen K, et al. Four themes to enhanced interprofessional integration: lessons learned from early implementation and curricular redesign. *Innov Pharm*. 2016;7(2):4.

14. Green B, Oeppen RS, Smith DW, Brennan PA. Challenging hierarchy in healthcare teams—ways to flatten gradients to improve teamwork and patient care. *Br J Oral Maxillofac Surg.* 2017;55(5):449-453.

15. Rural Health Information Hub. Rural aging. https://www.ruralhealthinfo.org/topics/aging. Updated October 30, 2018. Accessed March 1, 2020.

16. American Physical Therapy Association. Telehealth. http://www.apta.org/Telehealth/. Updated November 26, 2019. Accessed March 1, 2020.

17. Heuer A, Hector JR, Cassell V. An Update on Telehealth in Allied Health and Interprofessional Care. *J Allied Health.* 2019;48(2):140-147.

18. Ishani A, Christopher J, Palmer D, et al. Telehealth by an interprofessional team in patients with CKD: a randomized controlled trial. *Am J Kidney Dis.* 2016;68(1):41-49.

19. Ellison A. The rural hospital closure crisis: 15 key findings and trends. *Becker's Hospital Review.* https://www.beckershospitalreview.com/finance/the-rural-hospital-closure-crisis-15-key-findings-and-trends.html. Published February 11, 2016. Accessed March 1, 2020.

20. Rojas-Burke J. What happens when hospitals abandon inner cities. *Association of Health Care Journalists.* http://healthjournalism.org/blog/2014/07/what-happens-when-hospitals-abandon-inner-cities/. Published July 9, 2014. Accessed March 1, 2020.

21. Nguyen T, Hellebuyck M, Halperin M, Fritze D. The state of mental health in America 2018. Mental Health America. https://www.sprc.org/sites/default/files/resource-program/2018%20The%20State%20of%20MH%20in%20America%20-%20FINAL%20%28002%29.pdf. Published 2017. Accessed March 1, 2020.

22. Arora S, Geppert CM, Kalishman S, et al. Academic health center management of chronic diseases through knowledge networks: Project ECHO. *Acad Med.* 2007;82(2):154-160.

23. Gamble KH. Critical care network. ICU telehealth can ease the burden of caring for critically ill patients—provided all the right pieces are in place. *Healthc Inform.* 2009;26(12):26,28-30.

24. O'Connor M, Asdornwised U, Dempsey ML, et al. Using telehealth to reduce all-cause 30-day hospital readmissions among heart failure patients receiving skilled home health services. *Appl Clin Inform.* 2016;7(2):238-247.

25. Wasfy JH, Zigler CM, Choirat C, Wang Y, Dominici F, Yeh RW. Readmission rates after passage of the Hospital Readmissions Reduction Program: a pre-post analysis. *Ann Intern Med.* 2017;166(5):324-331.

26. Vaughn J, Shaw RJ, Molloy MA. A telehealth case study: the use of telepresence robot for delivering integrated clinical care. *J Am Psychiatr Nurses Assoc.* 2015;21(6):431-432.

27. Miller AG, Gentile MA, Davies JD, MacIntyre NR. Clinical management strategies for airway pressure release ventilation: a survey of clinical practice. *Respir Care.* 2017;62(10):1264-1268.

28. Allardet-Servent J, Lebsir M, Dubroca C, et al. Point-of-care versus central laboratory measurements of hemoglobin, hematocrit, glucose, bicarbonate and electrolytes: a prospective observational study in critically ill patients. *PLoS One.* 2017;12(1):e0169593.

29. Chan C, Yamabayashi C, Syed N, Kirkham A, Camp PG. Exercise telemonitoring and telerehabilitation compared with traditional cardiac and pulmonary rehabilitation: a systematic review and meta-analysis. *Physiother Can.* 2017;68(3):242-251.

30. Tenforde AS, Hefner JE, Kodish-Wachs JE, Iaccarino MA, Paganoni S. Telehealth in physical medicine and rehabilitation: a narrative review. *PM R.* 2017;9(5S):S51-S58.

31. Liu YM, Mathews K, Vardanian A, et al. Urban telehealth: the applicability of teleburns in the rehabilitative phase. *J Burn Care Res.* 2017;38(1):e235-e239.

32. Silva GS, Farrell S, Shandra E, Viswanathan A, Schwamm LH. The status of telestroke in the United States: a survey of currently active stroke telemedicine programs. *Stroke.* 2012;43(8):2078-2085.

33. Galiano-Castillo N, Cantarero-Villanueva I, Fernández-Lao C, et al. Telehealth system: a randomized controlled trial evaluating the impact of an internet-based exercise intervention on quality of life, pain, muscle strength, and fatigue in breast cancer survivors. *Cancer.* 2016;122(20):3166-3174.

34. National Clinical Care Commission Act, Pub L No. 115-80, 131 Stat 1261 (2017). https://www.congress.gov/115/plaws/publ80/PLAW-115publ80.pdf. Accessed April 6, 2020.

35. Center for Medicare & Medicaid Services. Telehealth services. https://www.cms.gov/Outreach-and-Education/Medicare-Learning-Network-MLN/MLNProducts/Downloads/TelehealthSrvcsfctsht.pdf. Published January 2019. Accessed February 21, 2020.

36. Shah VN, Garg SK. Managing diabetes in the digital age. *Clin Diabetes Endocrinol.* 2015;1:16.

37. American Diabetes Association. Standards of medical care in diabetes—2015. *Diabetes Care.* 2015;38:S1-S90.

38. Nicoll KG, Ramser KL, Campbell JD, et al. Sustainability of improved glycemic control after diabetes self-management education. *Diabetes Spectr.* 2014;27(3):207-211.

39. OnPoint Nutrition. https://www.onpoint-nutrition.com/. Accessed April 6, 2020.

40. Prieto-Egido I, González-Escalada A, García-Giganto V, Martínez-Fernández A. Design of new procedures for diagnosing prevalent diseases using a low-cost telemicroscopy system. *Telemed J E Health.* 2016;22(11):952-959.

41. FDA approves first telehealth option to program cochlear implants remotely. Press release. US Food and Drug Administration. https://www.fda.gov/news-events/press-announcements/fda-approves-first-telehealth-option-program-cochlear-implants-remotely. Published November 17, 2017. Accessed April 6, 2020.

42. Richmond T, Peterson C, Cason J, et al. American Telemedicine Association's principles for delivering telerehabilitation services. *Int J Telerehabil.* 2017;20;9(2):63-68.

43. Krupinski EA, Bernard J. Standards and guidelines in telemedicine and telehealth. *Healthcare (Basel).* 2014;2(1):74-93.

44. Trout KE, Rampa S, Wilson FA, Stimpson JP. Legal mapping analysis of state telehealth reimbursement policies. *Telemed J E Health.* 2017;23(10):805-814.

45. Centers for Medicare & Medicaid Services. Physician fee schedule 2019. https://www.cms.gov/Medicare/Medicare-Fee-for-Service-Payment/PhysicianFeeSched/PFS-Federal-Regulation-Notices-Items/CMS-1693-F.html. Published November 11, 2018. Accessed March 1, 2020.

46. Bierman RT, Kwong MW, Caloura C. State occupational and physical therapy telehealth laws and regulations: a 50-state survey. *Int J Telerehabil.* 2018;10(2):3-54.

47. AAP Division of Health Care Finance. Two new codes developed for interprofessional consultation. *AAP News.* https://www.aappublications.org/news/2019/01/04/coding010419. Published January 4, 2019. Accessed March 1, 2020.

48. Dalal AK, Bates DW, Collins S. Opportunities and challenges for improving the patient experience in the acute and postacute care setting using patient portals: the patient's perspective. *J Hosp Med.* 2017;12(12):1012-1016.

49. Wilson LS, Maeder AJ. Recent directions in telemedicine: review of trends in research and practice. *Healthc Inform Res.* 2015;21(4):213-222.

50. Yang J, Lee YS, Hong Y. Implementation of secure remote EMR medical information using encryption algorithm. *Journal of the Institute of Internet, Broadcasting and Communication.* 2014;14(4):133-139.

51. Stevenson L, Ball S, Haverhals LM, Aron DC, Lowery J. Evaluation of a national telehealth initiative in the Veterans Health Administration: factors associated with successful implementation. *J Telemed Telecare.* 2018;24(3):168-178.

Financial Disclosures

Dr. Rebecca A. Bates has no financial or proprietary interest in the materials presented herein.

Ms. Michele L. Bordelon has no financial or proprietary interest in the materials presented herein.

Dr. Susan V. Brammer has no financial or proprietary interest in the materials presented herein.

Mr. David Cattell-Gordon has no financial or proprietary interest in the materials presented herein.

Dr. Katherine E. Chike-Harris has no financial or proprietary interest in the materials presented herein.

Mr. Samuel Collins has no financial or proprietary interest in the materials presented herein.

Mr. Brian Gunnell has no financial or proprietary interest in the materials presented herein.

Dr. Tina Gustin has no financial or proprietary interest in the materials presented herein.

Dr. Kristi Henderson has no financial or proprietary interest in the materials presented herein.

Dr. Tonya L. Hensley has no financial or proprietary interest in the materials presented herein.

Ms. Allison Kirkner has no financial or proprietary interest in the materials presented herein.

Mr. Brian Myers has no financial or proprietary interest in the materials presented herein.

Index

Printed in the United States
by Baker & Taylor Publisher Services